Metabolic Alterations in Cancer

Metabolic Alterations in Cancer

Guest Editor

Paola Tucci

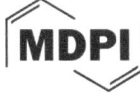

Basel • Beijing • Wuhan • Barcelona • Belgrade • Novi Sad • Cluj • Manchester

Guest Editor
Paola Tucci
Department of Pharmacy,
Health and Nutritional
Sciences
University of Calabria
Rende
Italy

Editorial Office
MDPI AG
Grosspeteranlage 5
4052 Basel, Switzerland

This is a reprint of the Special Issue, published open access by the journal *Cancers* (ISSN 2072-6694), freely accessible at: https://www.mdpi.com/journal/cancers/special_issues/metabolic_alterations.

For citation purposes, cite each article independently as indicated on the article page online and as indicated below:

Lastname, A.A.; Lastname, B.B. Article Title. *Journal Name* **Year**, *Volume Number*, Page Range.

ISBN 978-3-7258-3759-5 (Hbk)
ISBN 978-3-7258-3760-1 (PDF)
https://doi.org/10.3390/books978-3-7258-3760-1

© 2025 by the authors. Articles in this book are Open Access and distributed under the Creative Commons Attribution (CC BY) license. The book as a whole is distributed by MDPI under the terms and conditions of the Creative Commons Attribution-NonCommercial-NoDerivs (CC BY-NC-ND) license (https://creativecommons.org/licenses/by-nc-nd/4.0/).

Contents

About the Editor vii

Paola Tucci
Targeting Cancer Metabolism as a New Strategy to Enhance Treatment Efficacy and Overcome Resistance
Reprinted from: *Cancers* 2024, 16, 3629, https://doi.org/10.3390/cancers16213629 1

Vincent Tambay, Valérie-Ann Raymond, Corentine Goossens, Louise Rousseau, Simon Turcotte and Marc Bilodeau
Metabolomics-Guided Identification of a Distinctive Hepatocellular Carcinoma Signature
Reprinted from: *Cancers* 2023, 15, 3232, https://doi.org/10.3390/cancers15123232 4

Rida Iftikhar, Patricia Snarski, Angelle N. King, Jenisha Ghimire, Emmanuelle Ruiz, Frank Lau and Suzana D. Savkovic
Epiploic Adipose Tissue (EPAT) in Obese Individuals Promotes Colonic Tumorigenesis: A Novel Model for EPAT-Dependent Colorectal Cancer Progression
Reprinted from: *Cancers* 2023, 15, 977, https://doi.org/10.3390/cancers15030977 21

Elisabet Cuyàs, Salvador Fernández-Arroyo, Sara Verdura, Ruth Lupu, Jorge Joven and Javier A. Menendez
Metabolomic and Mitochondrial Fingerprinting of the Epithelial-to-Mesenchymal Transition (EMT) in Non-Tumorigenic and Tumorigenic Human Breast Cells
Reprinted from: *Cancers* 2022, 14, 6214, https://doi.org/10.3390//cancers14246214 32

César L. Ramírez-Tortosa, Rubén Alonso-Calderón, José María Gálvez-Navas, Cristina Pérez-Ramírez, José Luis Quiles, Pedro Sánchez-Rovira, et al.
Hypoxia-Inducible Factor-1 Alpha Expression Is Predictive of Pathological Complete Response in Patients with Breast Cancer Receiving Neoadjuvant Chemotherapy
Reprinted from: *Cancers* 2022, 14, 5393, https://doi.org/10.3390/cancers14215393 56

Haosheng Zheng, Guojie Long, Yuzhen Zheng, Xingping Yang, Weijie Cai, Shiyun He, et al.
Glycolysis-Related SLC2A1 Is a Potential Pan-Cancer Biomarker for Prognosis and Immunotherapy
Reprinted from: *Cancers* 2022, 14, 5344, https://doi.org/10.3390/cancers14215344 69

Muyang Li, Fredrick Philantrope, Alexandra Diot, Jean-Christophe Bourdon and Patricia Thompson
A Novel Role of SMG1 in Cholesterol Homeostasis That Depends Partially on p53 Alternative Splicing
Reprinted from: *Cancers* 2022, 14, 3255, https://doi.org/10.3390/cancers14133255 92

Cristina Banella, Gianfranco Catalano, Serena Travaglini, Elvira Pelosi, Tiziana Ottone, Alessandra Zaza, et al.
Ascorbate Plus Buformin in AML: A Metabolic Targeted Treatment
Reprinted from: *Cancers* 2022, 14, 2565, https://doi.org/10.3390/cancers14102565 110

Zoé Daverio, Aneta Balcerczyk, Gilles J. P. Rautureau and Baptiste Panthu
How Warburg-Associated Lactic Acidosis Rewires Cancer Cell Energy Metabolism to Resist Glucose Deprivation
Reprinted from: *Cancers* 2023, 15, 1417, https://doi.org/10.3390/15051417 130

Maurizio Ragni, Claudia Fornelli, Enzo Nisoli and Fabio Penna
Amino Acids in Cancer and Cachexia: An Integrated View
Reprinted from: *Cancers* 2022, 14, 5691, https://doi.org/10.3390/cancers14225691 144

Laura Di Magno, Fiorella Di Pastena, Rosa Bordone, Sonia Coni and Gianluca Canettieri
The Mechanism of Action of Biguanides: New Answers to a Complex Question
Reprinted from: *Cancers* **2022**, *14*, 3220, https://doi.org/10.3390/cancers14133220 . . . . **163**

Haosheng Zheng, Guojie Long, Yuzhen Zheng, Xingping Yang, Weijie Cai, Shiyun He, et al.
Correction: Zheng et al. Glycolysis-Related SLC2A1 Is a Potential Pan-Cancer Biomarker for Prognosis and Immunotherapy. *Cancers* 2022, *14*, 5344
Reprinted from: *Cancers* **2023**, *15*, 586, https://doi.org/10.3390/cancers15030586 . . . . **195**

About the Editor

Paola Tucci

Paola Tucci is an Associate Professor of Molecular Biology at the Department of Pharmacy, Health, and Nutritional Science, University of Calabria, Italy. She earned her Degree cum laude in 2003 from the University of Calabria. She subsequently obtained her Ph.D. in "Pharmacology and Biochemistry of Cell Death" in 2007, also at the University of Calabria, followed by a medical specialization in "Clinical Biochemistry" with honors in 2017 at the University of Rome "Tor Vergata." She gained valuable experience as a post-doctoral research fellow at the Medical Research Council (MRC) Toxicology Unit at the University of Cambridge (UK) and later worked as a research assistant at the University of Rome "Tor Vergata." In 2011, she returned to the University of Calabria, initially as an Assistant Professor of Biochemistry and then advancing to her current role as an Associate Professor of Molecular Biology.

With over 50 peer-reviewed publications in prestigious international journals such as *Blood*, *Cell Death and Differentiation*, *PNAS*, and *Oncogene*, Paola is recognized as a leading researcher in her field. She has been invited to speak at numerous international conferences and was awarded the Bioeconomy Rome 2013 prize by the Accademia Nazionale dei Lincei in recognition of her contributions to translational medicine in neurodegeneration.

Her research focuses on (i) identifying and validating new microRNAs involved in the pathogenesis of cancer and their role as potential biomarkers for early detection, diagnosis, and therapy; (ii) investigating the role of the p53 family members, including the p63 and p73 proteins, in tumorigenesis, metabolism, and neuronal development, particularly their regulation by microRNA; and (iii) evaluating the biological effects of natural compounds and their delivery systems on both normal and tumor cell lines.

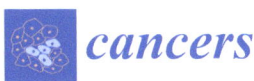

Editorial

Targeting Cancer Metabolism as a New Strategy to Enhance Treatment Efficacy and Overcome Resistance

Paola Tucci

Department of Pharmacy, Health and Nutritional Sciences, University of Calabria, 87036 Rende, CS, Italy; paola.tucci@unical.it; Tel.: +39-0984493185

Citation: Tucci, P. Targeting Cancer Metabolism as a New Strategy to Enhance Treatment Efficacy and Overcome Resistance. *Cancers* **2024**, *16*, 3629. https://doi.org/10.3390/cancers16213629

Received: 15 October 2024
Accepted: 19 October 2024
Published: 28 October 2024

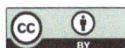

Copyright: © 2024 by the author. Licensee MDPI, Basel, Switzerland. This article is an open access article distributed under the terms and conditions of the Creative Commons Attribution (CC BY) license (https://creativecommons.org/licenses/by/4.0/).

The intricate relationship between metabolism and cancer has been a subject of growing interest in recent years, as metabolic reprogramming is recognized as one of the hallmarks of cancer [1–3]. Tumor cells exhibit profound alterations in their metabolic pathways that influence many, if not all, facets of tumor biology, including the growth, proliferation, and invasion of cancer cells as well as treatment resistance and metastasis [4–8]. These metabolic changes can be caused by mutations or modifications in the cancer cells, but the patient's metabolism also plays an important role. These metabolic alterations create unique vulnerabilities, which can be exploited for the development of new antitumoral strategies [9–12].

To this end, this Special Issue of *Cancers* brings together cutting-edge research on the metabolic alterations that occur in cancer, offering insights into novel therapeutic strategies targeting metabolic pathways to deprive cancer cells of the biochemical resources they have come to depend on.

This Special Issue opens with an article by Banella et al., which introduces a promising new approach for the treatment of Acute Myeloid Leukemia (AML). AML is a highly aggressive cancer with a poor prognosis, particularly in elderly patients who are often unfit for intensive chemotherapy. The study investigates the combination of ascorbate (vitamin C) with buformin, a biguanide that inhibits mitochondrial complex I. This combination leverages the metabolic peculiarities of AML cells, which are known to exhibit highly flexible and aggressive metabolic phenotypes. Ascorbate induces oxidative stress by interfering with the glycolytic pathway, while buformin blocks mitochondrial ATP production, effectively starving the cancer cells of energy. The study shows that this combination has a synergistic effect, significantly enhancing apoptosis in AML cells, particularly in primary blasts from elderly patients who are resistant to other treatments. Thus, this metabolic-targeted therapy offers a potential new avenue for treating a difficult-to-treat population.

Following this, Di Magno et al. present an in-depth review of biguanides, focusing on their mechanisms of action in cancer beyond their well-known inhibition of mitochondrial complex I. Biguanides such as metformin and buformin have garnered attention for their antitumor properties, which are believed to stem from their ability to induce energy stress in cancer cells. However, the review highlights that the concentrations of biguanides needed to inhibit complex I in vivo are much higher than what can be achieved in patients without toxicity. This discrepancy has led researchers to explore alternative mechanisms by which biguanides exert their effects. Di Magno and colleagues discuss emerging evidence suggesting that biguanides may affect other metabolic pathways, including redox balance, AMPK activation, and interference with the tumor microenvironment. They also examine the ongoing clinical trials investigating the use of biguanides in cancer therapy, emphasizing the importance of understanding the precise molecular targets of these drugs to maximize their therapeutic potential.

Li et al. take the exploration of metabolic pathways in a different direction, focusing on cholesterol metabolism. Their study investigates the role of SMG1, a kinase involved in nonsense-mediated RNA decay, in regulating cholesterol homeostasis through p53 alternative splicing. p53, a key tumor suppressor, has multiple isoforms, including p53β and p53γ, which have distinct roles in cancer metabolism. Li et al. demonstrate that inhibition of SMG1 increases the expression of these p53 isoforms, leading to altered cholesterol metabolism in cancer cells. This study is particularly important because cholesterol metabolism has been implicated in cancer progression, especially in aggressive tumors that rely on lipid biosynthesis for growth. By uncovering the link between SMG1, p53 isoforms, and cholesterol metabolism, the authors provide new insights into how metabolic reprogramming can be targeted in cancer therapy.

In the context of glycolysis, Zheng et al. present a pan-cancer analysis of the gene SLC2A1, which encodes the glucose transporter GLUT1. Enhanced glycolysis, also known as the Warburg effect, is a hallmark of cancer metabolism, and SLC2A1 plays a central role in this process by facilitating glucose uptake into cancer cells. Zheng et al. show that SLC2A1 is overexpressed in a wide range of cancers and is associated with poor prognosis. The study also highlights the role of SLC2A1 in modulating the tumor microenvironment, particularly in relation to immune evasion. SLC2A1 expression was found to correlate with biomarkers of T-cell exhaustion, such as PD-L1 and CTLA4, suggesting that it may play a role in suppressing the immune response against tumors. This finding positions SLC2A1 not only as a potential therapeutic target, but also as a biomarker for selecting patients who might benefit from immunotherapy.

Hypoxia is another critical aspect of the tumor microenvironment that drives metabolic reprogramming. In their study, Ramírez-Tortosa et al. investigate the role of Hypoxia-Inducible Factor-1 alpha (HIF-1α) in predicting the response to neoadjuvant chemotherapy in breast cancer. HIF-1α is a transcription factor that is stabilized under low oxygen conditions and regulates the expression of genes involved in glycolysis, angiogenesis, and survival under hypoxic conditions. The authors found that HIF-1α expression correlates with a higher likelihood of achieving a pathological complete response (pCR) following chemotherapy. Additionally, HIF-1α was associated with more aggressive tumor features, such as higher Ki-67 levels and hormone receptor negativity. These findings suggest HIF-1α could as a valuable biomarker for predicting treatment response and tailoring therapy in breast cancer patients.

Ragni et al. take a broader view of cancer metabolism, focusing on amino acids and their role in both tumor growth and cancer-associated cachexia. Cancer cells rely on amino acids not only for protein synthesis but also for energy production and signaling. The review discusses the potential of targeting amino acid metabolism in cancer therapy, either by depriving cancer cells of essential amino acids or by supplementing amino acids to support the host's metabolism in cases of cachexia. Cachexia is a debilitating syndrome characterized by extreme weight loss and muscle wasting, often seen in advanced cancer patients. Ragni et al. argue that while amino acid deprivation can be effective in slowing tumor growth, it may exacerbate cachexia, highlighting the need for a delicate balance in designing therapeutic strategies that consider both the tumor and the host.

Cuyàs et al. explore the metabolic changes associated with the epithelial-to-mesenchymal transition (EMT), a process that plays a key role in cancer metastasis and therapy resistance. Using breast cancer cells, the authors profile the metabolic and mitochondrial alterations that occur during EMT. They find that EMT is associated with increased mitochondrial utilization of glycolytic end-products, as well as a shift towards oxidative metabolism. These changes make EMT cells more resistant to mitochondrial inhibitors, which could explain why EMT-activated cancer cells are more resistant to conventional therapies. This study provides important insights into how targeting metabolic vulnerabilities in EMT cells could enhance the effectiveness of cancer treatments.

The role of obesity in cancer progression is highlighted in a novel study by Iftikhar et al., who examine how epiploic adipose tissue (EPAT) promotes colorectal cancer (CRC) in obese individuals. EPAT is a visceral fat deposit attached to the colon, and the authors show that in obese patients, EPAT creates a tumor-promoting microenvironment that enhances the migration and growth of colon cancer cells. Using a novel microphysiological system, they demonstrate that EPAT from obese individuals releases factors that drive cancer progression, linking obesity with increased CRC risk. This study opens up new avenues for exploring how targeting EPAT could mitigate obesity-associated cancer risks.

Daverio et al. review the phenomenon of lactic acidosis in the tumor microenvironment and how it helps cancer cells resist glucose deprivation. Lactic acidosis arises from the Warburg effect, where cancer cells produce lactate even in the presence of oxygen. The review discusses how lactic acidosis rewires cancer metabolism, promoting a switch from glycolysis to oxidative metabolism, allowing cancer cells to survive in glucose-limited environments. This metabolic flexibility is a key reason why tumors can resist therapies that target glycolysis, and the authors suggest lactic acidosis itself as a promising therapeutic target.

Finally, Tambay et al. use metabolomics to identify a distinctive metabolic signature for hepatocellular carcinoma (HCC). By comparing HCC tissue with adjacent non-tumoral liver tissue, they identify specific metabolites that are altered in cancer, including changes in glutathione, succinate, and alanine levels. These findings support the concept of metabolic reprogramming in HCC and highlight potential biomarkers for early detection and targets for therapy.

In conclusion, the articles (six research, one communication, and one review paper) collected in this Special Issue of *Cancers* highlight the central role of metabolism in cancer biology. The studies discussed here not only underline the impact of changes in metabolism in promoting the spread of cancer, but also create new avenues for targeted treatments that take advantage of the particular metabolic weaknesses in cancer cells. As the field of cancer metabolism continues to evolve, it holds great promise for improving patient outcomes through more effective and personalized treatment strategies.

Conflicts of Interest: The author declares no conflicts of interest.

References

1. Schulze, A.; Harris, A.L. How Cancer Metabolism is Tuned for Proliferation and Vulnerable to Disruption. *Nature* **2012**, *491*, 364–373. [CrossRef] [PubMed]
2. Locasale, J.W. Serine, Glycine and One-Carbon Units: Cancer Metabolism in Full Circle. *Nat. Rev. Cancer* **2013**, *13*, 572–583. [CrossRef] [PubMed]
3. Wettersten, H.; Abu Aboud, O.; Lara, P.N.; Weiss, R.H. Metabolic Reprogramming in Clear Cell Renal Cell Carcinoma. *Nat. Rev. Nephrol.* **2017**, *13*, 410–419. [CrossRef] [PubMed]
4. Schiliro, C.; Firestein, B.L. Mechanisms of Metabolic Reprogramming in Cancer Cells Supporting Enhanced Growth and Proliferation. *Cells* **2021**, *10*, 1056; Erratum in *Cells* **2022**, *11*, 3593. [CrossRef] [PubMed]
5. Lunt, S.Y.; Vander Heiden, M.G. Aerobic Glycolysis: Meeting the Metabolic Requirements of Cell Proliferation. *Annu. Rev. Cell Dev. Biol.* **2011**, *27*, 441–464. [CrossRef] [PubMed]
6. Makhov, P.; Joshi, S.; Ghatalia, P.; Kutikov, A.; Uzzo, R.G.; Kolenko, V.M. Resistance to Systemic Therapies in Clear Cell Renal Cell Carcinoma: Mechanisms and Management Strategies. *Mol. Cancer Ther.* **2018**, *17*, 1355–1364. [CrossRef] [PubMed]
7. Yang, M.; Vousden, K.H. Serine and one-carbon metabolism in cancer. *Nat. Rev. Cancer* **2016**, *16*, 650–662. [CrossRef] [PubMed]
8. Zaretsky, J.M.; Garcia-Diaz, A.; Shin, D.S.; Escuin-Ordinas, H.; Hugo, W.; Hu-Lieskovan, S.; Torrejon, D.Y.; Abril-Rodriguez, G.; Sandoval, S.; Barthly, L.; et al. Mutations Associated with Acquired Resistance to PD-1 Blockade in Melanoma. *N. Engl. J. Med.* **2016**, *375*, 819–829. [CrossRef] [PubMed]
9. Jin, J.; Byun, J.-K.; Choi, Y.-K.; Park, K.-G. Targeting Glutamine Metabolism as a Therapeutic Strategy for Cancer. *Exp. Mol. Med.* **2023**, *55*, 706–715. [CrossRef] [PubMed]
10. Siska, P.J.; Beckermann, K.E.; Rathmell, W.K.; Haake, S.M. Strategies to Overcome Therapeutic Resistance in Renal Cell Carcinoma. *Urol. Oncol. Semin. Orig. Investig.* **2017**, *35*, 102–110. [CrossRef] [PubMed]
11. Pellegrino, M.; Occhiuzzi, M.A.; Grande, F.; Pagani, I.S.; Aquaro, S.; Tucci, P. Modulation of Energetic and Lipid Pathways by Curcumin as a Potential Chemopreventive Strategy in Human Prostate Cancer Cells. *Biochem. Biophys. Res. Commun.* **2024**, *735*, 150477. [CrossRef] [PubMed]
12. Sánchez-Castillo, A.; Heylen, E.; Hounjet, J.; Savelkouls, K.G.; Lieuwes, N.G.; Biemans, R.; Dubois, L.J.; Reynders, K.; Rouschop, K.M.; Vaes, R.D.W.; et al. Targeting Serine/Glycine Metabolism Improves Radiotherapy Response in Non-Small Cell Lung Cancer. *Br. J. Cancer* **2024**, *130*, 568–584. [CrossRef] [PubMed]

Disclaimer/Publisher's Note: The statements, opinions and data contained in all publications are solely those of the individual author(s) and contributor(s) and not of MDPI and/or the editor(s). MDPI and/or the editor(s) disclaim responsibility for any injury to people or property resulting from any ideas, methods, instructions or products referred to in the content.

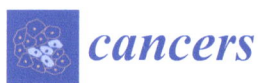 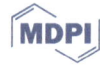

Article

Metabolomics-Guided Identification of a Distinctive Hepatocellular Carcinoma Signature

Vincent Tambay [1], Valérie-Ann Raymond [1], Corentine Goossens [1], Louise Rousseau [2], Simon Turcotte [2,3] and Marc Bilodeau [1,4,*]

[1] Laboratoire d'Hépatologie Cellulaire, Centre de Recherche du Centre Hospitalier de l'Université de Montréal, Montréal, QC H2X0A9, Canada; vincent.tambay@umontreal.ca (V.T.); valerie-ann.raymond.chum@ssss.gouv.qc.ca (V.-A.R.); corentine.goossens@gmail.com (C.G.)

[2] Biobanque et Base de Données Hépatobiliaire et Pancréatique, Centre Hospitalier de l'Université de Montréal, Montréal, QC H2X0C1, Canada; louise.rousseau.chum@ssss.gouv.qc.ca (L.R.); simon.turcotte.med@ssss.gouv.qc.ca (S.T.)

[3] Département de Chirurgie, Service de Transplantation Hépatique et de Chirurgie Hépatobiliaire et Pancréatique, Centre Hospitalier de l'Université de Montréal, Montréal, QC H2X0C1, Canada

[4] Département de Médecine, Université de Montréal, Montréal, QC H3T1J4, Canada

* Correspondence: marc.bilodeau@umontreal.ca

Simple Summary: Hepatocellular carcinoma is the third most prevalent cancer world-wide. This study aimed to reveal the metabolic signature of hepatocellular carcinoma compared to adjacent normal liver cells. To achieve this, metabolites were detected, analyzed, and quantified using targeted and non-targeted metabolomics. We found distinct metabolite signatures between both sample types. Targeted metabolomics identified distinct metabolites being specifically altered in hepatocellular tissue compared to adjacent liver, supporting the concept of metabolic reprogramming in hepatocellular carcinoma.

Abstract: Background: Hepatocellular carcinoma (HCC) is a major contributor to cancer-related morbidity and mortality burdens globally. Given the fundamental metabolic activity of hepatocytes within the liver, hepatocarcinogenesis is bound to be characterized by alterations in metabolite profiles as a manifestation of metabolic reprogramming. Methods: HCC and adjacent non-tumoral liver specimens were obtained from patients after HCC resection. Global patterns in tissue metabolites were identified using non-targeted ^{1}H Nuclear Magnetic Resonance (^{1}H-NMR) spectroscopy whereas specific metabolites were quantified using targeted liquid chromatography–mass spectrometry (LC/MS). Results: Principal component analysis (PCA) within our ^{1}H-NMR dataset identified a principal component (PC) one of 53.3%, along which the two sample groups were distinctively clustered. Univariate analysis of tissue specimens identified more than 150 metabolites significantly altered in HCC compared to non-tumoral liver. For LC/MS, PCA identified a PC1 of 45.2%, along which samples from HCC tissues and non-tumoral tissues were clearly separated. Supervised analysis (PLS–DA) identified decreases in tissue glutathione, succinate, glycerol-3-phosphate, alanine, malate, and AMP as the most important contributors to the metabolomic signature of HCC by LC/MS. Conclusions: Together, ^{1}H-NMR and LC/MS metabolomics have the capacity to distinguish HCC from non-tumoral liver. The characterization of such distinct profiles of metabolite abundances underscores the major metabolic alterations that result from hepatocarcinogenesis.

Keywords: liver; hepatocellular carcinoma; metabolic reprogramming; metabolomics; liquid chromatography–mass spectrometry; NMR spectroscopy; metabolites

Citation: Tambay, V.; Raymond, V.-A.; Goossens, C.; Rousseau, L.; Turcotte, S.; Bilodeau, M. Metabolomics-Guided Identification of a Distinctive Hepatocellular Carcinoma Signature. *Cancers* 2023, 15, 3232. https://doi.org/10.3390/cancers15123232

Academic Editor: Paola Tucci

Received: 27 April 2023
Revised: 14 June 2023
Accepted: 15 June 2023
Published: 18 June 2023

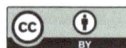

Copyright: © 2023 by the authors. Licensee MDPI, Basel, Switzerland. This article is an open access article distributed under the terms and conditions of the Creative Commons Attribution (CC BY) license (https://creativecommons.org/licenses/by/4.0/).

1. Introduction

Cancer is a complex disease characterized by the occurrence of a panoply of cellular alterations. Indeed, the neoplastic transformation of cells has been described by 10 hallmarks, which are attributable to genetic alterations and cellular adaptations to the tumor environment [1–3]. Metabolic reprogramming has become of major interest in cancer cell biology. Cancer cells require extensive modifications of cell metabolism to survive and proliferate in an array of environmental conditions [2]. Metabolic reprogramming has also been shown to be highly dynamic during carcinogenesis and cancer development, for example during the epithelial–mesenchymal transition (EMT) within the metastatic cascade [4,5]. The reprogramming of cell metabolism occurring in cancer cells encompasses all modifications of biosynthetic and bioenergetic pathways that allow sustained survival, optimal proliferation, as well as invasion and metastasis. Consequently, the fundamental implication of cell metabolism in the onset and progression of malignancy questions whether cancer is a metabolic disease.

Among the most deadly and prevalent malignancies world-wide is hepatocellular carcinoma (HCC) [6]. HCC is the most frequent primary liver cancer with a median five-year survival rate of approximately 20% [6]. This results mainly from the lack of strategies for early detection combined with limited curative therapeutic options, in addition to its association with chronic liver disease. Since the liver acts as the heart for systemic metabolism [7,8], it comes as no surprise that metabolic alterations are observed in the setting of HCC. Indeed, whereas normal hepatocytes are programmed to maintain normal metabolic homeostasis for the whole body, HCC cells need to maximize the availability of nutrients and metabolic substrates for their optimal growth and survival.

The Warburg effect is among the most widely accepted and studied metabolic phenomena in cancer cell metabolism. In the 1920s, Otto Warburg observed that cancer cells metabolized glucose through glycolysis and lactic acid fermentation rather than the mitochondrial pathway [9]. Since then, major studies have demonstrated the importance of metabolic plasticity and heterogeneity in cancer. For example, the avidity for exogenous glucose in HCC cells has been linked with tumorigenic potential in mice [10]. Lipid metabolism has also been shown to exhibit major alterations in cancer, where certain tumor types have enhanced free fatty acid uptake that has in turn been linked to tumor aggressiveness [11]. Understanding mitochondrial dysfunction is also of major interest in defining the deregulation of cancer cell energetics. In HCC, major modifications of the key enzymes involved in the tricarboxylic acid (TCA) cycle have been reported [12]. Mitochondrial fission within cancer cells has also been associated with an increase in the expression of lipogenic genes, with a concomitant decrease in fatty acid oxidation (FAO) genes [13]. Furthermore, alterations in mtDNA due to reactive oxygen species (ROS) accumulation have been proposed as the cause of mitochondrial dysfunction in hepatocarcinoma cells [14]. Distinct metabolic profiles have also been observed between tumors having high EMT activity compared to those with low EMT activity [15]. For example, in adrenocortical carcinoma, high levels of intratumor nucleotides correlate with enhanced EMT activity [15].

The origin of metabolic alterations in cancer cells is thought to arise from genetic alterations, including those that induce oncogenic signaling, as well as from adaptations to the cancer cell microenvironment. Hypoxia is a phenomenon not unknown to tumors: the rapid growth of cells frequently overcomes their vascular network, resulting in limited oxygen and nutrient availability [16]. Hypoxia-inducible factors (HIF) are transcription factors that respond to oxygen levels and act as major regulators of cell metabolism in addition to certain signaling pathways, including that of TGF-β through PI3K/Akt/mTOR [11]. The stabilization of HIF is thought to be key in promoting angiogenesis, invasion, and metastasis [16]. Under hypoxia, HIF1 has been shown to suppress fatty acid oxidation within mitochondria leading to a decrease in the burden of ROS accumulation from mitochondrial metabolism [17]. Nutrient availability has also been shown to impact the metabolic program of cancer cells: HCC cells have been shown to rewire energy metabolism toward FA oxidation under glucose deprivation [10]. Interestingly, in murine HCC, obesity has been linked with a net decrease in FA oxidation within HCC tumors with a resulting increase in dependence on glucose and glutamine in oxidative phosphorylation [18]. Furthermore, the downregulation of carnitine palmatoyltransferase II (CPT2) in HCC has been shown to limit lipotoxicity from microenvironments characterized by excessive lipids and thus allow cancer cell growth [18].

Moreover, distinct genetic alterations have distinct consequences on cancer cell metabolism. For example, p53, a major tumor suppressor often mutated in cancer cells, is an important regulator of glycolysis and glucose transporters [11]. p53 mutations have been shown to promote aberrant lipid metabolism by inducing sterol regulatory element binding protein (SREBP) activity [11]. Mutations of the PTEN tumor suppressor, which is linked to aberrant Akt activity and thus glucose uptake and metabolism, induce SREBP and subsequent lipid metabolism in cancer cells [11]. On the other hand, fundamental oncogenes have been associated with metabolic reprogramming in cancers. Namely, c-Myc, Kras, and mutations of EGFR have been linked with aberrant glycolysis, glutaminolysis, amino acid metabolism, and pentose phosphate pathway activities [11]. Oncogenic Ras and Src signaling have also been shown to promote normoxic activation of HIF1 by inhibiting prolyl hydroxylase domain (PHD) proteins, which could at least partially explain the development of anaerobic metabolism in the presence of oxygen [16]. In HCC, β-catenin mutations have been shown to drive CPT2 expression and an increase in FAO [17]. Additionally, transcriptomics of HCC tissues has identified molecular patterns of metabolism-related gene expression, which have even proposed metabolism-based molecular classifications of HCC [19–21]. Altogether, the current state of the literature suggests that metabolism is intimately linked with cancer onset and progression.

Hence, metabolomics has become a compelling novel tool for understanding cancer cell biology. Metabolomics has major potential in identifying novel clinical biomarkers for the screening, diagnosis, and monitoring of cancers and could aid in identifying cancer risk factors as well as developing novel metabolism-focused targeted therapies [22,23]. Indeed, metabolomics generates robust and highly specific metabolic information, which makes them potentially very useful in the context of personalized cancer medicine [24]. This study aimed to identify the metabolomic signatures of HCC by highlighting key changes in the metabolism of hepatocarcinoma compared to adjacent non-tumoral liver tissue as well as calling attention to the pertinence of metabolic reprogramming in HCC. To achieve this, both targeted and non-targeted metabolomics modalities were used in order to offer a comprehensive understanding of HCC metabolomics. Whereas ^{1}H-Nuclear Magnetic Resonance (^{1}H-NMR)-based non-targeted analyses allowed the identification of global patterns within the metabolite profiles of non-tumoral and neoplastic liver tissues, liquid chromatography/mass spectrometry (LC/MS)-based targeted analyses enabled the quantification of a specific set of metabolite alterations.

2. Materials and Methods

2.1. Patients and Sample Collection

Patients ($n = 5$) undergoing HCC tumor resection were recruited with written informed consent prior to surgery. For each participant, one specimen of tumoral tissue was collected and snap-frozen in liquid nitrogen, accompanied by the collection of one specimen of non-tumoral (normal) liver tissue at distance from the neoplastic foci. The time elapsed between the collection of samples and their cryopreservation is shown in Table S1. This research protocol was conducted in accordance with the Declaration of Helsinki and was approved by the "Comité d'éthique de la recherche du Centre de recherche du CHUM (CRCHUM)". All studied HCC tumors presented a trabecular pattern within livers devoid of underlying cirrhosis. Available clinical data are reported in Table 1.

Table 1. Clinical data of patients with HCC liver tumors and sample cryopreservation time. Collected clinical data of patients who participated for metabolomics analyses of HCC and adjacent non-cirrhotic liver. Time to cryopreservation was observed as the time elapsed between tissue resection and liquid nitrogen storage.

	Sexe	Age	Tissue Type	Grade (Edmonson-Steiner)	Sub-Type	Underlying Liver Condition	Time to Cryopreservation (m)
Patient 1	F	52	HCC Non-tumoral	2	Trabecular	Normal liver	25 25
Patient 2	M	73	HCC Non-tumoral	2	Trabecular	Normal liver	30 32
Patient 3	F	47	HCC Non-tumoral	1	Trabecular	Normal liver	28 30
Patient 4	M	57	HCC Non-tumoral	2	Trabecular	Normal liver	28 40
Patient 5	M	67	HCC Non-tumoral	2	Trabecular	Normal liver	45 47

2.2. Metabolite Extraction for Targeted LC/MS-Based Metabolomics

Water-soluble metabolites were extracted from tissue specimens using liquid–liquid extraction. Samples were homogenized in ice-cold metabolite extraction buffer (80% methanol, 2 mM ammonium acetate, pH 9.0; 20 µM [13C10,15N5]-AMP as an internal standard) using a Cryolis-cooled Precellys 24 Dual system (Bertin, France) with CK14 ceramic beads, for 2×25 s at 6000 rpm separated by a 15-second rest. Homogenates were centrifuged at $20,000 \times g$ for 10 min (4 °C); 183 µL of supernatant was transferred to 10×75 mm glass tubes and diluted with 367 µL of extraction buffer. Diluted supernatants were mixed and incubated on ice for 10 min. Then, 250 µL of water and 880 µL of chloroform:heptane (3:1) solution were added and samples were mixed thoroughly, followed by a 15-minute incubation on ice. Sample preparations were then centrifuged for 15 min at $4500 \times g$ (4 °C) and 500 µL of the aqueous/upper phase was transferred to polypropylene tubes for the concentration of extracted metabolites. Organic solvents were removed in a refrigerated CentriVap (Labconco, Kansas City, MO, USA; 90 min, 10 °C) and the remaining liquid (100 µL) was freeze-dried overnight. Prior to LC/MS processing and analysis, 40 µL of water was added to each sample followed by rapid 5-minute centrifugation (4 °C); re-suspended concentrated metabolite extracts were transferred to HPLC vials.

2.3. Metabolite Extraction for Non-Targeted ^{1}H-NMR-Based Metabolomics

For ^{1}H-NMR metabolomic profiling, extraction of liver specimen metabolites was performed by dual-phase methanol:water:chloroform (2:1:2) extraction. Tumor and non-tumoral specimens were ground and homogenized in 600 µL of extraction buffer (2:1 methanol:water) with ceramic beads in a Precellys Homogenizer (Bertin Technologies, Montigny-le-Bretonneux, France). Then, 400 µL of chloroform was added to each sample, followed by a 15-minute incubation (4 °C). Samples were centrifuged for 15 min at $15,000 \times g$ (4 °C). The upper polar phase was collected and dried overnight under nitrogen flow. Prior to ^{1}H-NMR processing and analysis, dried tissue extracts were dissolved in 600 µL of D2O-prepared phosphate buffer solution (pH 7.4) containing 0.4 mM of sodium trimethylsilyl-(2,2,3,3-d$_4$)-propionate (TSP) as an internal reference, and re-suspended samples transferred to 5 mm NMR tubes.

2.4. Targeted LC/MS Metabolite Detection and Data Acquisition

Liver specimen metabolites and standard analyte solutions were separated by liquid phase chromatography using a Nexera X2 Ultra-High-Performance Liquid Chromatography (UHPLC) system (Shimadzu, Kyoto, Japan) at 40 °C with 3 µL injections on a Poroshell 120 EC-C18 2.1 mm $\times$ 75 mm $\times$ 2.7 µm UHPLC column (Agilent Technologies, Santa Clara, CA, USA) following a Poroshell 120 EC-C18 2.1 mm $\times$ 5 mm $\times$ 2.7 µm UHPLC guard column (Agilent Technologies, USA). To perform this, gradient elution with an initial mobile phase was used, consisting of 95%: 10 mM tributylamine and 15 mM acetic acid in water, pH 5.2; 5%: acetonitrile:water (95:5, v/v) fortified with 0.1% formic acid; this was performed at a flow rate of 0.75 mL/min. Standard and sample metabolites were detected using negative electrospray ionization on a SCIEX 4000 Qtrap mass spectrometer (Framingham, MA, USA). MS/MS parameters were optimized for each metabolite and quantified using SCIEX MultiQuant 3.0.2 (Framingham, USA) according to calibration curves (0.15 to 12,000 pmol per injection) of pure analytes purchased from Sigma Aldrich (Oakville, ON, Canada), prepared in water. Values were normalized per mg of tissue.

2.5. Non-Targeted ^{1}H-NMR Metabolite Detection and Data Acquisition

The detection of liver sample metabolites for ^{1}H-NMR analysis was performed on an Ascend 700 MHz spectrometer (Bruker, Billerica, MA, USA) coupled to an AVANCE NEO console equipped with a 5-millimeter triple resonance probe (Bruker, USA) at 298 K. For each sample, a one-dimensional ^{1}H-NMR spectrum was acquired with water peak suppression using a nuclear Overhauser enhancement spectroscopy (NOESY) presaturation pulse sequence; 128 scans; 65,000 data points; an acquisition time of 2.4 s; a relaxation delay of 4 s; a mixing time of 10 milliseconds; and a spectral width of 20 ppm.

2.6. ^{1}H-NMR Spectral Processing and Analysis

After acquisition of ^{1}H-NMR spectra for each specimen, free induction decays were multiplied by an exponential function equivalent to a 0.3 Hz line-broadening factor before applying Fourier transform. The spectra were phased and the baseline was corrected and referenced to the TSP peak (at 0 ppm) using TopSpin 4.0.5 (Bruker, USA). One-dimensional spectra ranging from 0.5 to 9.5 ppm were binned by intelligent adaptive bucketing and the corresponding spectral areas were integrated using the NMRProcFlow tool (https://www.nmrprocflow.org/; accessed on 18 February 2020). The spectral region from 4.5 to 5 ppm was removed as this corresponded to residual water within samples. Total spectral areas were calculated using the remaining buckets and followed by constant sum normalization.

2.7. Statistical Analysis

Various statistical methods were used to analyze metabolomic datasets from LC/MS and ^{1}H-NMR metabolite profiling modalities. For both datasets, all samples were normalized according to each original specimen's wet weight, then metabolites/variables were mean-centered and divided by the square root of their standard deviation (Pareto scaling) prior to subsequent statistical analysis. To obtain a reduced dimensionality view of the metabolomic profiles of HCC and non-tumoral liver samples, principal component analysis (PCA) and partial least squares–discriminate analysis (PLS–DA) were performed using MetaboAnalyst 5.0 (https://metaboanalyst.ca/; accessed on 2 September 2022). PCA allowed the identification of global trends in metabolite signatures between study groups and of clusters and possible outliers within the metabolic data matrices in an unsupervised analytical manner. As a supervised statistical analysis, PLS–DA allowed the maximization of the covariance between the observed abundances of metabolites in liver samples and the sample type (tumoral and non-tumoral samples). In PLS–DA, the number of components was determined by "Leave One Out Cross-Validation" which yielded goodness-of-fit (R_2) and predictability (Q_2) of the regression. Loadings plots obtained from PLS–DA allowed the identification of metabolites greatly contributing to the metabolomic discrimination of liver samples between both study groups. The most weighted metabolites in this statistical classification of the analyzed samples were identified using the variable importance in projection (VIP) method. Student's t test was used to measure statistical differences in specific metabolite concentrations between both sample groups. Statistical differences were considered significant when $p < 0.05$.

3. Results

3.1. ^{1}H-NMR Profiling Identifies a Distinct Metabolomic Signature of HCC

To establish the metabolite makeup of HCC, we compared the global metabolomic profile of all liver specimens (tumoral and non-tumoral) using non-targeted ^{1}H-NMR. Through intelligent processing methodologies, a total of 450 metabolomic features were analyzed and subsequently compared between all samples. To reduce the dimensionality of the ^{1}H-NMR dataset and identify major trends in metabolomic feature abundance between samples, an initial Principal Component Analysis (PCA) was performed (Figure 1A,B). The PCA identified a primary principal component (PC1) explaining 56.5% of metabolic data variability within the 10 studied samples and a second principal component (PC2) explaining 22.3% of data variability (Figure 1A). Interestingly, the identification of individual samples (red: HCC tumors; blue: non-tumoral livers; shaded area: 95% confidence interval for each group) within the PCA scores plot revealed a distinct clustering of both groups along the primary principal component. The PCA loading plot represents all analyzed metabolomic features and their importance in positioning samples within the scores plot. As seen in Figure 1B, a select population of features corresponded to those whose abundances were characteristic of non-tumoral tissue, whereas the abundance of a more important proportion of liver metabolites was characteristic of HCC tumors. Observations made through PCA were further studied using PLS–DA to identify the metabolic discrimination of both sample groups using their respective metabolomic datasets (Figure 1C,D). PLS–DA cross-validation for one component revealed validation metrics with a goodness-of-fit of 0.855 and a model predictability of 0.716 (accuracy = 1.0) and, for two components, revealed a goodness-of-fit of 0.927 and a model predictability of 0.623 (accuracy = 0.9). In this supervised analysis of liver specimen metabolomic profiles, which maximizes covariance between the observed changes in metabolomic features and both study groups, the primary component explained 56.3% of data variability, whereas the second component explained 16.0% (Figure 1C). The PLS–DA loading plot represents all analyzed metabolomic features and their importance in positioning samples within the PLS–DA scores plot (Figure 1D). Interestingly, for both PCA and PLS–DA scores plots, non-tumoral liver samples were circumscribed within a relatively small region of the scores plots, whereas HCC tumor samples were much sparser within the plots and their 95% confidence interval region (Figure 1B,D). In Figure 1E, a volcano scatter plot shows the identified metabolomic features being significantly altered, either increased (red) or decreased (blue), in HCC compared to non-tumoral samples. Features that remained unaltered in hepatocarcinoma samples are identified in gray. For the visualization of the global metabolomic pattern of each studied sample, Figure 1F depicts a heatmap of the relative abundance of all 450 analyzed metabolite features. Clearly, this depiction shows that the identification of the metabolomic signatures of HCC tumors is completely distinct from those of non-tumoral liver.

3.2. Targeted HCC Metabolomics Identify Altered Amino Acid and TCA Cycle Profiles

Our initial non-targeted analysis of liver tissue metabolomics revealed distinctive metabolite signatures between HCC and non-tumoral liver tissues. This interesting finding, which showcased the capacity of liver metabolomics to successfully discriminate between HCC and non-tumoral liver through metabolite profiling, prompted us to study changes in the tissue abundance of specific metabolites; hence, 26 metabolites from distinct metabolic pathways were chosen for targeted screening of liver specimen metabolomics. Firstly, diverse amino acids were quantified in all samples having been analyzed through ^{1}H-NMR profiling. The non-essential amino acid arginine, an important intermediate of the urea cycle, was the only significantly altered amino acid between the two groups. Indeed, the concentration of arginine was higher in HCC (23.1 ± 4.5 pmol/mg$_{tissue}$) compared to non-tumoral specimens (12.5 ± 1.2 pmol/mg$_{tissue}$) ($p < 0.05$, Figure 2A). As seen in Figure 2B–D, no changes in aspartate, alanine, or leucine concentrations were observed in HCC tissues compared to their paired non-tumoral samples. The amino acid glutamine was marginally decreased in HCC specimens (Figure 2E), which was accompanied by an increase in glutamate abundance in certain tumor samples (Figure 2F), though not reaching statistical significance. In addition, we quantified lactate, the product of pyruvate fermentation following glycolysis: its tissue abundance was unchanged in tumors compared to control specimens (Figure 2G). Five intermediates of the tricarboxylic acid (TCA) cycle pathway were also measured in each sample to unveil potential disturbances in mitochondrial metabolism in hepatocarcinoma. The levels of (iso)citrate (Figure 2H) and α-ketoglutarate (Figure 2I) remained similar between HCC and non-tumoral tissue samples. On the other hand, succinate was significantly decreased from 2.29 ± 0.39 nmol/mg$_{tissue}$ in controls to 0.59 ± 0.15 nmol/mg$_{tissue}$ in HCC samples ($p < 0.01$, Figure 2J). Fumarate, another TCA cycle intermediate, was lower in tumors (191.9 ± 18.2 pmol/mg$_{tissue}$) in comparison to non-tumoral specimens (346.2 ± 26.7 pmol/mg$_{tissue}$) ($p < 0.01$, Figure 2K). A similar change was observed for malate, the level of which was greatly reduced in HCC (1.11 ± 0.078 nmol/mg$_{tissue}$) compared to surrounding liver tissue (0.36 ± 0.097 nmol/mg$_{tissue}$, $p < 0.001$, Figure 2L).

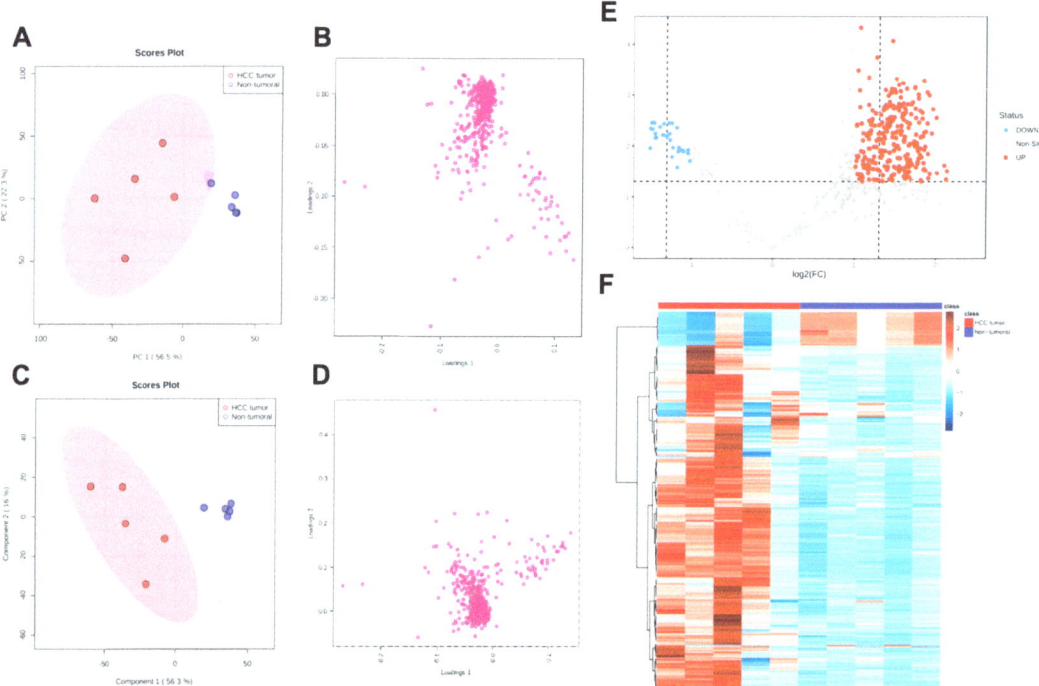

Figure 1. ^{1}H-NMR profiling of HCC compared to paired non-tumoral liver tissue. Non-targeted metabolomics was performed by ^{1}H-NMR after metabolite extraction. Processed spectra and binning with intelligent adaptive bucketing of 450 bins (metabolomic features) were integrated and analyzed with principal component analysis (PCA): PCA scores plot (**A**), PCA loadings plot (**B**). Metabolomic profiles between both sample groups were compared using partial least squares–discriminate analysis (PLS–DA): PLS–DA scores plot (**C**), PLS–DA loadings plot (**D**). Volcano scatter plot (**E**) of significantly altered ($p < 0.05$) features (increased, red; decreased, blue; unchanged, gray) in HCC specimens compared to non-tumoral specimens. Heatmap depiction (**F**) of the differential abundance of the 450 analyzed spectral features in all samples (red, HCC; blue, non-tumoral liver).

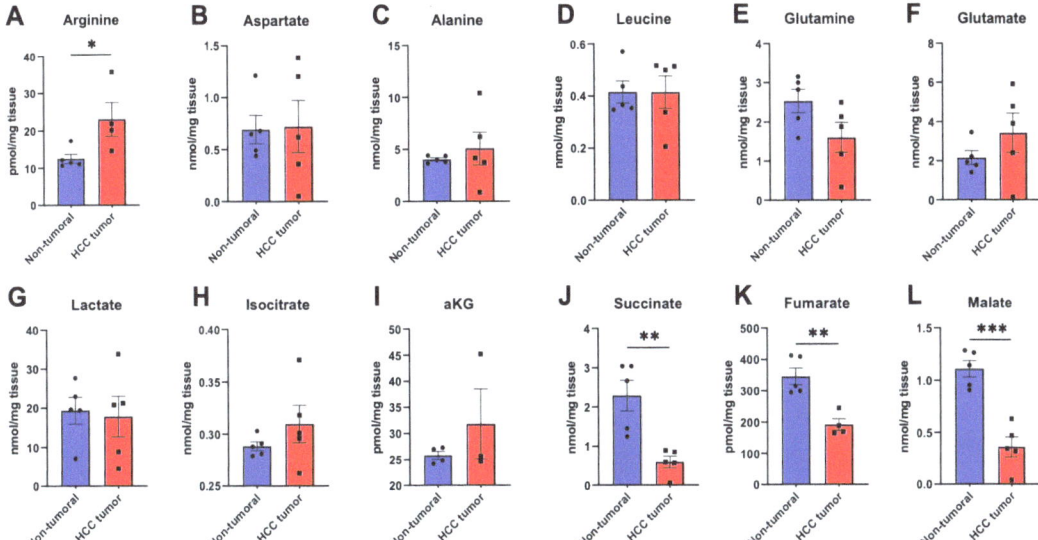

Figure 2. Targeted identification of amino acids and TCA cycle metabolites in hepatocellular carcinoma specimens and adjacent normal liver. HCC (red) and non-tumoral liver (blue) specimens were analyzed through targeted LC/MS metabolomics to characterize the tissue abundances of arginine (**A**), aspartate (**B**), alanine (**C**), leucine (**D**), glutamine (**E**), and glutamate (**F**) amino acids, as well as lactate (**G**), (iso)citrate (**H**), α-ketoglutarate (αKG, (**I**)), succinate (**J**), fumarate (**K**), and malate (**L**). *: $p < 0.05$, **: $p < 0.01$, ***: $p < 0.001$.

3.3. Metabolic Reprogramming of HCC Encompasses Major Changes in Energy Metabolism and the Glycerol-3-Phosphate/Dihydroxyacetone Phosphate Pathway

We then studied key metabolic intermediates at the crossroad between glycolysis and lipid metabolism such as dihydroxyacetone phosphate (DHAP) and glycerol-3-phosphate (glycerol-3P) as well as those involved in energy metabolism, such as ATP and the NADH cofactor. Interestingly, both DHAP and glycerol-3P were significantly lower in HCC samples compared to adjacent non-tumoral tissues (Figure 3A,B). Taken together, the calculated ratio of glycerol-3P-to-DHAP was significantly lower in HCC compared to non-tumoral samples (24.9 ± 6.7 vs. 71.7 ± 7.3, respectively; $p < 0.01$, Figure 3C). The concentration of NADH was found to be 0.18 ± 0.018 nmol/mg$_{tissue}$ in non-tumoral specimens and 0.048 ± 0.012 nmol/mg$_{tissue}$ in HCC specimens, which represents a 3.75-fold decrease in HCC samples ($p < 0.001$, Figure 3D). Though the oxidized form of NADH, NAD (Figure 3E), was only marginally lower in tumors, the calculated NADH/NAD ratio (Figure 3F) was significantly lower in HCC ($p < 0.05$). Given this important change in NADH, we studied ATP and its metabolites ADP and AMP to further understand the state of energy storage and metabolism in HCC. As shown in Figure 3G, AMP was significantly lower in HCC (467.0 ± 168.9 pmol/mg$_{tissue}$) compared to non-tumoral liver (1289.5 ± 103.8 pmol/mg$_{tissue}$, $p < 0.01$). A similar trend was observed for ADP, which was nearly three-fold lower (105.6 ± 31.8 pmol/mg$_{tissue}$) in HCC samples ($p < 0.01$, Figure 3H). Importantly, as shown in Figure 3I, ATP could not be detected (0.00 ± 0.00 pmol/mg$_{tissue}$) in HCC tumors in opposition to non-tumoral liver specimens (57.5 ± 10.3 pmol/mg$_{tissue}$) ($p < 0.001$). Finally, the calculated energy charge remained similar between both groups (Figure 3J).

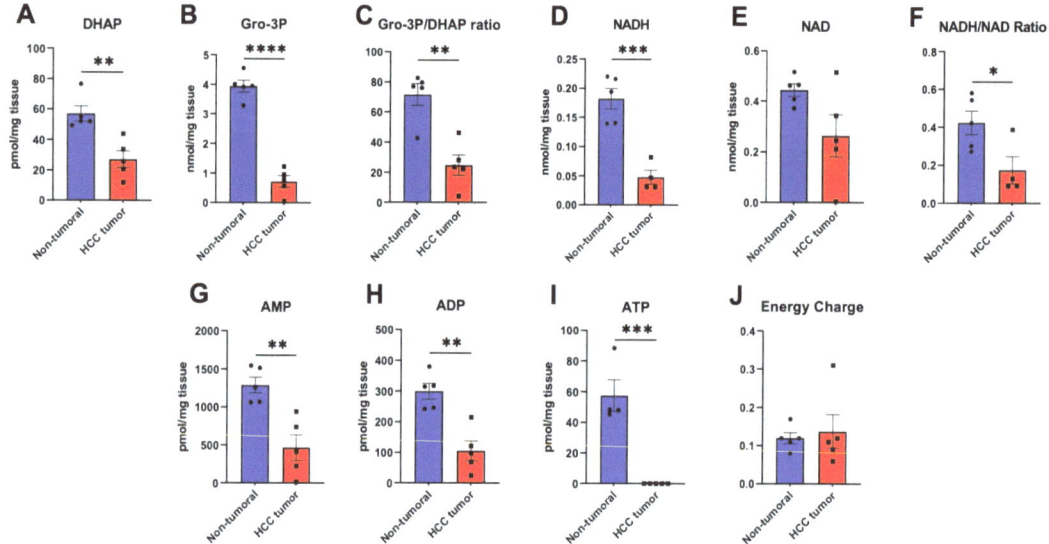

Figure 3. Metabolites and the glycerol-3-phosphate/dihydroxyacetone phosphate pathway in hepatocellular carcinoma specimens and adjacent normal liver. HCC (red) and non-tumoral (blue) specimens were analyzed through targeted LC/MS metabolomics to characterize the tissue abundances of dihydroxyacetone phosphate (DHAP, (**A**)), glycerol-3-phosphate (Gro-3P, (**B**)), and the resulting Gro-3P/DHAP ratio (**C**), NADH (**D**), NAD (**E**), the NADH/NAD ratio (**F**), AMP (**G**), ADP (**H**), and ATP (**I**). The adenylate energy charge was calculated as follows: [ATP + 1/2ADP]/[ATP + ADP + AMP] (**J**). *: $p < 0.05$, **: $p < 0.01$, ***: $p < 0.001$, ****: $p < 0.0001$.

3.4. Perturbations of Oxidative-Stress-Related Metabolites Glutathione and NADPH in Hepatocarcinoma Compared to Adjacent Non-Tumoral Tissue

Oxidative stress is thought to be a key component contributing to tumorigenesis as well as cancer progression. As such, we quantified glutathione, an important mediator of cellular redox homeostasis, in all liver specimens. The reduced form of glutathione, GSH, had a concentration of 3.20 ± 0.66 nmol/mg$_{tissue}$ in non-tumoral specimens and was significantly depleted in HCC tumors (0.24 ± 0.10 nmol/mg$_{tissue}$, $p < 0.01$, Figure 4A). Though the oxidized form of glutathione, GSSG, was relatively unchanged in HCC (Figure 4B), the calculated GSH/GSSG ratio plummeted 13.4-fold from 6.69 ± 1.15 in the non-tumoral liver to 0.50 ± 0.25 in HCC ($p < 0.01$, Figure 4C). Additionally, as glutathione recycling from GSSG to GSH requires NADPH, we quantified the abundance of the latter as well as its oxidized form NADP. NADPH marginally decreased in HCC (Figure 4D) whereas NADP, as depicted in Figure 4E, was significantly lower in HCC tumors ($p < 0.05$). Nonetheless, the NADPH/NADP ratio increased in tumors, though without reaching statistical significance (Figure 4F). Adenosine, cAMP, and GMP abundances remained similar between both study groups (Figure 4G–I). Altogether, targeted LC/MS metabolomics allowed the identification of major changes in the tissue abundance of diverse metabolic intermediates in HCC, supporting the global metabolite signature of hepatocarcinoma having been identified using non-targeted ^{1}H-NMR profiling.

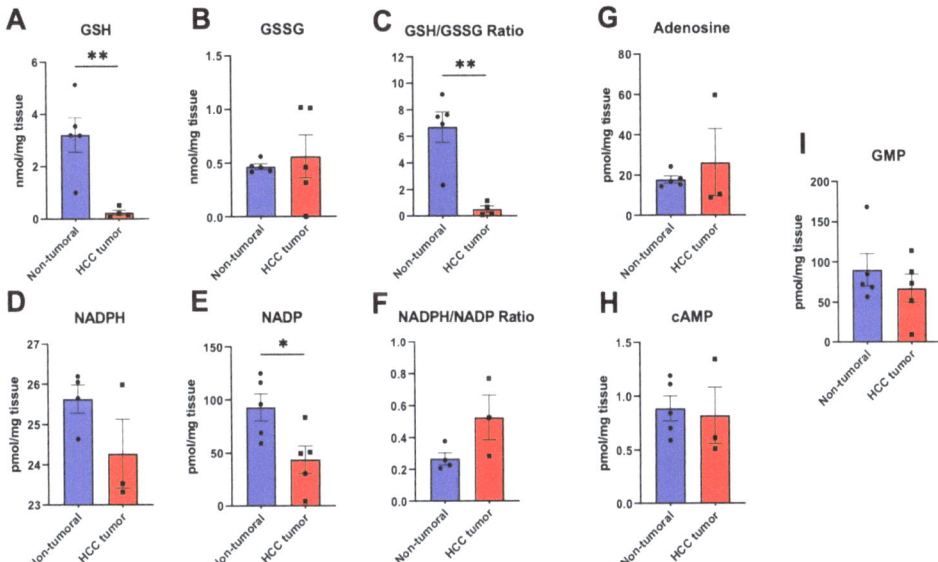

Figure 4. Oxidative stress-related metabolites glutathione and NADPH in hepatocellular carcinoma specimens and adjacent normal liver. HCC (red) and non-tumoral (blue) specimens were analyzed through targeted LC/MS metabolomics to characterize the tissue abundances of reduced glutathione (GSH) (**A**), oxidized glutathione (GSSG) (**B**), the GSH/GSSG ratio (**C**), NADPH (**D**), NADP (**E**), the resulting NADPH/NADP ratio (**F**), as well as adenosine (**G**), cyclic AMP (cAMP), (**H**), and GMP (**I**). *: $p < 0.05$, **: $p < 0.01$.

3.5. Ability of Targeted LC/MS to Characterize HCC and Metabolites Contributing to the HCC Metabolomic Signature

Given the identification of significant differences in the abundance of the many metabolites from various metabolic pathways between HCC and non-tumoral tissue, as observed in Figures 2–4, we analyzed our LC/MS metabolomics dataset using multivariate and descriptive statistics. The metabolomic profiles of all studied samples were analyzed through PCA, as shown in the scores plot in Figure 5A. Using the 26 quantified metabolites, unsupervised PCA identified a primary principal component (PC1) that explained 45.2% of metabolite quantification variability between the ten liver specimens; a second observed principal component (PC2) encompassed 16.8% of metabolomic data variability. Then, the labeling of positioned samples within the PCA scores plot according to their respective groups (red: HCC tumors; blue: non-tumoral liver; shaded area: 95% confidence interval for each group) allowed the identification of two well-segregated clusters along the primary principal component (PC1) that corresponded to both study groups (HCC and non-tumoral samples). Further decomposition of the PCA revealed that lactate and glutamate tended to be more abundant in HCC tumor samples, whereas higher levels of GSH, succinate, alanine, glycerol-3P, and AMP were rather distinctive of non-tumoral specimens (Figure 5B). Furthermore, we analyzed our LC/MS dataset using supervised PLS–DA (Figure 5C–E). PLS–DA cross-validation for one component revealed validation metrics with a goodness-of-fit of 0.827 and a model predictability of 0.669 (accuracy = 0.9) and revealed a goodness-of-fit of 0.968 and a model predictability of 0.707 (accuracy = 0.9) for two components. As shown in the scores plot of Figure 5C, PLS–DA component analysis revealed a component one explaining 44.6% and a component two explaining 12.3% of the observed variability of liver metabolomics. Given that PLS–DA is optimized to maximize the relationship between the observed variance of metabolite quantities and the descriptor sample group (tumor vs. non-tumoral), samples were clearly separated without any overlap between both groups along component one of the scores plot (Figure 5C). All studied metabolites and calculated metabolite ratios were depicted in a loadings plot (Figure 5D). In addition, as shown in Figure 5E, PLS–DA attributed variable importance in projection (VIP) scores to all studied features. Metabolites and ratios having a VIP greater than 1.000 were considered significant contributors to the metabolomic discrimination of liver specimens as either belonging to the HCC or the non-tumoral group. Namely, the decreased abundance of GSH, glycerol-3P, succinate, alanine, malate, and AMP, as well as the decrease in GSH/GSSG and glycerol-3P/DHAP ratios were the most discriminant features of the HCC metabolomic signature. The GSH/GSSG ratio had a VIP score of 3.155, and those of GSH, glycerol-3P, succinate, alanine, malate, the glycerol-3P/DHAP ratio, and AMP were 2.351, 1.998, 1.795, 1.319, 1.282, 1.281, and 1.236, respectively.

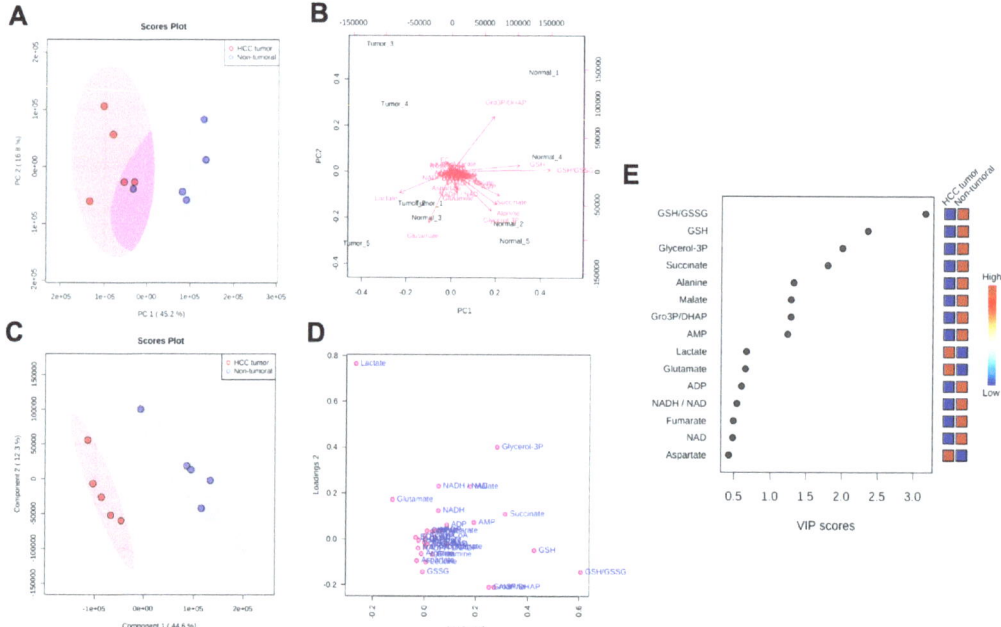

Figure 5. Ability of targeted LC/MS liver metabolomics to discriminate hepatocellular carcinoma specimens and adjacent normal liver. Targeted metabolomics of HCC and paired non-tumoral liver specimens were performed by LC/MS after metabolite extraction for a set of 26 chosen metabolites. Metabolomic profiles of liver specimens were compared using the specific tissue abundance (nmol/mg$_{tissue}$) of all metabolites. Metabolomic profiles were analyzed using principal component analysis (PCA): PCA scores plot (**A**), PCA scores plot with identification of metabolite positioning (**B**). Metabolomic profiles between both sample groups were compared using partial least squares–discriminate analysis (PLS–DA): PLS–DA scores plot (**C**), PLS–DA loadings plot (**D**), and attributed variable importance in projection (VIP) scores (**E**) to important metabolites in the PLS–DA model. Relative abundance of the important metabolites was classified as increased (red) or decreased (blue) in HCC samples compared to non-tumoral liver tissue.

4. Discussion

The phenomenon of altered metabolism within cancer cells emerged nearly one century ago. Nevertheless, much mystery still remains concerning the implication of metabolic reprogramming in cancer pathophysiology from onset to progression. Indeed, changes in biosynthetic metabolism and bioenergetics within cancer cells have yet to be demonstrated effective for cancer management, especially for HCC. From a metabolic point of view, the detection and treatment of neoplastic liver lesions are hindered by the important metabolic function of the normal liver. Targeting metabolism in HCC will need to be specific to pathways preferentially expressed in liver cancer cells and preferably absent or of low importance in functional, normal hepatocytes. The quest for discovering such metabolic targets for anti-neoplastic treatment begins with a better understanding of HCC pathophysiology. Although some studies have reported metabolomics analyses of fluids from HCC patients, the metabolomics of HCC tissue itself has yet to be better characterized and validated [25–27]. Nevertheless, metabolomics has become a crucial tool for characterizing cancer cell metabolic behavior [22,28]. This study characterized the metabolomic profiles of human HCC compared to adjacent non-tumoral liver tissue through the identification of metabolite signatures from liver specimens. To achieve this, complimentary metabolomics techniques were performed: non-targeted ^{1}H-NMR profiling detected all extracted tissue metabolites within samples whereas targeted metabolomics, through LC/MS, quantified the abundance of a specific ensemble of metabolites.

Our initial analysis of liver tissue metabolomics was performed through a non-targeted approach using five HCC samples and their paired non-tumoral adjacent tissues. The ^{1}H-NMR dataset enabled the detection of 450 metabolomic features, many of which were altered in HCC compared to adjacent liver tissue. Indeed, PCA, which aimed to reduce data dimensionality, revealed a PC1 explaining 56.5% of data variability. Further identification of samples in the PCA plot showed that the clusters of both groups, that is HCC or non-tumoral tissues, were clearly separated along the PC1 axis. This suggests that the main factor explaining changes in the abundance of all liver tissue metabolites is attributed to the type of tissue (HCC vs. non-tumoral). Similar observations were made using supervised PLS–DA statistical analyses. HCC and adjacent non-tumoral tissues also showed distinct profiles of metabolomic heterogeneity. Whereas non-tumoral liver samples were well circumscribed within a smaller 95% confidence interval region, samples belonging to the HCC group were scattered within a large 95% confidence interval region. These findings highlight the significance of inter-individual heterogeneity in HCC, which seems to be accordingly much greater than in normal livers [29,30]. Indeed, tumor heterogeneity is an important concept in cancer biology, and our untargeted metabolomics calls attention to cell metabolism as a key component of inter-tumoral heterogeneity in HCC; therefore, untargeted metabolomics has a powerful ability to discriminate whether a given sample is neoplastic or not. PCA of the targeted metabolomics dataset, which quantified 26 specific metabolites within the studied samples, revealed in turn a PC1 explaining 45.2% of data variability. This result is interesting, as specifically measuring only 26 metabolites within liver tissue, rather than detecting all metabolites, had a discriminative capacity nearly matching that of ^{1}H-NMR profiling. Indeed, both groups, HCC and adjacent non-tumoral tissues, were separated along the PC1, confirming with non-targeted metabolomics that metabolomic variations are a major hallmark of HCC. Distinct clustering of both groups was also clear along component one of the PLS–DA. Altogether, these findings highlight that changes in the metabolic program of hepatocytes occurring during hepatocarcinogenesis are so important that the study of the metabolite landscape within liver tissue is powerful enough to identify HCC. This discriminative ability of metabolomics has also been described by various groups in lung cancer compared to chronic obstructive pulmonary disease and pancreatic cancer compared to pancreatitis [31–33]. Furthermore, Kowalczyk et al. also discussed the ability of specific metabolites to precisely discriminate between subtypes of lung cancer [34].

Additionally, the heatmap depiction and volcano scatter plot of the 450 detected metabolomic features represented in Figure 1 highlight the presence of distinct metabolite patterns between non-tumoral and HCC tissues; hence, a specific population of metabolites is abundant in the normal liver whereas a large population of different metabolites tend to accumulate in HCC. Moreover, according to our targeted metabolomics analysis, the most significant alterations observed between the two groups were lower levels of specific metabolites in HCC. This is different to what was observed in ^{1}H-NMR, where many detected metabolites had increased levels in tumors: this could be explained by the fact that the chosen metabolites in the LC/MS targeted approach are indeed those that characterized the population of metabolomic features that specifically decreased in HCC tumors shown by ^{1}H-NMR. The important proportion of metabolites that were shown to be increased in HCC tumors compared to non-tumoral tissues by ^{1}H-NMR could potentially be waste products and metabolic by-products, which could emerge from rapid and likely inefficient metabolism in cancer cells [35]. Regarding the identity of the metabolites within this population, the profiling of liver sample metabolomic profiles using an initial non-targeted ^{1}H-NMR approach aimed to establish global changes in metabolite signatures between the two study groups, that is non-tumoral liver and HCC tumors, rather than specifically identify the detected metabolites within the dataset. Ulterior identification of such metabolite populations could reveal additional metabolic intermediates that belong to the class of oncometabolites, that is, metabolites that are either specific to cancer cells or are greater in abundance within tumoral tissues. An important example of such a phenomenon is the oncometabolite 2-hydroxyglutarate, which is abundant in isocitrate dehydrogenase-mutant cancers including glioma and acute myeloid leukemia [22,36].

Furthermore, our targeted metabolomics approach allowed the quantification of specific metabolites from an array of pathways central to cell and energy metabolism. First, arginine was the only significantly altered amino acid found in HCC, in which its abundance increased. This could possibly be explained should the urea cycle metabolism be shown to be decreased within HCC tumors, which is known to be highly functional in the normal liver [7]. Arginine is the final substrate of the urea cycle, its breakdown by arginase leading the release of urea and ornithine. As such, decreased urea cycle activity within HCC cells, in addition to increased arginine consumption, are plausible explanations for this increase in tissue arginine within tumors compared to adjacent tissue. Interestingly, contrary to the increase in arginine tissue abundance found in HCC, arginine levels have been shown to be decreased in the sera of HCC patients [37]. Together with metabolomic data from Morine et al. and He et al., our findings are complementary in highlighting the important metabolic changes occurring in HCC from the identification of metabolites in liver samples [26,27]. Indeed, our study not only shows that HCC metabolomics has a distinct profile to non-tumoral liver, as suggested in other studies, but ^{1}H-NMR analysis has also proven that non-cirrhotic liver exhibits very limited metabolomic variability between individuals, highlighting the importance of studying liver tissue metabolomics in HCC among other liver diseases.

Concentrations of important metabolic intermediates of the TCA cycle, such as succinate, fumarate, and malate, were found to be significantly lower in HCC samples compared to adjacent non-tumoral tissue. This finding could be linked with various aspects of hepatocarcinogenesis. Indeed, this decrease could be explained by the increased turnover of TCA cycle metabolites within HCC cells, namely those exhibiting oxidative metabolism. This turnover can in turn support biosynthetic demands for the genesis of lipids, proteins, and nucleic acids, as well as cellular energy. Another explanation of this interesting finding could be that HCC tumors exhibit increased hypoxic features, hypoxia being a well-known characteristic of cancer. As such, the presence of hypoxia as well as mitochondrial dysfunction within HCC cells could yield a decrease in the flux of cytosolic carbons through mitochondria and the TCA cycle. Though there exists insufficient evidence to support severe hypoxia in HCC, altered oxygen availability is bound to occur in HCC cells when tumor expansion surpasses its inherently irregular angiogenetic program [38,39]. Mitochondrial dysfunction, on the other hand, has been suggested to occur in HCC as a result of mtDNA mutations and copy number variations [14,40]. In a similar perspective, decreased glycerol-3-phosphate and DHAP could be explained by such a phenomenon. Indeed, decreased glycerol-3-phosphate shuttle activity and, as such, decreased flux of high energy electrons toward mitochondria, could be explained by increased tissue hypoxia in HCC tumors. Additionally, DHAP and glycerol-3-phosphate can be used as important bioenergetic and biosynthetic precursors, for example, lipid synthesis within cancer cells, which could explain their decreased abundance in tumors compared to adjacent liver. Nevertheless, an important finding of our targeted metabolomic analysis of HCC and adjacent liver tissues suggests an imbalance in the TCA cycle as a hallmark of the metabolic landscape of hepatocarcinoma. Interestingly, various studies have suggested succinate as an oncometabolite in other tumor types such as paraganglioma, pheochromocytoma, and renal cell carcinoma [41–43]. On the other hand, our current metabolomic analysis does not identify succinate, another important TCA cycle intermediate, as a significant oncometabolite in HCC as its abundance statistically decreases within the studied cancer tissues. In fact, the decrease in the abundance of succinate was among the most important features of the metabolomic profile of HCC according to the VIP analysis of the LC/MS dataset. This observation remains to be explained.

Our targeted metabolomic analysis also revealed a major perturbation in energy metabolites in tumors. Indeed, energy-related metabolites ATP, ADP, and AMP as well as the NADH cofactor and the resulting NADH/NAD ratio were all consistently decreased in hepatocarcinoma samples compared to adjacent liver tissue samples. These findings suggest an unbalanced utilization of energy metabolites by HCC cells, and that bioenergetic substrates such as ATP become limiting in such tumors. Strikingly, HCC seems devoid of ATP reserves, which is pertinent in the context of metabolic reprogramming as a response to rapid cell proliferation, a highly energy-demanding cellular process. Compared to previous metabolomics analyses performed on murine HCC cells, certain findings within this study overlap with those from cellular metabolomics, such as decreased glycerol-3P, NADH, NAD, and NADP [10]. Inversely, in murine HCC tissues, ATP, ADP/AMP, and NADH/NAD have been previously found to be decreased, opposing the findings within the human cohort [10]. Indeed, comparisons between cell cultures, murine liver tissue, and actual human liver tissue remain challenging, given their completely different natures. Murine hepatocarcinogenesis occurs in a highly regulated and reproductive environment, whereas HCC in patients is a multi-factorial disease occurring in a much less controlled manner.

Moreover, decreased reductive potential, characterized by a pronounced drop in the GSH/GSSG ratio, was the most important feature of the metabolomic signature of HCC tumors per VIP analysis. In fact, GSH was among the most significantly altered metabolites in HCC, its abundance being markedly lower in tumors than in adjacent non-tumoral tissue. The oxidized form of NADPH, NADP, was also significantly lower in HCC. Given that both GSH and NADPH are major agents involved in the control of cellular oxidative stress, and consequently redox homeostasis, these findings suggest that oxidative stress is likely exacerbated in HCC and that it surpasses the reductive capacity of HCC cells. Decreased GSH and NADP have also been reported previously in murine HCC, which only further highlight the possibility that oxidative stress could be a vulnerability of HCC [10].

Given the important findings of the reported metabolomics analyses of HCC compared to adjacent normal liver tissues, considered with previous findings of metabolomics in HCC and cirrhosis, studying paramount changes in metabolism occurring during liver disease and hepatocarcinogenesis is bound to lead to paramount discoveries for improving the clinical management of HCC [26,27]. Together with other LC/MS studies of HCC, the main overlapping metabolites considered as altered pathways in liver tumors include alanine, arginine, lactate, succinate, NADH, and NADP metabolites [26,27]. Likewise, convincing evidence of the molecular analysis suggests metabolic reprogramming in HCC [19–21]. As such, collaboration within the research community on HCC, with a multi-omics approach, is fundamental in the identification of holistic metabolism-based HCC classifications.

5. Conclusions

In conclusion, this study combining non-targeted and targeted metabolomics has revealed that the metabolite signatures of HCC and adjacent non-tumoral liver are constitutionally distinct. Through non-targeted ^{1}H-NMR analysis, we identified that HCC tumors exhibit much greater metabolomic variability than adjacent non-cancerous liver, which can be likely attributed to the high degree of heterogeneity observed in such cancers.

Through targeted LC/MS analysis, on the other hand, we specifically identified a number of metabolic intermediates that are found in lower concentrations in HCC tissues, such as ATP and GSH. Overall, these findings are paramount for the global objective to delineate HCC metabolism and pathophysiology. They could ultimately pave the way for the identification of precision biomarkers of this disease as well as, potentially, novel targets for HCC therapeutics.

Supplementary Materials: The following supporting information can be downloaded at: https://www.mdpi.com/article/10.3390/cancers15123232/s1, Table S1: Cryopreservation times of studied tumor and non-tumoral liver tissue specimens.

Author Contributions: Conceptualization, M.B.; methodology, V.-A.R., C.G. and L.R.; software, V.T. and C.G.; validation, V.T., V.-A.R. and C.G.; biobanking resources: L.R. and S.T.; sample collection: L.R. and S.T.; formal analysis, V.T.; investigation, V.-A.R. and C.G.; data curation, V.T., V.-A.R. and C.G.; writing—original draft preparation, V.T.; writing—review and editing, V.T., V.-A.R., C.G., L.R., S.T. and M.B.; supervision, V.-A.R. and M.B.; project administration, V.-A.R. and M.B.; funding acquisition, M.B. All authors have read and agreed to the published version of the manuscript.

Funding: This research was funded by the "Chaire de recherche en hépatologie Novartis—Fondation canadienne du foie de l'Université de Montréal. The CHUM hepatopancreatobiliary and colorectal biobank and prospective database is supported by the "Chaire Roger Des Groseillers d'oncologie chirurgicale hépato-biliaire et pancréatique de l'Université de Montréal". S. Turcotte was supported by the FRQS Young Clinician Scientist Seed Grant #32633, the FRQS Clinician Scientist Junior-one and two Salary Award (#30861, #298832), the Institut du Cancer de Montréal establishment award, and the Université de Montréal Roger Des Groseillers Research Chair in Hepatopancreatobiliary Surgical Oncology. The Structural Biology Platform of Université de Montréal was funded by a Canadian Foundation for Innovation Award #30574.

Institutional Review Board Statement: This study was conducted in accordance with the Declaration of Helsinki and approved by the "Comité d'éthique du Centre de recherche du Centre Hospitalier de l'Université de Montréal".

Informed Consent Statement: Written informed consent was obtained from all participants involved in this study prior to surgery.

Data Availability Statement: The data presented in this study are available in this article.

Acknowledgments: We thank J. Lamontagne from the Metabolomics core facility of the Centre de recherche du Centre Hospitalier de l'Université de Montréal as well as S. Beaulieu from the Regional Centre of NMR spectroscopy of the Department of Chemistry of Université de Montréal. We also thank S. Langevin, J. Bilodeau, and A. Aubourg from the CHUM hepatopancreatobiliary cancer and prospective registry for patient recruitment, biospecimen acquisition, and maintenance of clinicopathological data.

Conflicts of Interest: The authors declare no conflict of interest. The funders had no role in the design of this study; in the collection, analyses, or interpretation of data; in the writing of the manuscript; or in the decision to publish the results.

References

1. Hanahan, D.; Weinberg, R.A. Hallmarks of cancer: The next generation. *Cell* **2011**, *144*, 646–674. [CrossRef]
2. Wu, S.; Kuang, H.; Ke, J.; Pi, M.; Yang, D.H. Metabolic Reprogramming Induces Immune Cell Dysfunction in the Tumor Microenvironment of Multiple Myeloma. *Front. Oncol.* **2020**, *10*, 591342. [CrossRef]
3. Schiliro, C.; Firestein, B.L. Mechanisms of Metabolic Reprogramming in Cancer Cells Supporting Enhanced Growth and Proliferation. *Cells* **2021**, *10*, 1056. [CrossRef]
4. Ohshima, K.; Morii, E. Metabolic Reprogramming of Cancer Cells during Tumor Progression and Metastasis. *Metabolites* **2021**, *11*, 28. [CrossRef]
5. Roda, N.; Gambino, V.; Giorgio, M. Metabolic Constrains Rule Metastasis Progression. *Cells* **2020**, *9*, 2081. [CrossRef]
6. Chidambaranathan-Reghupaty, S.; Fisher, P.B.; Sarkar, D. Hepatocellular carcinoma (HCC): Epidemiology, etiology and molecular classification. *Adv. Cancer Res.* **2021**, *149*, 1–61. [CrossRef]
7. Gebhardt, R.; Matz-Soja, M. Liver zonation: Novel aspects of its regulation and its impact on homeostasis. *World J. Gastroenterol.* **2014**, *20*, 8491–8504. [CrossRef]

8. Han, H.S.; Kang, G.; Kim, J.S.; Choi, B.H.; Koo, S.H. Regulation of glucose metabolism from a liver-centric perspective. *Exp. Mol. Med.* **2016**, *48*, e218. [CrossRef] [PubMed]
9. Warburg, O.; Wind, F.; Negelein, E. The Metabolism of Tumors in the Body. *J. Gen. Physiol.* **1927**, *8*, 519–530. [CrossRef] [PubMed]
10. Cassim, S.; Raymond, V.A.; Dehbidi-Assadzadeh, L.; Lapierre, P.; Bilodeau, M. Metabolic reprogramming enables hepatocarcinoma cells to efficiently adapt and survive to a nutrient-restricted microenvironment. *Cell Cycle* **2018**, *17*, 903–916. [CrossRef] [PubMed]
11. Navarro, C.; Ortega, A.; Santeliz, R.; Garrido, B.; Chacin, M.; Galban, N.; Vera, I.; De Sanctis, J.B.; Bermudez, V. Metabolic Reprogramming in Cancer Cells: Emerging Molecular Mechanisms and Novel Therapeutic Approaches. *Pharmaceutics* **2022**, *14*, 1303. [CrossRef]
12. Todisco, S.; Convertini, P.; Iacobazzi, V.; Infantino, V. TCA Cycle Rewiring as Emerging Metabolic Signature of Hepatocellular Carcinoma. *Cancers* **2019**, *12*, 68. [CrossRef]
13. Wu, D.; Yang, Y.; Hou, Y.; Zhao, Z.; Liang, N.; Yuan, P.; Yang, T.; Xing, J.; Li, J. Increased mitochondrial fission drives the reprogramming of fatty acid metabolism in hepatocellular carcinoma cells through suppression of Sirtuin 1. *Cancer Commun.* **2022**, *42*, 37–55. [CrossRef]
14. Lee, H.Y.; Nga, H.T.; Tian, J.; Yi, H.S. Mitochondrial Metabolic Signatures in Hepatocellular Carcinoma. *Cells* **2021**, *10*, 1901. [CrossRef]
15. Sung, J.Y.; Cheong, J.H. Pan-Cancer Analysis Reveals Distinct Metabolic Reprogramming in Different Epithelial-Mesenchymal Transition Activity States. *Cancers* **2021**, *13*, 1778. [CrossRef]
16. Tarrado-Castellarnau, M.; de Atauri, P.; Cascante, M. Oncogenic regulation of tumor metabolic reprogramming. *Oncotarget* **2016**, *7*, 62726–62753. [CrossRef]
17. Nakagawa, H.; Hayata, Y.; Kawamura, S.; Yamada, T.; Fujiwara, N.; Koike, K. Lipid Metabolic Reprogramming in Hepatocellular Carcinoma. *Cancers* **2018**, *10*, 447. [CrossRef]
18. Fujiwara, N.; Nakagawa, H.; Enooku, K.; Kudo, Y.; Hayata, Y.; Nakatsuka, T.; Tanaka, Y.; Tateishi, R.; Hikiba, Y.; Misumi, K.; et al. CPT2 downregulation adapts HCC to lipid-rich environment and promotes carcinogenesis via acylcarnitine accumulation in obesity. *Gut* **2018**, *67*, 1493–1504. [CrossRef]
19. Nwosu, Z.C.; Megger, D.A.; Hammad, S.; Sitek, B.; Roessler, S.; Ebert, M.P.; Meyer, C.; Dooley, S. Identification of the Consistently Altered Metabolic Targets in Human Hepatocellular Carcinoma. *Cell Mol. Gastroenterol. Hepatol.* **2017**, *4*, 303–323.e301. [CrossRef]
20. Qi, F.; Li, J.; Qi, Z.; Zhang, J.; Zhou, B.; Yang, B.; Qin, W.; Cui, W.; Xia, J. Comprehensive Metabolic Profiling and Genome-wide Analysis Reveal Therapeutic Modalities for Hepatocellular Carcinoma. *Research* **2023**, *6*, 0036. [CrossRef]
21. Yang, C.; Huang, X.; Liu, Z.; Qin, W.; Wang, C. Metabolism-associated molecular classification of hepatocellular carcinoma. *Mol. Oncol.* **2020**, *14*, 896–913. [CrossRef]
22. Schmidt, D.R.; Patel, R.; Kirsch, D.G.; Lewis, C.A.; Vander Heiden, M.G.; Locasale, J.W. Metabolomics in cancer research and emerging applications in clinical oncology. *CA Cancer J. Clin.* **2021**, *71*, 333–358. [CrossRef]
23. Armitage, E.G.; Southam, A.D. Monitoring cancer prognosis, diagnosis and treatment efficacy using metabolomics and lipidomics. *Metabolomics* **2016**, *12*, 146. [CrossRef]
24. Andrisic, L.; Dudzik, D.; Barbas, C.; Milkovic, L.; Grune, T.; Zarkovic, N. Short overview on metabolomics approach to study pathophysiology of oxidative stress in cancer. *Redox. Biol.* **2018**, *14*, 47–58. [CrossRef]
25. Guo, W.; Tan, H.Y.; Wang, N.; Wang, X.; Feng, Y. Deciphering hepatocellular carcinoma through metabolomics: From biomarker discovery to therapy evaluation. *Cancer Manag. Res.* **2018**, *10*, 715–734. [CrossRef]
26. Morine, Y.; Utsunomiya, T.; Yamanaka-Okumura, H.; Saito, Y.; Yamada, S.; Ikemoto, T.; Imura, S.; Kinoshita, S.; Hirayama, A.; Tanaka, Y.; et al. Essential amino acids as diagnostic biomarkers of hepatocellular carcinoma based on metabolic analysis. *Oncotarget* **2022**, *13*, 1286–1298. [CrossRef]
27. He, M.J.; Pu, W.; Wang, X.; Zhong, X.; Zhao, D.; Zeng, Z.; Cai, W.; Liu, J.; Huang, J.; Tang, D.; et al. Spatial metabolomics on liver cirrhosis to hepatocellular carcinoma progression. *Cancer Cell Int.* **2022**, *22*, 366. [CrossRef] [PubMed]
28. Beger, R.D. A review of applications of metabolomics in cancer. *Metabolites* **2013**, *3*, 552–574. [CrossRef]
29. Barcena-Varela, M.; Lujambio, A. The Endless Sources of Hepatocellular Carcinoma Heterogeneity. *Cancers* **2021**, *13*, 2621. [CrossRef]
30. Chan, L.K.; Tsui, Y.M.; Ho, D.W.; Ng, I.O. Cellular heterogeneity and plasticity in liver cancer. *Semin. Cancer Biol.* **2022**, *82*, 134–149. [CrossRef]
31. Deja, S.; Porebska, I.; Kowal, A.; Zabek, A.; Barg, W.; Pawelczyk, K.; Stanimirova, I.; Daszykowski, M.; Korzeniewska, A.; Jankowska, R.; et al. Metabolomics provide new insights on lung cancer staging and discrimination from chronic obstructive pulmonary disease. *J. Pharm. Biomed. Anal.* **2014**, *100*, 369–380. [CrossRef]
32. Di Gangi, I.M.; Mazza, T.; Fontana, A.; Copetti, M.; Fusilli, C.; Ippolito, A.; Mattivi, F.; Latiano, A.; Andriulli, A.; Vrhovsek, U.; et al. Metabolomic profile in pancreatic cancer patients: A consensus-based approach to identify highly discriminating metabolites. *Oncotarget* **2016**, *7*, 5815–5829. [CrossRef]
33. Lindahl, A.; Heuchel, R.; Forshed, J.; Lehtio, J.; Lohr, M.; Nordstrom, A. Discrimination of pancreatic cancer and pancreatitis by LC-MS metabolomics. *Metabolomics* **2017**, *13*, 61. [CrossRef]

34. Kowalczyk, T.; Kisluk, J.; Pietrowska, K.; Godzien, J.; Kozlowski, M.; Reszec, J.; Sierko, E.; Naumnik, W.; Mroz, R.; Moniuszko, M.; et al. The Ability of Metabolomics to Discriminate Non-Small-Cell Lung Cancer Subtypes Depends on the Stage of the Disease and the Type of Material Studied. *Cancers* **2021**, *13*, 3314. [CrossRef] [PubMed]
35. Judge, M.T.; Wu, Y.; Tayyari, F.; Hattori, A.; Glushka, J.; Ito, T.; Arnold, J.; Edison, A.S. Continuous in vivo Metabolism by NMR. *Front. Mol. Biosci.* **2019**, *6*, 26. [CrossRef]
36. Parker, S.J.; Metallo, C.M. Metabolic consequences of oncogenic IDH mutations. *Pharm. Ther.* **2015**, *152*, 54–62. [CrossRef]
37. Bai, C.; Wang, H.; Dong, D.; Li, T.; Yu, Z.; Guo, J.; Zhou, W.; Li, D.; Yan, R.; Wang, L.; et al. Urea as a By-Product of Ammonia Metabolism Can Be a Potential Serum Biomarker of Hepatocellular Carcinoma. *Front. Cell Dev. Biol.* **2021**, *9*, 650748. [CrossRef]
38. Cramer, T.; Vaupel, P. Severe hypoxia is a typical characteristic of human hepatocellular carcinoma: Scientific fact or fallacy? *J. Hepatol.* **2022**, *76*, 975–980. [CrossRef] [PubMed]
39. Muz, B.; de la Puente, P.; Azab, F.; Azab, A.K. The role of hypoxia in cancer progression, angiogenesis, metastasis, and resistance to therapy. *Hypoxia. Auckl.* **2015**, *3*, 83–92. [CrossRef] [PubMed]
40. Hsu, C.C.; Lee, H.C.; Wei, Y.H. Mitochondrial DNA alterations and mitochondrial dysfunction in the progression of hepatocellular carcinoma. *World J. Gastroenterol.* **2013**, *19*, 8880–8886. [CrossRef]
41. Nowicki, S.; Gottlieb, E. Oncometabolites: Tailoring our genes. *FEBS J.* **2015**, *282*, 2796–2805. [CrossRef] [PubMed]
42. Eijkelenkamp, K.; Osinga, T.E.; Links, T.P.; van der Horst-Schrivers, A.N.A. Clinical implications of the oncometabolite succinate in SDHx-mutation carriers. *Clin. Genet.* **2020**, *97*, 39–53. [CrossRef] [PubMed]
43. Liu, Y.; Yang, C. Oncometabolites in Cancer: Current Understanding and Challenges. *Cancer Res.* **2021**, *81*, 2820–2823. [CrossRef] [PubMed]

Disclaimer/Publisher's Note: The statements, opinions and data contained in all publications are solely those of the individual author(s) and contributor(s) and not of MDPI and/or the editor(s). MDPI and/or the editor(s) disclaim responsibility for any injury to people or property resulting from any ideas, methods, instructions or products referred to in the content.

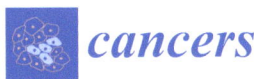

Communication

Epiploic Adipose Tissue (EPAT) in Obese Individuals Promotes Colonic Tumorigenesis: A Novel Model for EPAT-Dependent Colorectal Cancer Progression

Rida Iftikhar [1,†], Patricia Snarski [1,†], Angelle N. King [1], Jenisha Ghimire [1], Emmanuelle Ruiz [1], Frank Lau [2] and Suzana D. Savkovic [1,*]

[1] Department of Pathology and Laboratory Medicine, Tulane University School of Medicine, New Orleans, LA 70112, USA
[2] Department of Surgery, Louisiana State University Health Sciences Center, New Orleans, LA 70112, USA
* Correspondence: ssavkovi@tulane.edu; Tel.: +1-504-988-1409
† These authors contributed equally to this manuscript.

Simple Summary: The role of epiploic adipose tissue (EPAT), understudied fat appendages attached to the colon, in obesity-facilitated colorectal cancer (CRC) is unexamined. In our novel microphysiological system, EPAT obtained from obese individuals, unlike EPAT from lean, attracts colon cancer cells' intrusion and enhances their migration and growth. Conditioned media from this model mediated gene expression in colon cancer cells that are linked to metabolic and tumorigenic remodeling. This EPAT-mediated transcriptional signature defines transcriptomes of human colon cancer. These findings highlight a tumor-promoting role of EPAT, a metabolic tissue, in the colon of obese individuals and establishes a platform for exploration of involved mechanisms and development of effective treatments.

Abstract: The obesity epidemic is associated with increased colorectal cancer (CRC) risk and progression, the mechanisms of which remain unclear. In obese individuals, hypertrophic epiploic adipose tissue (EPAT), attached to the colon, has unique characteristics compared to other fats. We hypothesized that this understudied fat could serve as a tumor-promoting tissue and developed a novel microphysiological system (MPS) for human EPAT-dependent colorectal cancer (CRC-MPS). In CRC-MPS, obese EPAT, unlike lean EPAT, considerably attracted colon cancer HT29-GFP cells and enhanced their growth. Conditioned media (CM) from the obese CRC-MPS significantly increased the growth and migration of HT29 and HCT116 cells ($p < 0.001$). In HT29 cells, CM stimulated differential gene expression ($hOEC_{867}$) linked to cancer, tumor morphology, and metabolism similar to those in the colon of high-fat-diet obese mice. The $hOEC_{867}$ signature represented pathways found in human colon cancer. In unsupervised clustering, $hOEC_{867}$ separated transcriptomes of colon cancer samples from normal with high significance (PCA, $p = 9.6 \times 10^{-11}$). These genes, validated in CM-treated HT29 cells ($p < 0.05$), regulate the cell cycle, cancer stem cells, methylation, and metastasis, and are similarly altered in human colon cancer (TCGA). These findings highlight a tumor-promoting role of EPAT in CRC facilitated with obesity and establishes a platform to explore critical mechanisms and develop effective treatments.

Keywords: obesity; epiploic adipose tissue (EPAT); colon cancer

1. Introduction

The obesity epidemic affects half a billion individuals worldwide [1]. Obesity is directly associated with increased colorectal cancer (CRC) risk, progression, recurrence, resistance to therapy, and mortality [2,3]. CRC, the second leading cause of cancer-related deaths worldwide, is initiated and driven by complex intracellular and extracellular remodeling [4,5]. We have demonstrated that colonic tumorigenesis augmented by obesity is

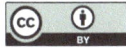

mediated by increased lipid metabolism in colonic cells and surroundings [6–8]. Understanding these obesity-driven tumorigenic processes will promote further exploration of critical mechanisms and the development of more effective treatments.

Emerging findings revealed that epiploic adipose tissue (EPAT), visceral fat appendages attached to the colon, is linked to obesity-mediated systemic pathobiology [9]. Adult individuals have about 50–100 of these EPAT appendages, which are ~1.5 cm thick and 3.5 cm long [10]. EPAT provides blood supply for the colon, supports colonic absorption, and delivers nutrition to the colon during starvation [11,12]. It has been speculated that EPAT is involved in host–microbe interactions and may be regulated by paracrine factors [13]. In obese individuals, EPAT is enlarged and is linked to colonic pathobiology such as diverticulitis and epiploic appendagitis [14,15]. Recently, Krieg et al. assessed abdominal fat in a large number of obese individuals undergoing gastric bypass surgery and demonstrated unique characteristics of EPAT compared to other adipose tissue [9]. Given these lines of evidence, we hypothesized that this understudied fat serves as a tumor-promoting tissue in the colon of obese individuals. In order to study the role of EPAT in colorectal cancer progression, it was necessary to establish a novel model since neither in vitro nor in vivo models specific to this fat are available. A recently developed microphysiological system (MPS) appeared to be suitable for studying the role of adipose tissues in obesity processes [16–18]; thereby, we utilized this platform to establish a novel MPS specific for EPAT-dependent colorectal cancer.

2. Materials and Methods

2.1. Human Samples

Human epiploic adipose tissue (EPAT) samples were obtained from local patients undergoing surgery unrelated to colonic inflammation and cancer from the larger New Orleans metropolitan area. Patients (ages 16–67) were a mix of female and male, African American and Caucasian, with Body Mass Index (BMI, as calculated (kilograms/meters^2), ranging from 17.6 to 40.7. The de-identified patient samples used in this study were approved by the institutional review board (IRB, protocol number 867) at Tulane University, which waived the requirement for informed consent for sample collection.

Publicly available transcriptomes from human colon cancer patients comprised control ($n = 23$) and colonic tumor samples ($n = 198$) (GSE4183; GSE141174). Additionally, publicly available TCGA transcriptomic data was obtained from colon cancer patients (normal colon ($n = 41$) and tumor ($n = 457$)). These data were acquired using NCBI's GEO2R.

2.2. Mouse Model for High-Fat Diet Obesity and Colonic Tumorigenesis (Transcriptomic Data)

C57BL/6J mice (6 weeks old) were housed at Tulane University School of Medicine according to the guidelines of the Tulane Institutional Animal Care and Use Committee (protocol number 1161). One group of mice was maintained on a standard chow diet (RD), and the other on a high-fat chow diet (HFD) (60% kcal/fat) (D12492, Research Diets, New Brunswick, NJ). In addition, colonic tumors were induced in experimental mice by a single azoxymethane (AOM, Sigma, St. Louis, MO, USA) intraperitoneal injection of 10 mg/kg, followed by three separate 5-day cycles of 2.5% dextran sulfate sodium (DSS, MP Biomedicals, San Diego, CA, USA) added to drinking water, as we described before [8]. Transcriptomic analysis was performed after RNA-seq from the colons of these mice ($n = 3$ for each group) and is available through NCBI's Sequence Read Archive (SRP093363) [8].

2.3. Cells

Human colon cancer cells HT29 (ATCC, Manassas, VA, USA), GFP-tagged HT29 (Genecopoeia, Rockville, MD, USA), and HCT116 (ATCC, Manassas, VA) were propagated in complete McCoy's 5A media (Sigma, St. Louis, MO) containing 10% fetal bovine serum (FBS) (Peak Serum, Wellington, CO, USA). EPAT-derived stromal cells (ESC) from human EPAT were isolated by collagenase digestion of tissue, vigorous washing, and selection via cell adherence [19,20]. ESC were propagated using DMEM containing 10% fetal bovine serum and 10% penicillin/streptomycin (Gibco, Waltham, MA, USA). Cancer cells were serum-starved overnight prior to experimental procedures and were serum-starved for three days to synchronize cells in the cell cycle prior to treatments.

2.4. Epiploic Colonic Microphysiological System (CRC-MPS) and Conditioned Media

EPAT was obtained from obese or lean patients undergoing abdominal surgery unrelated to colonic diseases (inflammation or cancer). From EPAT, isolated adipose stromal cells (ESC) were used to sandwich CRC-MPS (containing EPAT-isolated adipocytes and human colonic cells) (Figure 1A). Fresh EPAT was physically minced, and 200 µL of their cell suspension was used for each CRC-MPS well. HT29-GFP cells, cultured independently, were trypsinized, and 200,000 cells were added to each CRC-MPS well. Two ESC sheets are needed for each CRC-MPS well. On the first ESC sheet, grown on a 6-well plate, EPAT and HT29-GFP cells were added. A second ESC monolayer was grown on a thermosensitive polymer (poly(N-isopropylacrylamide), Nunc UpWell 6-well dish, 174902). 3D-printed plungers loaded with a hydrogel (12% Gelatin B, ~225 bloom, G9382, Sigma, St. Louis, MO) were gently pressed onto the ESC monolayer, and incubated at room temperature, then at 4 °C, allowing the ESC layer to be lifted off the plate. The plunger carrying these ESC was then placed on top of EPAT and HT29-GFP cells that were added to the first ESC monolayer to create a sandwich (Figure 1A). Colon cancer cell status in CRC-MPS was assessed daily under the microscope, and GFP signal from acquired images was quantified by pixel area per field of view. These CRC-MPS, kept in DMEM and 10% FBS at 37 °C, were maintained for 5 days. Their 24 h growth media, diluted 1:5 with serum-free McCoy's 5A media, was used as a conditioned media (CM) to treat colon cancer cells. Two cell lines were used to increase rigor and reproducibility.

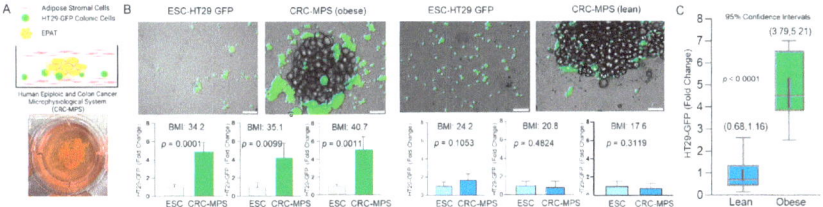

Figure 1. (**A**) Cross-sectional model of Epiploic (EPAT) Colorectal Cancer Microphysiological System (CRC-MPS). (**B**) Representative images of CRC-MPS with HT29-GFP cells and EPAT obtained from obese (BMI 34.2) or lean (BMI 24.2) individuals vs. HT29-GFP grown with EPAT-derived stromal cells (ESC) only (48 h). Graphs represent the intensity of GFP pixels from CRC-MPS images, three independent wells for each EPAT, obtained from three obese or three lean individuals relative to ESC (Scale bar = 100 µm, BMI = Body Mass Index). (**C**) All individual values from CRC-MPS were normalized to matched ESC-only GFP signal, then normalized to lean average. Box and whisker plot represents the median, 25% and 75% quartiles, and highest and lowest values of each group. Thick dark grey bar within the box and whisker plot reports confidence interval (CI, 95%) with range in brackets above each box.

2.5. BrdU and EdU Staining and Migration Assays

Human colon cancer cells were grown on coverslips incubated with SFM, oleic acid, or conditioned media from ESC alone or obese CRC-MPS and in the presence of BrdU (10 µM, Sigma, St. Louis, MO, USA). We visualized and quantified as we described before [7]. A parallel experiment utilizing EdU to visualize the proliferation of cells was performed according to the manufacturer's instructions (C10639, Invitrogen, Waltham, MA, USA). Colon cancer cell migration confluency disruption and transwell assays were performed as described before [7].

2.6. RNA Isolation and cDNA Synthesis

RNA isolation (miRNeasy kit, Qiagen, Germany) and cDNA synthesis (SuperMix synthesis system, Thermo Fisher, Waltham, MA, USA) were performed according to the manufacturers' protocols, as we described before [8].

2.7. Quantitative PCR

cDNA generated from human colon cancer cells and colonospheres was utilized for qPCR as previously described [8]. Independent experiments were performed 3 times by different investigators. The primers for amplification of human cDNA were: for hSNAI1 (F: 5'-GGTTCTTCTGCGCTACTGCT-3', R: 5'-TGCTGGAAGGTAAACTCTGGATT-3'), hTRIB2 (F: 5'-AGCTGGTGTGCAAGGTGTT-3', R: 5'-GAGCAGACAGGCAAAAGCAC-3'), hCENPE (F: 5'-AGCCTGCAAGAAACCAAAGC-3', R: 5'-TCTGTCGGTCCTGCTTTTTCT-3'), hBCCIP (F: 5'-ATGTACCAGCAGCTTCAGAAAGA-3', R: 5'-AGTAGCACTTCCCACATGGC-3'), hNNMT (F: 5'-TGATTGACATCGGCTCTGGC-3', R: 5'-TCTGGACCCTTGACTCTGTTC-3'), and hOAS1 (F: 5'-CTCCTGGATTCTGCTGACCC-3', R: 5'-GTGCAGGTCCAGTCCTCTTC-3'). The relative levels of mRNA were determined by the comparative Ct method using actin and GAPDH as housekeeping controls as previously described [7,8].

2.8. RNA Sequencing and Differential Expression

RNA sequencing (RNAseq) of experimental colon cancer cells was accomplished as described previously [7,8]. Transcriptomic data and differentially expressed genes (DEGs) were analyzed by using Ingenuity Pathway Analysis (IPA, Qiagen, Germany). Principal component analysis (PCA) and unsupervised hierarchal clustering were performed as we described before [7,8].

2.9. Statistical Analysis

All experiments were repeated independently by the same or different researchers, and data are represented as mean ± S.D. for a series of experiments. Investigators were blinded during experimentation. Student's unpaired t-test or one-way analysis of variance (ANOVA) and a Student–Newman–Keuls post-test were each calculated as we described before [7,8]. Confidence intervals (95%) were calculated for human samples as well.

3. Results and Discussion

The role of EPAT in homeostasis and pathobiology of the colon is understudied, primarily due to the lack of models and challenges in obtaining biopsies. We established a novel microphysiological system (MPS) utilizing human EPAT and colonic cells sandwiched between tissue-engineered sheets of EPAT-derived stromal cells (ESC) (Figure 1A). It is important to highlight that in this EPAT-dependent colorectal cancer model (CRC-MPS), which is stable in culture for a week, wholesale EPAT tissue is used, not isolated nor differentiated adipocytes. As human white adipose tissue sandwiched between sheets of stromal cells maintained physiologic tissue characteristics [16], the CRC-MPS provides a reliable ex vivo model to study EPAT-mediated processes in colonic cells. EPAT was obtained from obese (Body Mass Index (BMI) > 29.9) and lean (BMI < 24.9) patients undergoing surgery unrelated to colonic inflammation or cancer. Initially, in this CRC-MPS, we utilized HT29-GFP cells, as a reporter and stable colon cancer cell line, to establish a reliable model. In the CRC-MPS model, we found significantly increased growth of HT29-GFP cells when co-cultured with obese EPAT compared to the control, represented by HT29-GFP sandwiched between the ESC sheets alone (Figure 1B). When co-cultured with EPAT obtained from lean individuals, HT29-GFP growth remained unaffected compared to ESC alone (Figure 1B). Further, confidence intervals (CI, 95%) and a box and whisker plot demonstrated a 4.895-fold increase in colon cancer HT29-GFP cell growth by obese EPAT (relative to lean) normalized to ESC-only negative controls (CI, obese: (3.79, 5.21), lean: (0.68, 1.16)) (Figure 1C). Moreover, this finding was supported using conditioned media (CM) from obese CRC-MPS and two colon cancer cell lines (HT29 and HCT116). Specifically, this CM significantly stimulated BrdU or EdU incorporation into newly synthesized DNA in both HT29 and HCT116 cells relative to CM from ESC alone (Figure 2A,B). Additionally, we noticed in the CRC-MPS model that HT29-GFP cells were closely associated with obese—relative to lean—EPAT (Figure 1A). We assessed this migratory signal in CM from the obese EPAT to colon cancer cells using HT29 and HCT116 cells in confluency disruption and transwell migration assays. After the confluency disruption of HT29 cells, CM presence led to a smaller distance between their migratory fronts (Figure 2C). Further, it increased HCT116 colon cancer cell migration from the upper chamber to the lower chamber of transwells (Figure 2D). These findings revealed the important role of EPAT in augmenting colon cancer cell growth and migration with obesity (directly and indirectly). Utilization of two colon cancer cell lines may limit interpretation; hence, different colonic cells will be considered in further expansion of the CRC-MPS. Further, metabolic remodeling has a profound effect on the transcriptomes of colonic cells compared to underlying mutations [21]; thus, we speculate that parental gene mutations will have a secondary effect on metabolic remodeling, requiring further exploration of critical mechanisms driving tumorigenesis.

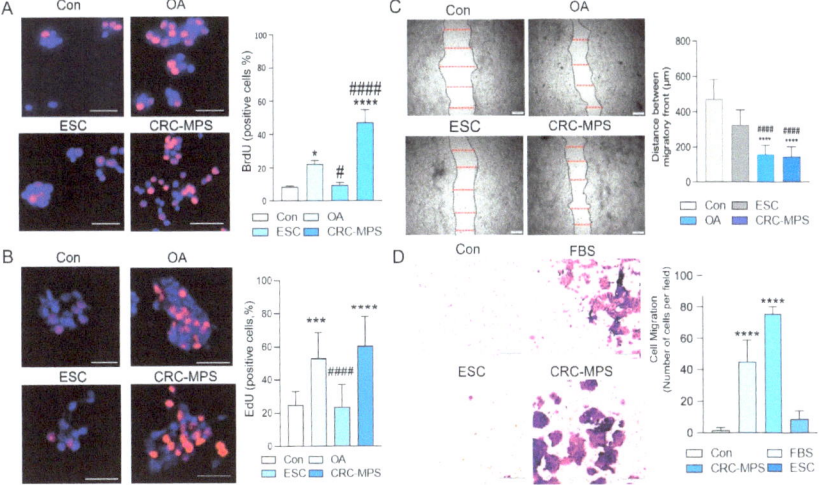

Figure 2. (**A**) Representative images and quantification of BrdU incorporation during DNA synthesis in HT29 cells treated with conditioned media (CM) from CRC-MPS (obese) vs. CM from ESC. Oleic acid (OA) treatment represents positive control and serum-free media (Con) represents negative control (24 h, $n = 3$, **** $p < 0.0001$, * $p < 0.05$ vs. Con; #### $p < 0.0001$, # $p < 0.05$ vs. OA, scale bar = 50 μm). (**B**) Representative images and quantification of EdU incorporation during DNA synthesis in HCT116 cells treated with CM from CRC-MPS (obese) vs. CM from ESC. Oleic acid (OA) treatment represents positive control and serum-free media (Con) represents negative control (24 h, $n = 3$ wells in 2 independent experiments, **** $p < 0.0001$, *** $p < 0.001$ vs. Con; #### $p < 0.0001$ vs. OA, scale bar = 50 μm). (**C**) Representative images and quantification of confluency disruption of HT29 monolayers via scratch assay (24 h, $n = 3$, **** $p < 0.0001$ vs. Con; #### $p < 0.0001$ vs. ESC, scale bar 200 = μm). (**D**) Transwell migration assay of HCT116 cells, with CM from CRC-MPS (obese), ESC, fetal bovine serum (FBS) as a positive control, and serum-free media as a negative control (Con) (24 h, $n = 3$, **** $p < 0.0001$ vs. Con, scale bar 100 = μm).

Next, we sought to determine how EPAT mediates growth and migratory behavior by systematically surveying the gene expression in colon cancer cells (RNA-seq). We identified 867 differentially expressed genes (DEGs) altered in HT29 cells by CM from obese CRC-MPS (>|1.5|-fold change, FDR < 0.05 and meeting stringent differential expression and statistical thresholds of $\log_2$ fold-change > |1.5| and an adjusted p-value < 0.001). These DEGs, representing a transcriptional signature mediated by human obese EPAT in colon cancer cells (hOEC$_{867}$), are linked to cancer, gastrointestinal diseases, metabolic processes, and growth (Figure 3A). Moreover, the pathways representing hOEC$_{867}$ were compared with pathways representing transcriptomes of the colon of high-fat-diet (HFD) obese mice and colonic tumors of HFD obese mice with AOM/DSS-induced tumors. In this mouse model, we demonstrated that HFD obese mice had increased colonic tumor burden and pathways associated with metabolic and tumorigenic remodeling [8]. We found that pathways representing hOEC$_{867}$ were similar to the pathways in the colon of HFD obese mice in colonic tissue (Figure 3B, IPA) and tumors (and when compared to the colon of mice fed with a regular diet) (Figure 3C, IPA). Further, we determined the significance of these hOEC$_{867}$ pathways in human colonic tumorigenesis using publicly available transcriptomic data from tumor tissue samples obtained from two colon cancer patient cohorts. Pathways representing hOEC$_{867}$ were similar to those characterizing human colon cancer (GSE4183, GSE141174) (Figure 3D, IPA). Next, we determined the significance of hOEC$_{867}$ in human colonic tumorigenesis using publicly available transcriptomes from a large patient population (TCGA). Principal component analysis (PCA) and unsupervised hierarchal clustering showed that hOEC$_{867}$ separated the transcriptomes of human colon cancer samples from normal with a high degree of significance ($p = 9.6 \times 10^{-11}$) (TCGA, Figure 3E,F). These findings demonstrated the importance of EPAT-mediated gene expression in colonic cells in obesity-augmented metabolic and tumorigenic remodeling.

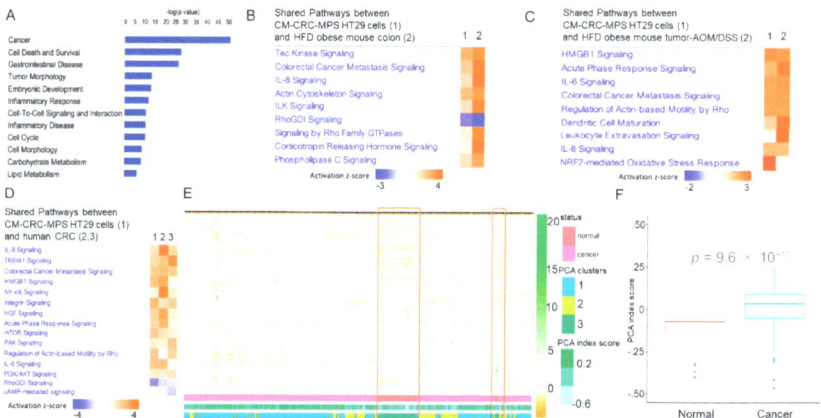

Figure 3. (**A**) Top diseases representing differentially expressed genes (DEGs) in colon cancer HT29 cells mediated by CM from CRC-MPS from obese patients relative to control ($p < 0.05$, IPA). (**B**,**C**) Top canonical pathways representing these DEGs compared to DEGs from colon and colonic tumors (AOM/DSS) of HFD obese mice ($n = 3$ for each group, FC > |1.5|, FDR < 0.05, IPA). In (**B**), Column 1 contains pathways representing DEGs in HT29 cells treated with CM from CRC-MPS (vs. ESC), and Column 2 contains pathways in HFD obese mouse colon (vs. RD colon). In (**C**) Column 1 contains pathways representing DEGs in HT29 cells treated with CM from CRC-MPS (vs. ESC), and Column 2 contains pathways in HFD obese mouse tumors (AOM/DSS model vs. RD normal colon). (**D**) Shared pathways representing DEGs from HT29 cells treated with CM from CRC-MPS (Column 1) and human colon cancer relative to normal colon (Column 2, GSE4183, $n = 23$; Column 3, GSE141174, $n = 198$; fold change > |1.5|, FDR < 0.05, IPA). (**E**,**F**) Unsupervised hierarchical clustering and heatmap showing hOEC$_{867}$ signature separating transcriptome of colon cancer samples from normal. Orange boxes highlight normal samples. Principal Component Analysis (PCA) of hOEC$_{867}$ signature and significance of PCA index score (TCGA), normal colon ($n = 41$), and tumors ($n = 457$).

Finally, we validated selected obese EPAT-mediated DEGs for expression in HT29 cells treated with CM from obese CRC-MPS vs. ESC (Figure 4A). Transcriptional levels of these genes were similarly altered in the human colon cancer samples relative to normal

(TCGA, Figure 4A). These genes regulate diverse cellular functions, and limited data implicated them in cancer. Specifically, SNAI1 is linked to the epithelial-to-mesenchymal transition (EMT), while TRIB2 is associated with colon cancer stem cells [22,23]. Further, several of these genes regulate the cell cycle and migration, such as CENPE, a kinesin-like motor protein required for stable spindle microtubule capture, and BCCIP, which modulates CDK2 kinase activity [24,25]. OAS1 was recently detected in pancreatic and breast cancer [26,27]. Moreover, NNMT regulates methylation and has been linked to gastric and colon cancer [28]. Next, we analyzed the distribution of these genes' expression according to the BMI status of colon cancer patients, utilizing cancer stage subsets based on clinical parameters associated with tumor dissemination [29]. In boxplots corresponding to significant and close-to-significant differential gene expression, we found increased levels of TRIB2 and CENP2 corresponding with obesity (BMI > 30) and lymph node metastasis (Figure 4B). Similarly, increased NNMT levels correspond to obesity in late stages of solid colonic and metastatic tumors (lymph nodes, perineural invasion, and distant metastasis) (Figure 4B). These findings demonstrated that in obese individuals, EPAT mediates the expression of genes in colonic cells associated with growth, cancer stem cells, and epigenetic changes (methylation). Further, increased levels of several of these genes regulating cancer stem cells, migration, and methylation, corresponding to obesity, are linked to metastasis, which establishes a platform to determine novel biomarkers representing obese EPAT-mediated colorectal tumorigenesis.

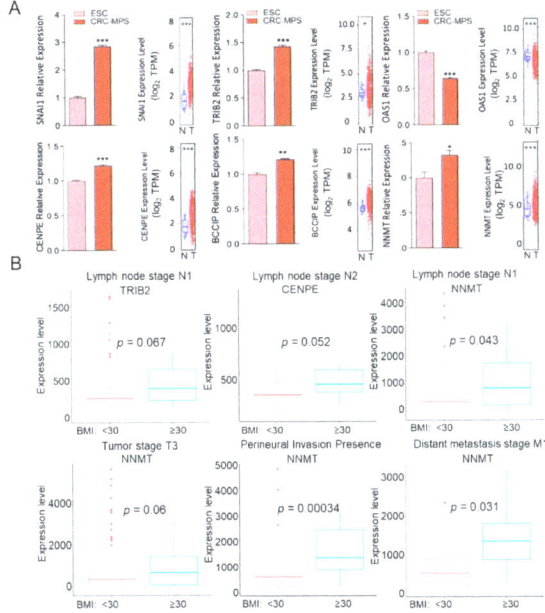

Figure 4. (**A**) Validation of DEGs in HT29 cells treated with CM from CRC-MPS (obese) and ESC (24 h) by qPCR. The following transcripts were assessed: SNAI1, TRIB2, OAS1, CENPE, BCCIP, and NNMT (qPCR, $n = 3$, * $p < 0.05$, ** $p < 0.01$, *** $p < 0.001$). Similar significant alterations of these transcripts were found in colon cancer patient tissue (grey box plots) (TCGA: normal colon ($n = 41$) and tumors ($n = 457$)). (**B**) Transcriptomic data of samples from colon cancer patients that included both weight and height information (TCGA) were further classified by BMI (obese: BMI > 30, $n = 84$, and non-obese: BMI < 30, $n = 198$). Selected genes were analyzed for expression levels (log$_2$ TPM) in various clinical cancer stage subsets associated with tumor dissemination (Box plots).

Here, we demonstrated a tumor-promoting role of human EPAT in obesity-facilitated colorectal cancer utilizing our novel model. Emerging findings demonstrated that EPAT in obese individuals differs from mesenteric, omental, and subcutaneous fats in methylome, transcriptome, and proteome [9]. Further, EPAT has uniquely altered pathways in obese individuals with insulin resistance compared to insulin sensitivity [9], suggesting its systemic metabolic role. This adipose tissue is understudied due to lack of a mouse model and the difficulty of obtaining human EPAT tissue biopsies. Our novel ex vivo model will allow us to further elucidate mechanisms of EPAT-mediated processes in the colon. Utilization of wholesale EPAT tissue gives us an advantage for future understanding of the EPAT cell landscape (adipose, non-adipose, and stromal cells) and their released mediators in processes involving the colon. As the initial utilization of colon cancer cells in this model can be extended to human organoids, it is important to keep in mind that the complexity of colonic tissue is underrepresented, primarily as other non-colonic cells are not considered.

Moreover, our findings revealed that EPAT may indirectly and directly augment tumorigenic processes in colonic cells, in part, by impacting the tumor microenvironment. Onogi and Ussar suggested a possible role of EPAT in the regulation of host–microbe interaction [13]. In the small intestine, microbiota translocate to mesenteric adipose tissue, which promotes M2 macrophage activation [30]. Therefore, it is plausible that in the colon, interactions between EPAT and microbiota may be one of the mechanisms driving tumorigenesis in obesity. Moreover, microbiota and obesity facilitate inflammatory signaling in the colon, which may be essential for EPAT function, as studies have shown that inflammation is required for physiological adipose tissue remodeling [31]. Additionally, released mediators from EPAT (adipocytes and non-adipocytes), such as TNF and leptin, as well as metabolites, such as fatty acids [8,9,32,33], may further drive tumorigenesis in the colon. Together, EPAT and microbiota axes could create a microenvironment that is further augmented with obesity in promoting tumorigenesis in the colon. Along with these complex changes in the colonic environment, EPAT may directly affect colonic cells, such as their gene expression and epigenetic changes. We found that methylation via NNMT is augmented in colonic cells by EPAT. Further, EPAT-mediated growth of colon cancer cells may be, in part, due to CENPE- and BCCIP-dependent cell cycle dysregulation. Our findings further revealed that EPAT may affect cancer stem cells, in part, via TRIB2, which can lead to resistance to therapy and tumor recurrence in colon cancer patients. Moreover, EPAT may accelerate the metastatic characteristics of colon cancer cells by promoting EMT and the spread of cancer cells. It is possible that EPAT drives EMT through increased expression of SNAI1, which may involve loss of FOXO3 in colonic cells mediated by obesity. In the colon, loss of FOXO3 is one of the mechanisms by which obesity mediates metabolic reprogramming linked to tumorigenic processes [6,34,35]. In renal cell carcinoma, loss of FOXO3 facilitates EMT by increasing SNAI1 [36]. Moreover, increased expression of genes regulating cancer stem cells, migration, and methylation (TRIB2, CENP2, NNMT) corresponded to metastatic tumors in obese colon cancer patients. Therefore, it is tempting to speculate that EPAT may aid escaped metastatic colon cancer through lymph nodes to distant organs. These findings highlight the critical role of EPAT in obesity-facilitated colonic tumorigenesis, thus establishing a platform to identify novel markers and to develop effective treatment options.

4. Conclusions

The obesity epidemic, affecting half a billion individuals worldwide, is associated with increased CRC risk, progression, recurrence, resistance to therapy, and mortality [1,3]. Further, CRC incidence has been on the rise globally among young adults, mainly due to this epidemic [37,38]. This poses an urgent, unmet demand to understand the mechanisms driving obesity-mediated tumorigenesis in the colon. Here, we demonstrated that fat outpouchings attached to the colon, known as EPAT, have a tumor-promoting role in obesity-facilitated colonic tumorigenesis, especially in metastatic processes. These findings provide conceptual advances in our understanding of how obesity facilitates CRC. Establishing this platform will further drive the exploration of critical mechanisms of EPAT-mediated processes in colonic cells and identify novel biomarkers needed for the development of effective treatment options for CRC.

Author Contributions: Conceptualization, S.D.S. and F.L.; methodology, R.I., P.S., and A.N.K.; software, E.R.; validation, A.N.K. and J.G.; formal analysis, R.I. and P.S.; investigation, R.I., P.S., and A.N.K.; resources, S.D.S.; data curation, S.D.S., R.I., and P.S.; writing—original draft preparation, S.D.S.; writing—review and editing, S.D.S., F.L., J.G., and P.S.; visualization, S.D.S. and P.S.; supervision, S.D.S.; project administration, S.D.S.; funding acquisition, S.D.S. All authors have read and agreed to the published version of the manuscript.

Funding: This work is supported by the NIH award R01CA252055 and by the Crohn's & Colitis Foundation award 663445.

Institutional Review Board Statement: The study was conducted according to the guidelines approved by the Institutional Review Board (Ethics Committee) of Tulane University (Protocol number 867, approved on 25 August 2021).

Informed Consent Statement: For publicly available transcriptomic data from different colon cancer patient cohorts, consent statements were not applicable. Tulane's IRB waived patient consent in the collection of EPAT because this tissue is considered waste tissue during abdominal surgeries.

Data Availability Statement: The data presented in this study are available on request from the corresponding author. RNA sequencing of experimental colon cancer cells will be submitted to NCBI's Archive to be publicly available.

Conflicts of Interest: The authors declare no conflict of interest.

References

1. Bluher, M. Obesity: Global epidemiology and pathogenesis. *Nat. Rev. Endocrinol.* **2019**, *15*, 288–298. [CrossRef]
2. Rawla, P.; Sunkara, T.; Barsouk, A. Epidemiology of colorectal cancer: Incidence, mortality, survival, and risk factors. *Gastroenterol. Rev.* **2019**, *14*, 89–103. [CrossRef]
3. Duraiyarasan, S.; Adefuye, M.; Manjunatha, N.; Ganduri, V.; Rajasekaran, K. Colon Cancer and Obesity: A Narrative Review. *Cureus* **2022**, *14*, e27589. [CrossRef]
4. Shah, S.C.; Itzkowitz, S.H. Colorectal Cancer in Inflammatory Bowel Disease: Mechanisms and Management. *Gastroenterology* **2022**, *162*, 715–730 e713. [CrossRef] [PubMed]
5. Nenkov, M.; Ma, Y.; Gassler, N.; Chen, Y. Metabolic Reprogramming of Colorectal Cancer Cells and the Microenvironment: Implication for Therapy. *Int. J. Mol. Sci.* **2021**, *22*, 6262. [CrossRef] [PubMed]
6. Qi, W.; Fitchev, P.S.; Cornwell, M.L.; Greenberg, J.; Cabe, M.; Weber, C.R.; Roy, H.K.; Crawford, S.E.; Savkovic, S.D. FOXO3 growth inhibition of colonic cells is dependent on intraepithelial lipid droplet density. *J. Biol. Chem.* **2013**, *288*, 16274–16281. [CrossRef]
7. Iftikhar, R.; Penrose, H.M.; King, A.N.; Samudre, J.S.; Collins, M.E.; Hartono, A.B.; Lee, S.B.; Lau, F.; Baddoo, M.; Flemington, E.F.; et al. Elevated ATGL in colon cancer cells and cancer stem cells promotes metabolic and tumorigenic reprogramming reinforced by obesity. *Oncogenesis* **2021**, *10*, 82. [CrossRef]
8. Penrose, H.M.; Heller, S.; Cable, C.; Nakhoul, H.; Baddoo, M.; Flemington, E.; Crawford, S.E.; Savkovic, S.D. High-fat diet induced leptin and Wnt expression: RNA-sequencing and pathway analysis of mouse colonic tissue and tumors. *Carcinogenesis* **2017**, *38*, 302–311. [CrossRef] [PubMed]
9. Krieg, L.; Didt, K.; Karkossa, I.; Bernhart, S.H.; Kehr, S.; Subramanian, N.; Lindhorst, A.; Schaudinn, A.; Tabei, S.; Keller, M.; et al. Multiomics reveal unique signatures of human epiploic adipose tissue related to systemic insulin resistance. *Gut* **2021**, *71*, 2179–2193. [CrossRef]
10. Giannis, D.; Matenoglou, E.; Sidiropoulou, M.S.; Papalampros, A.; Schmitz, R.; Felekouras, E.; Moris, D. Epiploic appendagitis: Pathogenesis, clinical findings and imaging clues of a misdiagnosed mimicker. *Ann. Transl. Med.* **2019**, *7*, 814. [CrossRef]
11. Devos, H.; Goethals, L.; Belsack, D.; Brucker, Y.; Allemeersch, G.J.; Ilsen, B.; Vandenbroucke, F.; de Mey, J. Fat misbehaving in the abdominal cavity: A pictorial essay. *Pol. J. Radiol.* **2020**, *85*, e32–e38. [CrossRef]
12. Sand, M.; Gelos, M.; Bechara, F.G.; Sand, D.; Wiese, T.H.; Steinstraesser, L.; Mann, B. Epiploic appendagitis-clinical characteristics of an uncommon surgical diagnosis. *BMC Surg.* **2007**, *7*, 11. [CrossRef]
13. Onogi, Y.; Ussar, S. Is epiploic fat the dermal fat of the intestine? *Gut* **2021**, *71*, 2147–2148. [CrossRef]
14. Choi, Y.I.; Woo, H.S.; Chung, J.W.; Shim, Y.S.; Kwon, K.A.; Kim, K.O.; Kim, Y.J.; Park, D.K. Primary epiploic appendagitis: Compared with diverticulitis and focused on obesity and recurrence. *Intest. Res.* **2019**, *17*, 554–560. [CrossRef] [PubMed]
15. Nugent, J.P.; Ouellette, H.A.; O'Leary, D.P.; Khosa, F.; Nicolaou, S.; McLaughlin, P.D. Epiploic appendagitis: 7-year experience and relationship with visceral obesity. *Abdom. Radiol.* **2018**, *43*, 1552–1557. [CrossRef]

16. Lau, F.H.; Vogel, K.; Luckett, J.P.; Hunt, M.; Meyer, A.; Rogers, C.L.; Tessler, O.; Dupin, C.L.; St Hilaire, H.; Islam, K.N.; et al. Sandwiched White Adipose Tissue: A Microphysiological System of Primary Human Adipose Tissue. *Tissue Eng. Part C Methods* **2018**, *24*, 135–145. [CrossRef]
17. Gurrala, R.; Byrne, C.E.; Brown, L.M.; Tiongco, R.F.P.; Matossian, M.D.; Savoie, J.J.; Collins-Burow, B.M.; Burow, M.E.; Martin, E.C.; Lau, F.H. Quantifying Breast Cancer-Driven Fiber Alignment and Collagen Deposition in Primary Human Breast Tissue. *Front. Bioeng. Biotechnol.* **2021**, *9*, 618448. [CrossRef] [PubMed]
18. Scahill, S.D.; Hunt, M.; Rogers, C.L.; Lau, F.H. A Microphysiologic Platform for Human Fat: Sandwiched White Adipose Tissue. *J. Vis. Exp.* **2018**, *138*, e57909. [CrossRef]
19. Strong, A.L.; Strong, T.A.; Rhodes, L.V.; Semon, J.A.; Zhang, X.; Shi, Z.; Zhang, S.; Gimble, J.M.; Burow, M.E.; Bunnell, B.A. Obesity associated alterations in the biology of adipose stem cells mediate enhanced tumorigenesis by estrogen dependent pathways. *Breast Cancer Res.* **2013**, *15*, R102. [CrossRef] [PubMed]
20. Bourin, P.; Bunnell, B.A.; Casteilla, L.; Dominici, M.; Katz, A.J.; March, K.L.; Redl, H.; Rubin, J.P.; Yoshimura, K.; Gimble, J.M. Stromal cells from the adipose tissue-derived stromal vascular fraction and culture expanded adipose tissue-derived stromal/stem cells: A joint statement of the International Federation for Adipose Therapeutics and Science (IFATS) and the International Society for Cellular Therapy (ISCT). *Cytotherapy* **2013**, *15*, 641–648. [CrossRef]
21. Penrose, H.M.; Heller, S.; Cable, C.; Nakhoul, H.; Ungerleider, N.; Baddoo, M.; Pursell, Z.F.; Flemington, E.K.; Crawford, S.E.; Savkovic, S.D. In colonic rho(0) (rho0) cells reduced mitochondrial function mediates transcriptomic alterations associated with cancer. *Oncoscience* **2017**, *4*, 189–198. [CrossRef] [PubMed]
22. Pena, C.; Garcia, J.M.; Larriba, M.J.; Barderas, R.; Gomez, I.; Herrera, M.; Garcia, V.; Silva, J.; Dominguez, G.; Rodriguez, R.; et al. SNAI1 expression in colon cancer related with CDH1 and VDR downregulation in normal adjacent tissue. *Oncogene* **2009**, *28*, 4375–4385. [CrossRef]
23. Hou, Z.; Guo, K.; Sun, X.; Hu, F.; Chen, Q.; Luo, X.; Wang, G.; Hu, J.; Sun, L. TRIB2 functions as novel oncogene in colorectal cancer by blocking cellular senescence through AP4/p21 signaling. *Mol. Cancer* **2018**, *17*, 172. [CrossRef] [PubMed]
24. Mirzaa, G.M.; Vitre, B.; Carpenter, G.; Abramowicz, I.; Gleeson, J.G.; Paciorkowski, A.R.; Cleveland, D.W.; Dobyns, W.B.; O'Driscoll, M. Mutations in CENPE define a novel kinetochore-centromeric mechanism for microcephalic primordial dwarfism. *Hum. Genet.* **2014**, *133*, 1023–1039. [CrossRef]
25. Huhn, S.C.; Liu, J.; Ye, C.; Lu, H.; Jiang, X.; Feng, X.; Ganesan, S.; White, E.; Shen, Z. Regulation of spindle integrity and mitotic fidelity by BCCIP. *Oncogene* **2017**, *36*, 4750–4766. [CrossRef] [PubMed]
26. Lu, L.; Wang, H.; Fang, J.; Zheng, J.; Liu, B.; Xia, L.; Li, D. Overexpression of OAS1 Is Correlated With Poor Prognosis in Pancreatic Cancer. *Front. Oncol.* **2022**, *12*, 944194. [CrossRef]
27. Zhang, Y.; Yu, C. Prognostic characterization of OAS1/OAS2/OAS3/OASL in breast cancer. *BMC Cancer* **2020**, *20*, 575. [CrossRef]
28. Zhang, L.; Song, M.; Zhang, F.; Yuan, H.; Chang, W.; Yu, G.; Niu, Y. Accumulation of Nicotinamide N-Methyltransferase (NNMT) in Cancer-associated Fibroblasts: A Potential Prognostic and Predictive Biomarker for Gastric Carcinoma. *J. Histochem. Cytochem.* **2021**, *69*, 165–176. [CrossRef]
29. Amin, M.B.; Greene, F.L.; Edge, S.B.; Compton, C.C.; Gershenwald, J.E.; Brookland, R.K.; Meyer, L.; Gress, D.M.; Byrd, D.R.; Winchester, D.P. The Eighth Edition AJCC Cancer Staging Manual: Continuing to build a bridge from a population-based to a more "personalized" approach to cancer staging. *CA Cancer J. Clin.* **2017**, *67*, 93–99. [CrossRef]
30. Ha, C.W.Y.; Martin, A.; Sepich-Poore, G.D.; Shi, B.; Wang, Y.; Gouin, K.; Humphrey, G.; Sanders, K.; Ratnayake, Y.; Chan, K.S.L.; et al. Translocation of Viable Gut Microbiota to Mesenteric Adipose Drives Formation of Creeping Fat in Humans. *Cell* **2020**, *183*, 666–683 e617. [CrossRef]
31. Wernstedt Asterholm, I.; Tao, C.; Morley, T.S.; Wang, Q.A.; Delgado-Lopez, F.; Wang, Z.V.; Scherer, P.E. Adipocyte inflammation is essential for healthy adipose tissue expansion and remodeling. *Cell Metabolism* **2014**, *20*, 103–118. [CrossRef]
32. Liu, Z.; Brooks, R.S.; Ciappio, E.D.; Kim, S.J.; Crott, J.W.; Bennett, G.; Greenberg, A.S.; Mason, J.B. Diet-induced obesity elevates colonic TNF-alpha in mice and is accompanied by an activation of Wnt signaling: A mechanism for obesity-associated colorectal cancer. *J. Nutr. Biochem.* **2012**, *23*, 1207–1213. [CrossRef]
33. Drew, J.E. Molecular mechanisms linking adipokines to obesity-related colon cancer: Focus on leptin. *Proc. Nutr. Soc.* **2012**, *71*, 175–180. [CrossRef] [PubMed]
34. Iftikhar, R.; Penrose, H.M.; King, A.N.; Kim, Y.; Ruiz, E.; Kandil, E.; Machado, H.L.; Savkovic, S.D. FOXO3 Expression in Macrophages Is Lowered by a High-Fat Diet and Regulates Colonic Inflammation and Tumorigenesis. *Metabolites* **2022**, *12*, 250. [CrossRef] [PubMed]
35. Penrose, H.M.; Cable, C.; Heller, S.; Ungerleider, N.; Nakhoul, H.; Baddoo, M.; Hartono, A.B.; Lee, S.B.; Burow, M.E.; Flemington, E.F.; et al. Loss of Forkhead Box O3 Facilitates Inflammatory Colon Cancer: Transcriptome Profiling of the Immune Landscape and Novel Targets. *Cell. Mol. Gastroenterol. Hepatol.* **2019**, *7*, 391–408. [CrossRef] [PubMed]
36. Ni, D.; Ma, X.; Li, H.Z.; Gao, Y.; Li, X.T.; Zhang, Y.; Ai, Q.; Zhang, P.; Song, E.L.; Huang, Q.B.; et al. Downregulation of FOXO3a promotes tumor metastasis and is associated with metastasis-free survival of patients with clear cell renal cell carcinoma. *Clin. Cancer Res.* **2014**, *20*, 1779–1790. [CrossRef]

37. Collaborative, R.; Zaborowski, A.M.; Abdile, A.; Adamina, M.; Aigner, F.; d'Allens, L.; Allmer, C.; Alvarez, A.; Anula, R.; Andric, M.; et al. Characteristics of Early-Onset vs Late-Onset Colorectal Cancer: A Review. *JAMA Surg.* **2021**, *156*, 865–874. [CrossRef]
38. Vuik, F.E.; Nieuwenburg, S.A.; Bardou, M.; Lansdorp-Vogelaar, I.; Dinis-Ribeiro, M.; Bento, M.J.; Zadnik, V.; Pellise, M.; Esteban, L.; Kaminski, M.F.; et al. Increasing incidence of colorectal cancer in young adults in Europe over the last 25 years. *Gut* **2019**, *68*, 1820–1826. [CrossRef]

Disclaimer/Publisher's Note: The statements, opinions and data contained in all publications are solely those of the individual author(s) and contributor(s) and not of MDPI and/or the editor(s). MDPI and/or the editor(s) disclaim responsibility for any injury to people or property resulting from any ideas, methods, instructions or products referred to in the content.

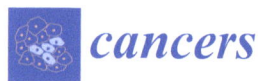

Article

Metabolomic and Mitochondrial Fingerprinting of the Epithelial-to-Mesenchymal Transition (EMT) in Non-Tumorigenic and Tumorigenic Human Breast Cells

Elisabet Cuyàs [1,2,*], Salvador Fernández-Arroyo [3], Sara Verdura [1,2], Ruth Lupu [4,5,6], Jorge Joven [7] and Javier A. Menendez [1,2,*]

1. Metabolism and Cancer Group, Program Against Cancer Therapeutic Resistance (ProCURE), Catalan Institute of Oncology, 17005 Girona, Spain
2. Girona Biomedical Research Institute, 17190 Girona, Spain
3. Eurecat, Centre Tecnològic de Catalunya, Centre for Omic Sciences, Joint Unit Eurecat-Universitat Rovira I Virgili, Unique Scientific and Technical Infrastructure (ICTS), 43204 Reus, Spain
4. Department of Laboratory Medicine and Pathology, Division of Experimental Pathology, Mayo Clinic, Rochester, MN 55905, USA
5. Department of Biochemistry and Molecular Biology Laboratory, Mayo Clinic Minnesota, Rochester, MN 55905, USA
6. Mayo Clinic Cancer Center, Rochester, MN 55905, USA
7. Unitat de Recerca Biomèdica (URB-CRB), Hospital Universitari de Sant Joan, Institut d'Investigació Sanitaria Pere Virgili, Universitat Rovira I Virgili, 43204 Reus, Spain
* Correspondence: ecuyas@idibgi.org (E.C.); jmenendez@idibgi.org (J.A.M.)

Simple Summary: Epithelial-to-mesenchymal transition (EMT) is a cellular program that enables epithelial cells to transition toward a mesenchymal phenotype with augmented cellular motility. Although EMT is a fundamental, non-pathological process in embryonic development and tissue repair, it also confers biological aggressiveness to cancer cells, including invasive behavior, tumor- and metastasis-initiating cancer stem cell activity, and greater resistance to all the cancer treatment modalities. Whereas alterations in the metabolic microenvironment are known to induce EMT, it is also true that the EMT process involves a very marked metabolic remodeling. However, whether there is a causal or merely an ancillary relationship between metabolic rewiring and the EMT phenomenon has not yet been definitively clarified. Here, we combined several technology platforms to assess whether the accompanying changes in the metabolic profile and mitochondria functioning that take place during the EMT process are independent or not of the non-tumorigenic versus tumorigenic nature of epithelial cells suffering a mesenchymal conversion. Understanding the metabolic basis of the non-tumorigenic and tumorigenic EMT provides fundamental insights into the causation and progression of cancer and may, in the long run, lead to new therapeutic strategies.

Abstract: Epithelial-to-mesenchymal transition (EMT) is key to tumor aggressiveness, therapy resistance, and immune escape in breast cancer. Because metabolic traits might be involved along the EMT continuum, we investigated whether human breast epithelial cells engineered to stably acquire a mesenchymal phenotype in non-tumorigenic and H-Ras^{V12}-driven tumorigenic backgrounds possess unique metabolic fingerprints. We profiled mitochondrial–cytosolic bioenergetic and one-carbon (1C) metabolites by metabolomic analysis, and then questioned the utilization of different mitochondrial substrates by EMT mitochondria and their sensitivity to mitochondria-centered inhibitors. "Upper" and "lower" glycolysis were the preferred glucose fluxes activated by EMT in non-tumorigenic and tumorigenic backgrounds, respectively. EMT in non-tumorigenic and tumorigenic backgrounds could be distinguished by the differential contribution of the homocysteine-methionine 1C cycle to the transsulfuration pathway. Both non-tumorigenic and tumorigenic EMT-activated cells showed elevated mitochondrial utilization of glycolysis end-products such as lactic acid, β-oxidation substrates including palmitoyl–carnitine, and tricarboxylic acid pathway substrates such as succinic acid. Notably, mitochondria in tumorigenic EMT cells distinctively exhibited a significant alteration in the electron flow intensity from succinate to mitochondrial complex III as they were highly refractory to

Citation: Cuyàs, E.; Fernández-Arroyo, S.; Verdura, S.; Lupu, R.; Joven, J.; Menendez, J.A. Metabolomic and Mitochondrial Fingerprinting of the Epithelial-to-Mesenchymal Transition (EMT) in Non-Tumorigenic and Tumorigenic Human Breast Cells. *Cancers* **2022**, *14*, 6214. https://doi.org/10.3390/cancers14246214

Academic Editor: Paola Tucci

Received: 5 November 2022
Accepted: 13 December 2022
Published: 16 December 2022

Publisher's Note: MDPI stays neutral with regard to jurisdictional claims in published maps and institutional affiliations.

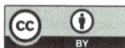

Copyright: © 2022 by the authors. Licensee MDPI, Basel, Switzerland. This article is an open access article distributed under the terms and conditions of the Creative Commons Attribution (CC BY) license (https://creativecommons.org/licenses/by/4.0/).

the inhibitory effects of antimycin A and myxothiazol. Our results show that the bioenergetic/1C metabolic signature, the utilization rates of preferred mitochondrial substrates, and sensitivity to mitochondrial drugs significantly differs upon execution of EMT in non-tumorigenic and tumorigenic backgrounds, which could help to resolve the relationship between EMT, malignancy, and therapeutic resistance in breast cancer.

Keywords: metabolism; mitochondria; phenotypic screening; breast cancer; therapy resistance; complex III

1. Introduction

Epithelial-to-mesenchymal transition (EMT), a developmental program that primes cells for subsequent cell fate conversion, was proposed as a key requirement for invasion and metastasis to distant organs more than 10 years ago [1–7]. This conceptual framework has been challenged by fate-mapping studies suggesting that EMT might be dispensable for metastatic outgrowth [8–10]. Indeed, cancer cells can metastasize via stable hybrid E/M phenotypes possessing higher stem-like tumor initiation properties and metastatic potential as compared to cells on either end of the EMT spectrum [11–14]. However, the evidence supporting a role for EMT in conferring therapeutic resistance is clear and compelling [15–21]. The correlation of lower survival with an activated EMT program in patients with residual disease is now viewed as the consequence of the capacity of EMT cells to resist a broad spectrum of therapeutic interventions such as hormonal therapy, chemotherapy, radiotherapy, and many targeted therapies including immunotherapy [22–27]. Accordingly, the successful therapeutic manipulation of EMT has tremendous clinical potential, and different approaches have been proposed to reprogram EMT, including the unlock of fully differentiated mesenchymal states, promotion of (re)epithelial differentiation, and targeting of EMT markers [24–27]. These strategies might involve inhibition of both cell-autonomous EMT drivers (e.g., growth factor signaling, epigenetic reprogramming, transcription factors, and microRNAs) and non-cell autonomous EMT-driving factors such as non-malignant stromal cells and non-cellular elements [24–27]. However, pharmacological inhibition of EMT-associated effectors at the molecular level remains challenging, and none of the aforementioned strategies have translated into approved therapies.

A growing number of studies have provided examples of how specific metabolic traits might represent integral parts of the EMT program [28–40]. A causal relationship between metabolic rewiring and EMT induction has been mostly explored in cancers with genetic deficiencies in metabolic enzymes such as fumarate hydratase (FH), isocitrate dehydrogenase (IDH), and succinate dehydrogenase (SDH) [30,32,34]. Genetic approaches to identifying the metabolic determinants of the EMT process have revealed the requirement of reprogrammed gluconeogenesis (via suppression of the gluconeogenesis rate-limiting enzyme fructose-1,6-bisphosphatase [41] and the key glycolytic enzyme phosphofructokinase-1 [42]) and nucleotide (via promotion of the pyrimidine-degrading enzyme dihydropyridine dehydrogenase [43]) pathways to support the mesenchymal phenotype. We previously reported that EMT-activated cells acquire the ability to metabolize high-energy nutrients such as glycolysis end-products and ketone bodies to support mitochondrial energy production [29]. Given that mitochondria are increasingly recognized as key signaling regulators of cell fate in physiological and pathological conditions [44], it is reasonable to suggest that shifts in mitochondrial function and dynamics might mechanistically resolve the causative versus bystander nature of the established correlation between metabolic reprogramming and EMT [45–50]. Moreover, metabolic targeting of EMT might be possible if the vulnerabilities in the distinct utilization of cellular metabolites between the epithelial and mesenchymal cellular state can be identified. Indeed, an underexplored possibility is that the mechanistic coupling between metabolism, (re)programming, and EMT also involves resistance to metabolic poisons with well-characterized mechanisms of action.

Here, we aimed to provide a comprehensive metabolomic and mitochondrial fingerprinting of the EMT phenomenon in human breast cells. We performed targeted metabolomics characterization coupled to functional mitochondrial phenotyping of the human breast EMT in non-tumorigenic and oncogenic H-Ras^{V12}-driven tumorigenic backgrounds (Figure 1). One phenotypic dimension was based on targeted analyses of metabolites representative of the catabolic/anabolic status of mitochondrial nodes and of the methionine/folate one-carbon (1C) cycle. A second phenotypic dimension was based on mitochondria-focused functional assays (MitoPlate™) that measures the rate of electron flow into and through the electron transport chain (ETC) from 31 different mitochondrial substrates that produce NAD(P)H or FADH$_2$ as well as the mitochondrial sensitivity to a panel of 22 diverse mitochondria-centered inhibitors. We provide evidence that non-tumorigenic and tumorigenic EMT cell fate conversion is accompanied by a conspicuous but distinctive rewiring of metabolic and mitochondria functioning.

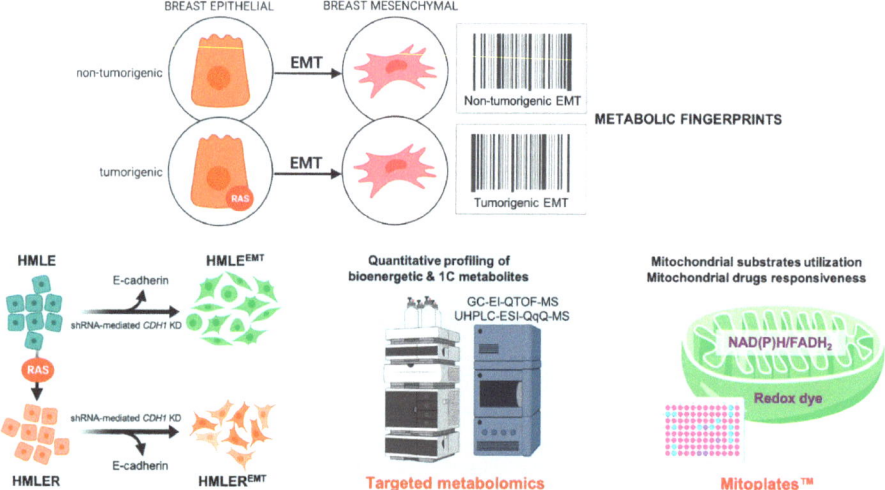

Figure 1. Metabolic fingerprinting of non-tumorigenic and tumorigenic EMT: a metabolomic and mitochondrial phenotyping approach. HMLE/HMLER cells induced for EMT upon loss of E-cadherin and their parental counterparts (HMLE/HMLER) were simultaneously subjected to quantitative screening for bioenergetic (n = 30) and 1C (n = 14) metabolites and qualitative phenotyping of multiple mitochondria energy substrates (n = 31, at low millimolar concentrations (2–5 mmol/L)) and mitochondrial drugs (n = 22) using the Mitoplate™ S-1 and I-1 assays, respectively. (shRNA: small hairpin RNA; KD: knock-down).

2. Materials and Methods

2.1. Cell Lines and Culture

HMLE^{shControl}, HMLE^{shECad}, HMLER^{shCntrol}, and HMLER^{shEcad} cells were gifts from Prof. Robert A. Weinberg (Whitehead Institute for Biomedical Research, Cambridge, MA). Cells were cultured in a 1:1 mixture of MEGM (Mammary Epithelial Bullet Kit, ref. H3CC-3150; Lonza, Basel, Switzerland) and DMEM/F12 supplemented with 10% fetal bovine serum (FBS), insulin (10 µg/mL), hydrocortisone (0.5 µg/mL), hEGF (10 ng/mL), 1% L-glutamine, and penicillin/streptomycin (Sigma, Madrid, Spain). All cells were tested for mycoplasma contamination using a PCR-based assay prior to experimentation and were intermittently tested thereafter.

2.2. Mammosphere Culture and Mammosphere-Forming Efficiency (MSFE)

For mammosphere formation, single cell suspensions of HMLER^{shCntrol} and HMLER^{shEcad} cells were seeded at 1000 cells/cm^2 in six-well ultralow attachment plates (Corning Inc.,

New York, NY, USA). Mammosphere medium consisted of serum-free F12/DMEM containing 5 mg/mL insulin, 0.5 mg/mL hydrocortisone, 2% B27 supplement (Invitrogen Ltd., Carslbad, CA, USA), and 20 ng/mL epidermal growth factor (Sigma, Madrid, Spain). The medium was made semi-solid by the addition of 0.5% methylcellulose (R&D Systems, Minneapolis, MN, USA) to prevent cell aggregation. The tumorsphere-forming efficiency (TFE) was calculated after 7 days using the following equation:

$$\text{TFE}(\%) = \frac{\text{\# of tumorspheres (large diameter} > 50 \text{ μm) per well}}{\text{\# of cells seeded per well}} \times 100$$

2.3. Flow Cytometry

Cells were washed once with phosphate-buffered saline (PBS) and then harvested with 0.05% trypsin/0.025% EDTA into single cell suspensions. Detached cells were washed with PBS containing 1% FBS and 1% penicillin/streptomycin (wash buffer), counted and resuspended in the wash buffer (10^6 cells/100 μL). Combinations of fluorochrome-conjugated monoclonal antibodies obtained from BD Pharmingen against human CD44 (PerCP-Cy™ 5.5, Mouse anti-human, ref. No. 560531) and CD24 (PE Mouse Anti-Human, ref. No. 555428) or their respective isotype controls (PerCP-Cy™ 5.5 Mouse IgG2b, κ Isotype Control, ref. No. 558304; PE Mouse IgG2a, κ Isotype Control, ref. No. 556653) were added to the cell suspensions at concentrations recommended by the manufacturer and incubated at 4 °C in the dark for 30–40 min. Labeled cells were washed in the wash buffer to eliminate unbound antibodies, then fixed in PBS containing 1% paraformaldehyde, and then analyzed no longer than 1 h post-staining on a Becton Dickinson Accuri C6 flow cytometer. Data were analyzed using Accuri C6 Flow software.

2.4. Targeted Metabolomics and Data Analysis

For targeted metabolomic experiments, HMLE^{shControl}, HMLE^{shECad}, HMLER^{shCntrol}, and HMLER^{shEcad} cells were plated in 6-well plates with normal growth medium, which was replaced after 18 h with complete fresh medium; cells were then incubated under standard cell culture conditions for additional 48 h (n = 5 biological replicates in triplicate). Quantitative measurement of up to 30 selected bioenergetic metabolites representative of the catabolic and anabolic status of mitochondria-related metabolic nodes was performed by employing a previously described GC-EI-QTOF-MS method [51–54]. Quantitative measurement of up to 14 selected metabolites representative of the methionine/folate bi-cyclic 1C metabolome was performed by employing a previously described UHPLC-ESI-QqQ-MS/MS method [55–57]. To measure energy metabolism-related metabolites, cell pellets were resuspended in 200 μL methanol/water (8:2) and D4-succinic acid and then lysed with three cycles of freezing and thawing using liquid N_2 and sonicated with three cycles of 30 s. Samples were maintained in ice for 1 min between each sonication step. Proteins were precipitated, samples were centrifuged, and supernatant was collected. After metabolite extraction, samples were dried under N_2 and derivatized to rapidly form silyl derivatives using methoxyamine hydrochloride dissolved in pyridine (40 mg/mL) and N-methyl-N-trimethylsilyl trifluoroacetamide. We used a 7890A gas chromatograph coupled with an electron impact source to a 7200 quadrupole time-of-flight mass spectrometer (Agilent Technologies, Santa Clara, CA, USA). For measuring 1C metabolites, extraction was carried out by resuspending the cell pellets in 200 μL of methanol/water (8:2) containing 1% ascorbic acid (m/v) and 0.5% β-mercaptoethanol (v/v). Cells were lysed using the same lysis procedure described above; after protein precipitation, samples were centrifuged, and the supernatants were dried under N_2 and then resuspended in ultrapure water containing 50 mmol/L ammonium acetate and 0.2% formic acid. The analysis was performed with an ultra-high pressure liquid chromatography-quadrupole time-of-light mass spectrometer (Agilent Technologiesm, Santa Clara, CA, USA). Raw data were processed, and compounds were detected and quantified using the Qualitative and Quantitative Analysis B.06.00 software (Agilent Technologies), respectively. Multivariate analysis was applied to pattern recognition, including supervised PLS-DA. The relative magnitude of observed changes was evaluated using VIP scores. Statistical significance was set at $p \leq 0.05$. MetaboAnalyst 4.0 program (available on the web: http://www.metaboanalyst.ca/ accessed on 1 June 2022) was used to generate scores/loading plots, heatmaps, and multivariate random forest analyses [58].

2.5. Mitochondrial Function Phenotyping

Mitochondrial activity was measured in triplicate using 96-well MitoPlate™ S-1 plates (Cat. #14105, Biolog, Hayward, CA, USA). Wells containing the different cytoplasmic and mitochondrial metabolic substrates (n = 31) were rehydrated with a solution containing mitochondrial assay solution (MAS) (Biolog cat. #72303), redox dye MC (Biolog cat. # 74353), and 30 µg/mL saponin (Sigma, cat. #84510) in sterile water. Cells were washed with PBS and resuspended in $1\times$ Biolog MAS and added to each well at a final cell density of 30,000 cells/well. Metabolism of substrates was assessed by monitoring colorimetric change of the terminal electron acceptor tetrazolium redox dye at a wavelength of 590 nm on a kinetic microplate reader (2 h).

2.6. Mitochondrial Drug Phenotyping

Responsiveness to mitochondria-centered drugs was measured using 96-well MitoPlate™ I-1 plates (Cat. #14104, Biolog, Hayward, CA, USA) following the manufacturer's instructions. Briefly, wells containing the different mitochondrial inhibitors were rehydrated with a solution containing redox dye MC, 30 µg/mL saponin, and 96 mmol/L succinate (Sigma, cat. #S2378) for 1 h at 37 °C. Cells were washed with PBS ($1\times$) and resuspended at a density of 10^5 cells/30 µL using $1\times$ Biolog MAS and added to each well. The MitoPlate™ I-1 plate was then loaded on a microplate reader for kinetic reading every 2 h. Alternatively, we omitted the saponification step and cells were cultured for 48 h in white DMEM medium before assessing cell viability by monitoring colorimetric changes at 590 nm for 2 h.

2.7. Statistical Analysis

Results from targeted metabolomics were compared by one-way ANOVA with Dunnett's multiple pair-wise comparison tests using a significance threshold of 0.05. Other calculations including comparisons with the Mann–Whitney U test and/or correlations were made using GraphPad Prism software 6.01 (GraphPad Software, San Diego, CA, USA).

3. Results

To avoid the confounding effects of significant differences in genetic backgrounds when employing non-EMT versus EMT-like cancer cell lines, or the possibility of generating "artificial phenotypes" by forced overexpression of EMT-driving transcription factors, we took advantage of two well-characterized models of EMT generated from mammary epithelial cells [59]. The experimental system is based on primary human mammary epithelial cells (HMECs) with sequential retroviral-mediated expression of the telomerase catalytic subunit (generating HMEC/hTERT cells), SV40 large T and small t antigens (generating HMLE cells), and the oncogenic H-Ras allele H-Ras^{V12} (generating HMLER cells). Non-tumorigenic HMLE and tumorigenic HMLER cells were modified by short hairpin RNA-mediated inhibition of *CDH1* encoding E-cadherin, triggering EMT and resulting in the stable acquisition of a mesenchymal phenotype with significantly increased drug resistance [59,60]. Before using the pairs of HMLE^{shControl}/HMLE^{shECad} (hereinafter named HMLE/HMLE-EMT) and HMLER^{shControl}/HMLER^{shECad} (hereinafter named HMLER/HMLER-EMT) for targeted metabolomic characterization and functional mitochondrial phenotyping of the breast EMT program in non-tumorigenic and tumorigenic backgrounds, we aimed to confirm the presence of their originally described EMT-like phenotypic traits [59–61] (Figure 2).

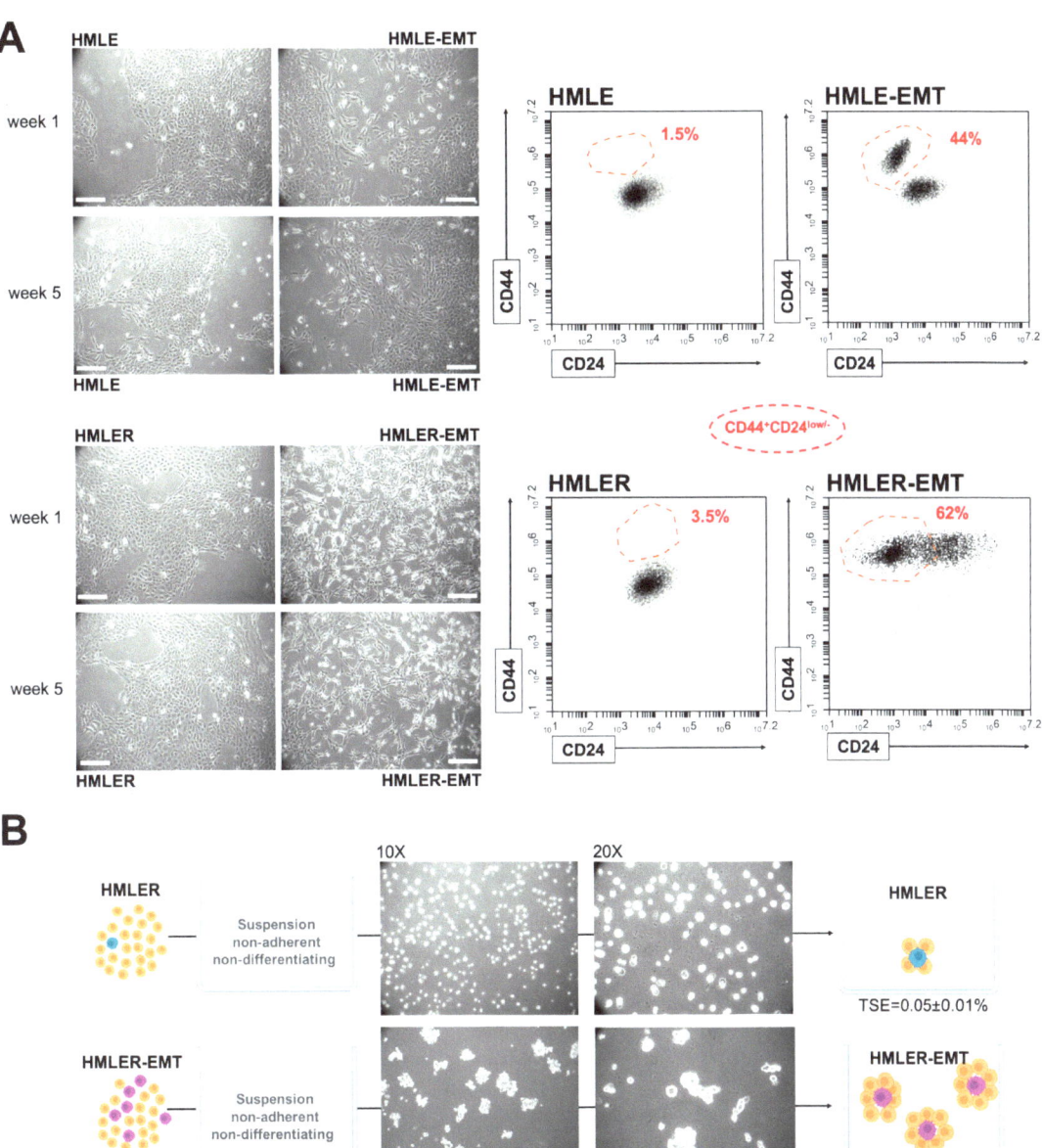

Figure 2. Mesenchymal and tumorigenic traits in HMLE/HMLER cells induced to undergo EMT. (**A**) Left: Representative phase contrast microphotographs of HMLE and HMLER cells modified by shRNA-mediated inhibition of the human *CDH1* gene. Scale bar, 100 µm. Right: Representative flow cytometry plots of CD44 and CD24 expression in HMLE/HMLE-EMT and HMLER/HMLER-EMT pairs (n = 3). Red dashed line indicates the distribution of the CD44$^+$CD24$^{-/low}$ subpopulation; percentage is indicated for each model. (**B**) Representative light microscope microphotographs of tumorspheres formed by HMLER and HMLER-EMT cells growing in sphere medium for 7 days (10X and 20X magnifications). MSFE was calculated as the number of tumorspheres (diameter > 50 µm) formed in 7 days divided by the original number of cells seeded and expressed as percentage means ± SD (n = 5 in triplicate).

When expanded in adherent conditions, phase contrast images confirmed that HMLE and HMLER cells grew in monolayer culture as tightly packed epithelial clusters with typical cobblestone morphology. Knock-down of E-cadherin in HMLE-EMT cells resulted in a more elongated shape and cell scattering in cell subpopulations that acquired a spindle-like morphology (Figure 2A). Fluorescence-activated cell sorting (FACS) using CD44 and CD24 as markers revealed that HMLE-EMT cultures likewise contained a distinct subpopulation of cells carrying the $CD44^+CD24^{low/-}$ antigenic phenotype associated with so-called mesenchymal cancer stem cells (CSC) [62,63]. An extreme elongated fibroblast-like morphology and almost complete loss of cell–cell contacts was observed in a majority of HMLER-EMT cells. This gaining of a mesenchymally transdifferentiated phenotype was accompanied by notorious acquisition of the $CD44^+CD24^{low/-}$ antigenic phenotype (Figure 2A). Because an increase in the proportion of HMLE cells that display a mesenchymal morphology has been reported to occur upon serial passaging (>8 weeks) [64], all the metabolomic/mitochondrial characterizations were carried out with HMLE/HMLE-EMT and HMLER/HMLER-EMT pairs cultured for less than 6 weeks to prevent spontaneous conversion of epithelial to mesenchymal cells during prolonged culture. The tumorigenicity of HMLER cells was originally confirmed by the Weinberg group following subcutaneous or orthotopic injection into the mammary glands of immunocompromised mice [61]. To verify an enhanced tumorigenic behavior of HMLER-EMT cells, we compared the capabilities of HMLER and HMLER-EMT cells to form multicellular "microtumors" in non-adherent and non-differentiations conditions (i.e., tumorspheres), a property associated with the presence of mammary stem/progenitor cells with tumor-initiating capacity [65,66]. HMLER-EMT cells showed a highly-significant increase (>30-fold) in the tumorsphere-forming capacity relative to HMLER parental cells (Figure 2B).

3.1. Carbon Metabolites in the Upper and Lower Chains of the Glycolytic–Gluconeogenic Reaction Pathway Are Differentially Affected by EMT in Non-Tumorigenic and Tumorigenic Background

We utilized an in-house targeted metabolomics platform coupling gas chromatography to quadrupole time-of-flight mass spectrometry and an electron impact source (GC-EI-QTOF-MS) to simultaneously measure up to 30 selected metabolites representative of the catabolic and anabolic status of mitochondria-related metabolic nodes [51–54]. The metabolites included representatives of glycolysis and the mitochondrial tricarboxylic acid (TCA) cycle, in addition to other biosynthetic routes such as the pentose phosphate pathway, amino acid metabolism, and de novo fatty acid biogenesis.

We performed a quantitative, comparative assessment of metabolites in HMLE-EMT and HMLER-EMT cells and in HMLE and HMLER parental counterparts (Table S1). A schematic view of the mean fold-change is presented in Figure 3 (left panels). Analysis of significant metabolic changes occurring post-EMT revealed that the levels of glucose-6-phosphate and fructose 1,6-bisphosphate were significantly higher in HMLE-EMT cells than in HMLE controls. Likewise, we found a significant increase in phosphoenolpyruvate accompanied by decreases in fructose 1,6-bisphosphate, succinate, and citrate in HMLER-EMT cells as compared with HMLER control cells (Table S1; Figure 3, left panels).

To better analyze our findings, we embedded the metabolic data from pre-/post-EMT pairs into a partial least squares discriminant analysis (PLS-DA) model to use the power of metabolite abundance in group discrimination and prevent type 2 statistical errors when analyzing data at the specific metabolite level. Metabolite-based clustering obtained by PLS-DA using two-dimensional score plots revealed a clear, non-overlapping differentiation of both HMLE-EMT and HMLER-EMT cells from HMLE and HMLER controls (Figure 3, middle panels). To identify the metabolites with the most relevant changes post-EMT, we calculated the variable importance of projection (VIP) scores as a measure of the variable's degree-of-alteration associated with the acquired EMT status: a higher VIP score was considered more relevant in mesenchymal versus epithelial status classification. When VIP scores ≥ 1.5 in the PLD-DA model were chosen to maximize the difference of metabolic profiles between post-EMT and epithelial parental counterparts, all "6-carbon" metabolites connecting glucose to glyceraldehyde-3-phosphate (G3P) in the upper chain of the glycolytic–gluconeogenic reaction pathway (i.e., glucose-6-phosphate, fructose-6-phosphate, and fructose 1,6-bisphosphate) showed the most relevant post-EMT changes in the non-tumorigenic HMLE/HMLE-EMT pair (Figure 3, right panels). The "3-carbon" metabolites connecting G3P to pyruvate in the lower chain of the glycolytic–gluconeogenic pathway (i.e., 3-phospho-glycerate, phosphoenolpyruvate, and pyruvate) showed the greatest impact by EMT in the tumorigenic HMLER/HMLER-EMT pair (Figure 3, right panels).

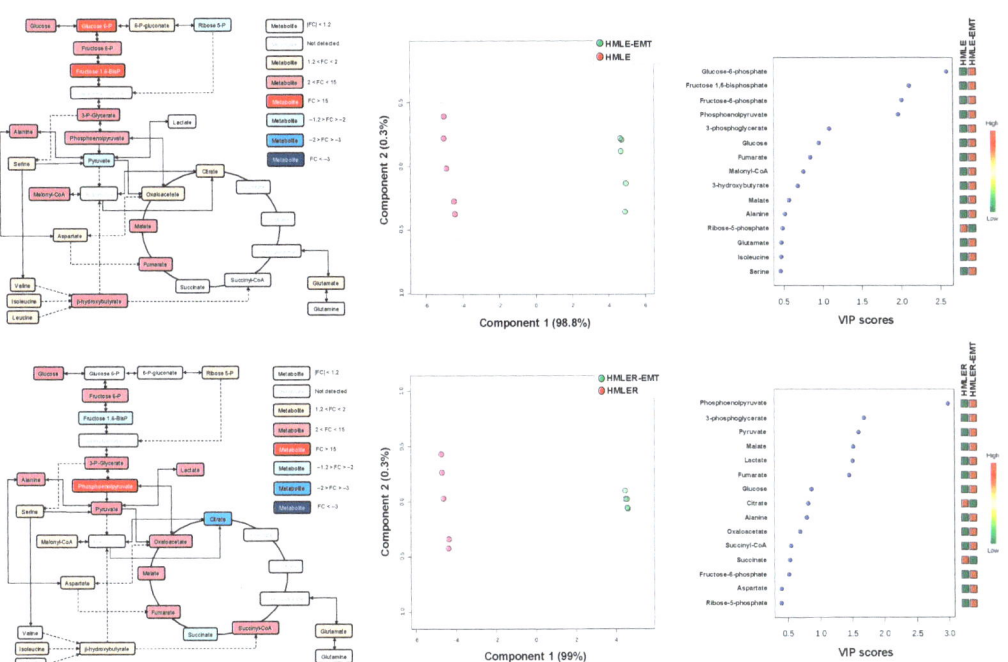

Figure 3. Bioenergetic fingerprints of non-tumorigenic and tumorigenic EMT (I). Left panels: Bioenergetic metabolites from non-tumorigenic HMLE-EMT and tumorigenic HMLER-EMT mesenchymal cells were extracted and quantitatively analyzed by GC-EI-QTOF-MS and compared with those in non-tumorigenic HMLE and tumorigenic HMLER parental counterparts. Significantly increased and decreased metabolites (EMT vs. epithelial controls) are shown using brown-red and light blue-dark blue color scales, respectively. Middle panels: Two-dimensional score plots of the partial least square discriminant analysis (PLS-DA) models of the GC-EI-QTOF-MS-based bioenergetic metabolomic profiling of HMLE/HMLE-EMT and HMLER/HMLER-EMT cells. The X and Y axes represent the combinations of the different bioenergetic metabolites analyzed, showing the maximum separation between groups. Right panels: Key bioenergetic metabolites separating the metabolomic profiles of HMLE/HMLE-EMT and HMLER/HMLER-EMT cells based on variable importance in projection (VIP) in PLS-DA analysis described in the middle panels. The VIP score, which is calculated as a weighted sum of the squared correlations between PLS-DA components and the original variable, summarizes the contribution of the metabolites' importance in the PLS-DA model. The number of terms in the sum depends on the number of PLS-DA components found to be significant in distinguishing the classes.

We next constructed two-dimensional PLS-DA models to simultaneously view how the clusters of HMLE, HMLER, HMLE-EMT, and HMLER-EMT cells behaved based on the similarity of their patterns of bioenergetic/anabolic metabolites. Whereas parental HMLE and HMLER cells grouped separately but closely, the EMT process was associated with changes in metabolite levels in such a manner that data samples from non-tumorigenic HMLE-EMT and tumorigenic HMLER-EMT cells mapped far apart (Figure 4, top panels). We then generated PLS-DA variable loading plots to evaluate how strongly each metabolic trait influenced a principal component. Taking a value >0.4 to indicate strong loading, phosphoenolpyruvate, fumarate, and 3-phosphoglycerate explained the separation between the groups in principal component 1, whereas leucine, 6-phospho-gluconate, and fructose-1,6-bisphosphate explained the separation between the groups in principal component 2 (Figure 4, top panels).

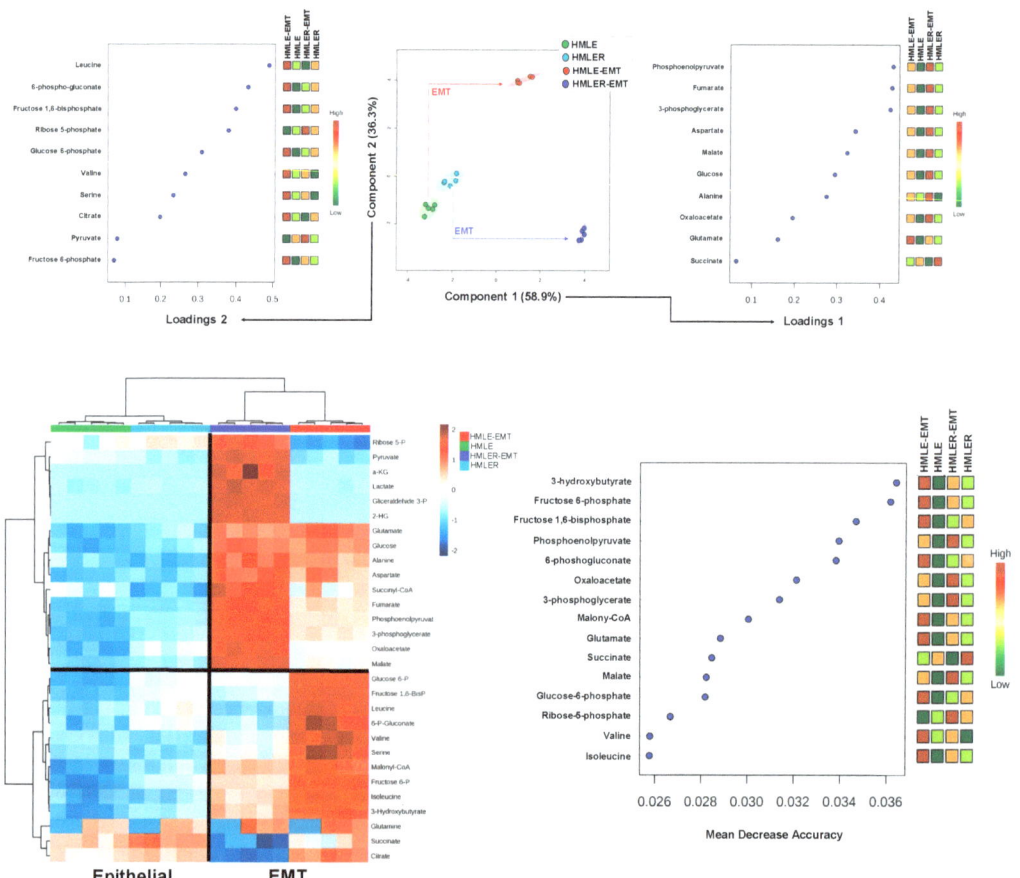

Figure 4. Bioenergetic fingerprints of non-tumorigenic and tumorigenic EMT (II). Top panels: PLS-DA showing four clusters and loading plots based on targeted bioenergetic metabolite profile data derived from HMLE/HMLE-EMT and HMLER/HMLER-EMT cells. Bottom panels: Heatmap visualization, hierarchical analyses, and random forest analysis, of the bioenergetic metabolome of HMLE/HMLE-EMT and HMLER/HMLER-EMT cells. Rows: metabolites; columns: samples; color key indicates metabolite expression value (blue: lowest; red: highest). The list of the first 15 bioenergetic metabolites highlighted by their mean decrease accuracy value is presented for each cell model. Mean decrease accuracy is the measure of the performance of the model without each metabolite. A higher value indicates the importance of such metabolite in predicting each cell line group; removal of that metabolite causes the models to lose accuracy in prediction.

To further explore the metabolites discriminating between epithelial and EMT states, the standardized metabolite concentrations were represented in a heatmap for unsupervised clustering. Changes in catabolic and anabolic metabolites segregated epithelial cells from EMT-activated cells irrespective of their background (Figure 4, bottom panels). Indeed, epithelial-to-EMT sample variation was clearly discernible, and the grouped metabolic differences (upper and bottom clusters) were also visible. To evaluate how much accuracy the model loses by excluding each metabolite, we constructed a mean decrease accuracy plot to infer which metabolites were more important for the successful epithelial versus EMT classification. Results showed that 3-hydroxybutyrate, fructose 6-phosphate, fructose 1,6-bisphosphate, phosphoenolpyruvate, and 6-phosphogluconate exhibited the highest values of mean decrease accuracy (or mean decrease Gini score), and therefore were of greater importance in the epithelial *versus* EMT model (Figure 4, bottom panels). Using a metabolite–metabolite Pearson correlation approach, we noted the occurrence of two distinct EMT-related clusters formed from the pool of quantified metabolites in the heat map (Figure S1, left panel).

3.2. One Carbon (1C) Metabolites Informing SAM/SAH (re)Methylation and/or Transsulfuration Activities Are Differentially Affected by EMT in Non-Tumorigenic and Tumorigenic Backgrounds

We applied a second inhouse targeted metabolomics platform using ultra-high pressure liquid chromatography coupled to an electrospray ionization source and a triple-quadrupole mass spectrometer (UHPLC-ESI-QqQ-MS/MS) [55–57] to quantitatively examine how the folate/methionine bicyclic 1C metabolome might be altered by EMT in non-tumorigenic and tumorigenic breast epithelial cells.

A quantitative, comparative assessment of 1C metabolite concentrations in HMLE-EMT and HMLER-EMT cells and in HMLE and HMLER parental counterparts is shown in Table S2, and a schematic view of the mean fold changes in 1C metabolite concentrations is presented in Figure 5 (left panels). Analysis of significant 1C metabolic changes occurring post-EMT revealed that the EMT process caused a significant build-up of methionine and homocysteine, accompanied by decreases in 5-adenosyl-methionine (SAM), 5-adenosyl-homocysteine (SAH), and cystathionine in HMLE-EMT cells when compared with HMLE control cells. Conversely, a significant elevation of SAM, SAH, and cystathionine, was found in HMLER-EMT cells when compared with HMLER control cells (Table S2; Figure 5, left panels). Sample clustering patterns provided by PLS-DA showed a clear separation of both HMLE-EMT and HMLER-EMT cells from HMLE and HMLER controls (Figure 5, middle panels). Considering VIP scores ≥ 1.5 in the PLD-DA model to maximize the difference in 1C metabolic profiles between post-EMT and epithelial parental cells, SAM and homocysteine showed the most relevant post-EMT alterations in the non-tumorigenic HMLE/HMLE-EMT pair, and SAH, cysteine, SAM, and NADH were the subset of 1C metabolites most strongly affected by EMT in the tumorigenic HMLER/HMLER-EMT pair (Figure 5, right panels).

Two-dimensional PLS-DA models simultaneously informing about the behavior of HMLE, HMLER, HMLE-EMT, and HMLER-EMT clusters based on the similarity of their 1C metabolite patterns revealed that the EMT process associated with changes in 1C metabolite levels in such a manner that data samples from non-tumorigenic HMLE-EMT and tumorigenic HMLER-EMT cells apparently mapped far apart (Figure 6, top panels). Loading plots >0.4 to weigh how strongly each 1C metabolic trait influenced a principal component revealed that homocysteine and serine largely explained the separation between the groups in principal component 1, whereas SAH, NADH, and cysteine explained the separation between the groups in principal component 2 (Figure 6, top panels). Unsupervised hierarchical clustering analysis revealed that variations in 1C metabolites segregated epithelial versus EMT cells irrespective of their non-tumorigenic/tumorigenic background (Figure 6, bottom panels). Similar to the bioenergetic/anabolic metabolites, epithelial-to-EMT sample variation was clearly discernible in terms of 1C metabolites, and the grouped metabolic differences (upper and bottom clusters) were also discernible. SAH, cystathionine, and cysteine exhibited the highest values of mean decrease accuracy (or mean decrease Gini score) and, therefore, were of greater importance in the epithelial versus EMT model (Figure 6, bottom panels). Two distinct EMT-related clusters formed from the pool of quantified 1C metabolites in the heat map were observed when using a metabolite–metabolite Pearson correlation approach (Figure S1, right panel).

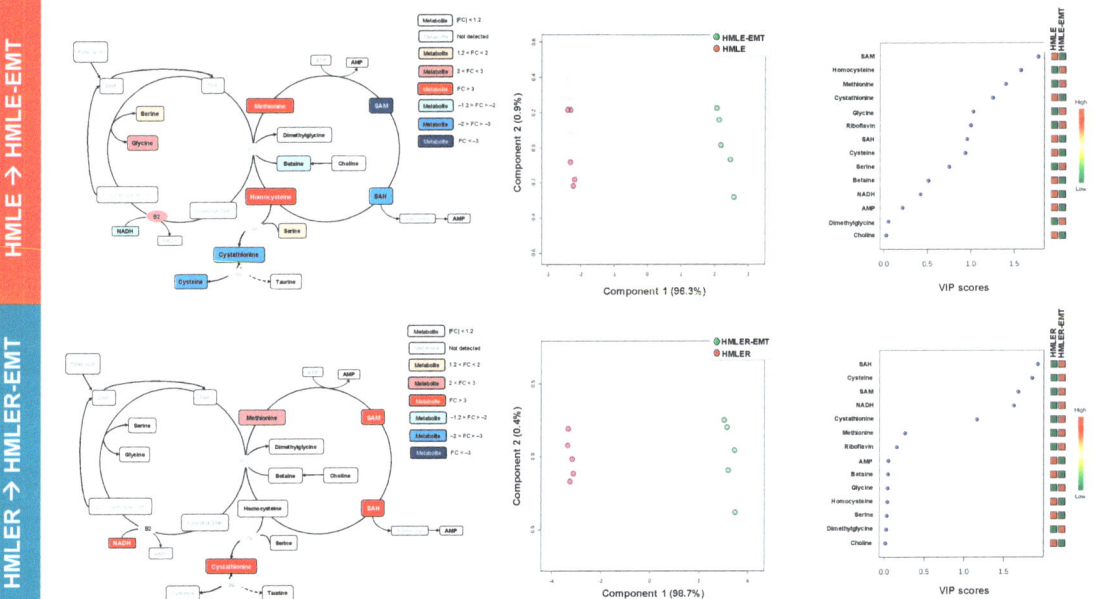

Figure 5. Homocysteine–methionine 1C metabolism fingerprints of non-tumorigenic and tumorigenic EMT (I). Left panels: Homocysteine–methionine 1C metabolites from non-tumorigenic HMLE-EMT and tumorigenic HMLER-EMT mesenchymal cells were extracted and quantitatively analyzed by UHPLC-ESI-QqQ-MS/MS and compared with those of non-tumorigenic HMLE and tumorigenic HMLER parental counterparts. Significantly increased and decreased metabolites (EMT vs. epithelial controls) are shown using brown-red and light blue-dark blue color scales, respectively. Middle panels: Two-dimensional score plots of the partial least square discriminant analysis (PLS-DA) models of the UHPLC-ESI-QqQ-MS/MS-based homocysteine–methionine 1C metabolomic profiling of HMLE/HMLE-EMT and HMLER/HMLER-EMT cells. The X and Y axes represent the combinations of the different 1C metabolites analyzed, showing the maximum separation between groups. Right panels: Key 1C metabolites separating the homocysteine–methionine 1C metabolomic profiles of HMLE/HMLE-EMT and HMLER/HMLER-EMT cells based on variable importance in projection (VIP) in PLS-DA analysis described in the middle panels. The VIP score, which is calculated as a weighted sum of the squared correlations between PLS-DA components and the original variable, summarizes the contribution of the metabolites' importance in the PLS-DA model. The number of terms in the sum depends on the number of PLS-DA components found to be significant in distinguishing the classes.

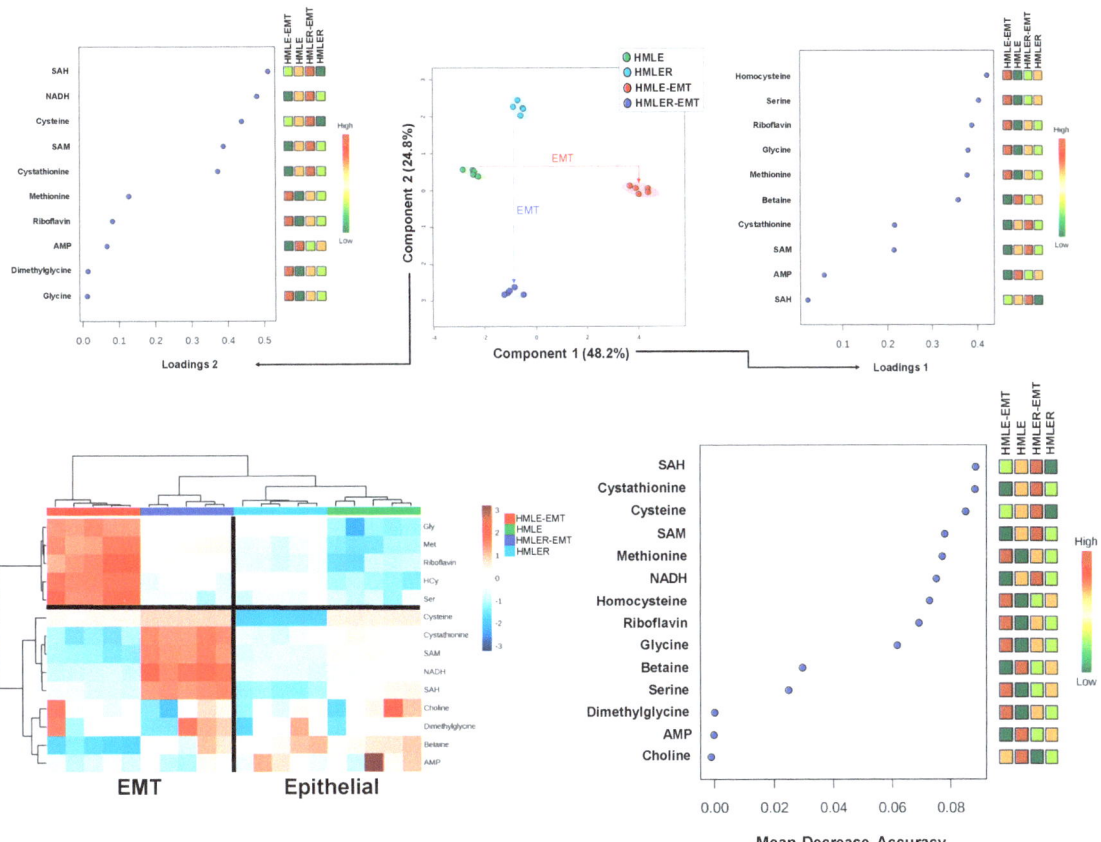

Figure 6. Homocysteine–methionine 1C metabolism fingerprints of non-tumorigenic and tumorigenic EMT (II). Top panels: PLS-DA showing four clusters and loading plots based on targeted homocysteine–methionine 1C metabolite profile data derived from HMLE/HMLE-EMT and HMLER/HMLER-EMT cells. Bottom panels: Heatmap visualization, hierarchical analyses, and random forest analysis of the homocysteine–methionine 1C metabolome of HMLE/HMLE-EMT and HMLER/HMLER-EMT cells. Rows: metabolites; columns: samples; color key indicates metabolite expression value (blue: lowest; red: highest). The list of the first 15 homocysteine–methionine 1C metabolites highlighted by their mean decrease accuracy value is presented for each cell model. Mean decrease accuracy is the measure of the performance of the model without each metabolite. A higher value indicates the importance of such metabolite in predicting each cell line group; removal of that metabolite causes the models to lose accuracy in prediction.

3.3. Mitochondrial Functioning in the Breast Cancer EMT Program Involves Changes in the Utilization of Pathway-Specific Substrates

We next employed MitoPlate™ technology, a novel phenotypic metabolic array, to measure the rates of production of NADH and $FADH_2$ from 31 potential mitochondrial energy substrates (https://www.biolog.com/products-portfolio-overview/mitochondrial-function-assays/ 1 December 2022) (Figure 7).

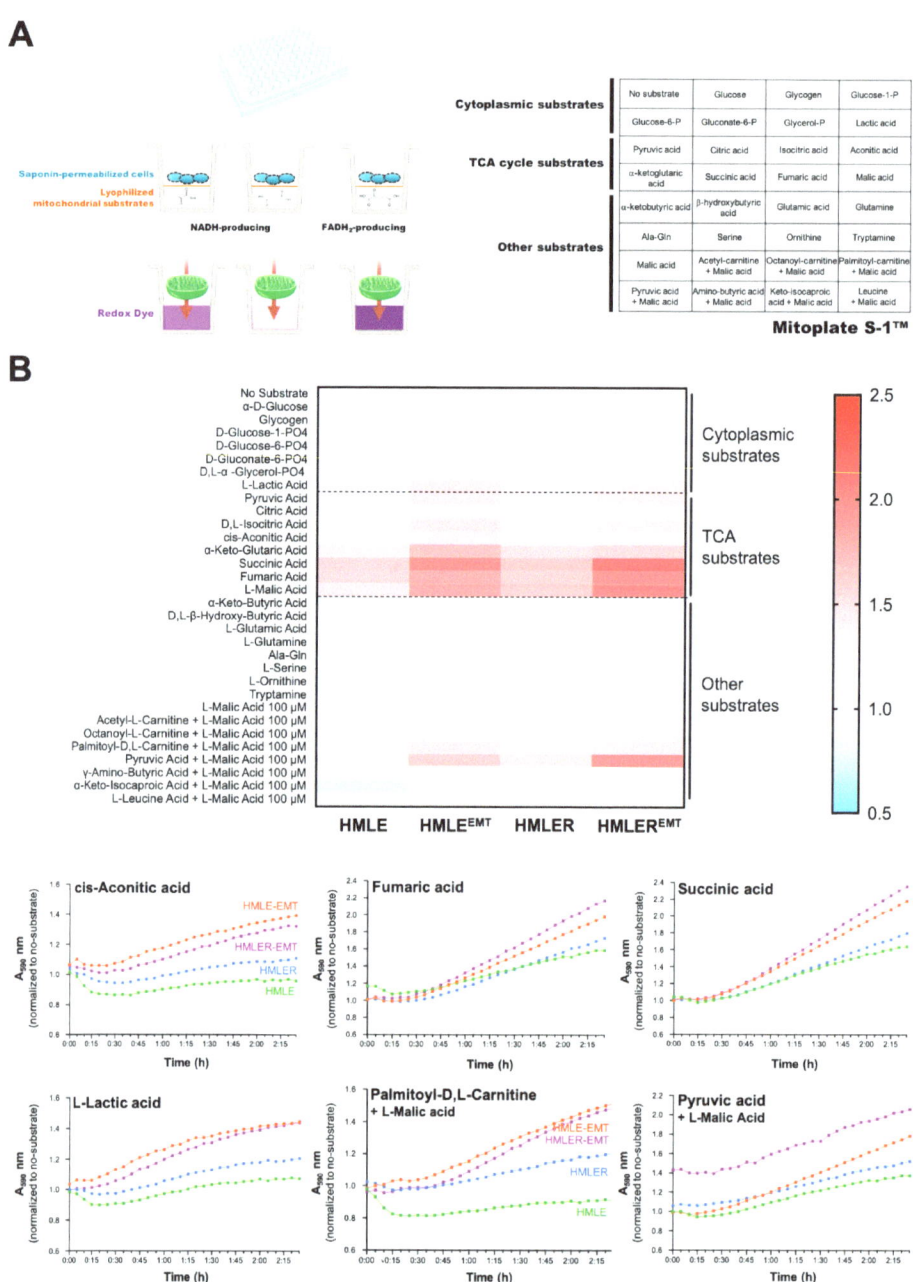

Figure 7. Mitochondrial functioning of non-tumorigenic and tumorigenic EMT. (**A**) Mitochondrial phenotyping of HMLE/HMLE-EMT and HMLER/HMLER-EMT cells using mitochondrial function assays with Biolog MitoPlate S-1 ($n = 3$). (**B**) Top: Representative heatmap of the metabolic substrate consumption (2 h) of fatty acids, glycolysis, amino acids, and TCA cycle intermediates in HMLE/HMLE-EMT and HMLER/HMLER-EMT cells ($n = 3$). Bottom: Representative reduction dynamics of the dye over time measured as absorbance at 590 nm for 2 h at 5-min intervals ($n = 3$).

By using saponin-permeabilized cells and a redox dye added to 96-well microplates containing triplicate samples of a panel of substrates (Figure 7A), we assayed the mitochondrial function of HMLE/HMLE-EMT and HMLER/HMLER-EMT pairs by measuring the rates of dye reduction from electrons flowing through the ETC from substrates whose oxidation produces NADH (e.g., pyruvate, L-malate, α-ketoglutarate, D-isocitrate, L-glutamate, D-β-hydroxy-butyrate) or $FADH_2$ (e.g., succinate, α-glycerol-3-P). Cytoplasmic substrates included glucose, glycogen, glucose-1-P, glucose-6-P, gluconate-6-P, glycerol-P, and lactic acid; TCA cycle substrates included pyruvic acid, citric acid, isocitric acid, aconitic acid, α-ketoglutaric acid, β-hydroxybutyric acid, glutamic acid, glutamine, alanine–glutamine, serine, ornithine, tryptamine, and malic acid; and other mitochondrial substrates included acetyl–carnitine + malic acid, octanoyl–carnitine + malic acid, palmitoyl–carnitine + malic acid, pyruvic acid + malic acid, amino-butyric acid + malic acid, ketoisocaproic acid + malic acid, leucine + malic acid.

The electrons donated to complex I or complex II travel to the distal end of the ETC where a tetrazolium redox dye acts as a terminal electron acceptor and changes from colorless to a purple formazan upon reduction. Thus, each of the 96 assays concurrently run in the MitoPlate S-1™ provides different information as substrates follow different metabolic routes using various transporters to enter the mitochondria, and different dehydrogenases to produce NADH or $FADH_2$. Heatmap analysis of the metabolic substrate consumption in HMLE/HMLE-EMT and HMLER/HMLER-EMT pairs is presented in Figure 7B. Results revealed a significant augmentation in the utilization of TCA cycle substrates such as cis-aconitic acid, fumaric acid, and succinic acid, in both non-tumorigenic HMLE-EMT and tumorigenic HMLER-EMT cells. Both HMLE-EMT and HMLER-EMT cells utilized other substrates including lactic acid and malic acid-containing combinations such as malic acid + the fatty acid ester palmitoyl–carnitine and malic acid + pyruvic acid, with the latter particularly utilized by mitochondria of HMLER-EMT cells.

3.4. Execution of the EMT Program in a Tumorigenic Background Promotes Resistance to Mitochondrial Complex III Inhibitors

Finally, we explored whether and how EMT execution modified the sensitivity of HMLE/HMLE-EMT and HMLER/HMLER-EMT pairs to mitochondrial-centered poisons. To do this, we used the MitoPlate™ I-1, which can measure the sensitivity of mitochondria to 22 diverse mitochondrial inhibitors that directly or indirectly inhibit the ETC. These included complex I inhibitors (rotenone, pyridaben, phenformin), complex II inhibitors (malonate and carboxin), complex III inhibitors (antimycin A and myxothiazol), uncoupling agents (trifluoromethoxy carbonylcyanide phenylhydrazone (FCCP) and 2,4-dinitrophenol), ionophores (valinomycin and calcium chloride), and other chemicals (gossypol, nordihydroguaiaretic acid, polymyxin B, amitriptyline, meclizine, berberine, alexidine, diclofenac, celastrol, trifluoperazine, and papaverine).

We first omitted the saponification step to convert a mitochondrial function assay into a conventional chemotherapeutic screen, and we measured the effects of the agents (each at four graded concentrations) via assessment of tetrazolium dye-based cell viability 48 h after initiation of drug treatment. After normalization of the optical density at 590 nm (purple color) obtained with each agent to those of the (no-drug) positive-control wells included in the MitoPlate™ I-1 plate, a qualitative overview of the fold change results showed that several mitochondrial agents (e.g., amitriptyline, alexidine, diclofenac, celastrol) indiscriminately reduced viability of all cell types irrespective of the non-EMT/EMT phenotype or non-tumorigenic/tumorigenic background when compared with no-drug controls (Figure 8A). To quantify the occurrence of EMT-related changes in responsiveness to mitochondrial agents, we also calculated a comparison score as the absolute ratio between the EMT and non-EMT parental counterparts (Figure 8B).

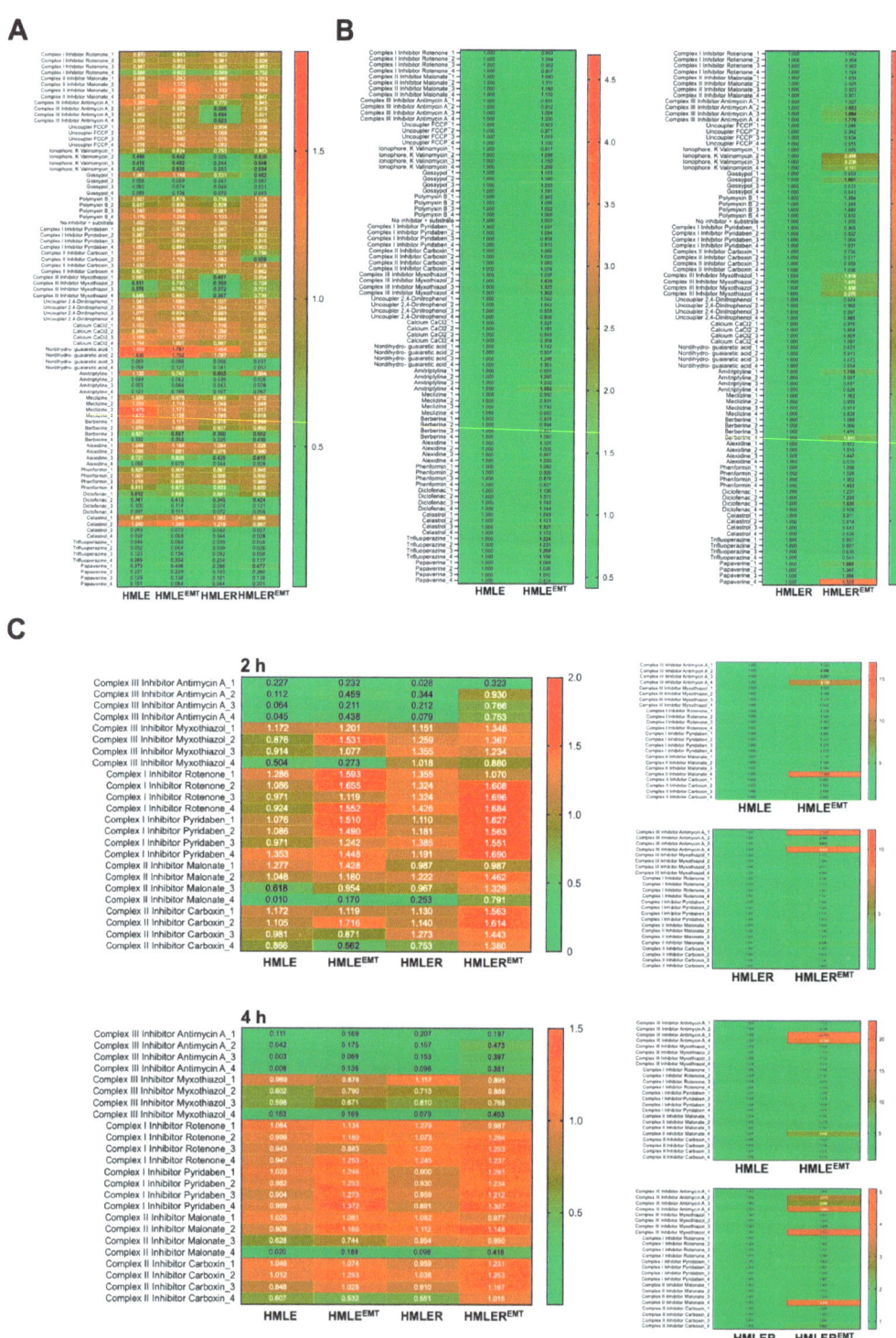

Figure 8. Responsiveness of non-tumorigenic and tumorigenic EMT to mitochondrial-centered drugs.

Representative phenetic maps of HMLE/HMLE-EMT and HMLER/HMLER-EMT cells growing in the presence of graded concentrations of mitochondria-centered drugs during 48 h, generated after normalization of the optical density values of each drug concentration at 590 nm (purple color) to those of the positive-control wells included in the MitoPlate™ I-1 plates (**A**) or calculating the absolute ratio between the optical densities at 590 nm of HMLE (=1.0) vs. HMLE-EMT and HMLER (=1.0) vs. HMLER-EMT cells (n = 3) (**B**,**C**) Representative phenetic maps of the 2 h (top) and 4 h (bottom) mitochondrial activity in saponin-permeabilized HMLE/HMLE-EMT and HMLER/HMLER-EMT cells in the presence of succinate and complex I, II, and III inhibitors (n = 3).

Non-tumorigenic HMLE-EMT cells were slightly more sensitive than HMLE controls to the anti-emetic meclizine, whereas HMLER-EMT cells were (at least 1.5-fold) more sensitive than epithelial HMLER counterparts to the natural phenol gossypol, the phenolic lignan nordihydroguaiaretic acid (NDGA), and the antipsychotic phenothiazine trifluoperazine. Remarkably, HMLER-EMT cells were significantly more resistant than HMLER counterparts to the complex III inhibitors antimycin A and myxothiazol, and to the ionophore valinomycin. HMLER-EMT cells were also partly resistant to the FDA-approved drug papaverine, an inhibitor of mitochondrial complex I that was highly cytotoxic against HMLE, HMLE-EMT, and HMLER cells.

As resistance phenotypes to complex III inhibitors in 48 h lasting cytotoxic assays can be argued to arise from adaptive metabolic reprogramming leading to activation of pro-survival processes, we decided to directly assess mitochondrial function in saponin-permeabilized cells using succinate as substrate (Figure 8C). A metabolic substrate that feeds complex II such as succinate will result in a strong flow of electrons via succinate dehydrogenase, which is expected to be inhibited by complex II and III (antimycin A and myxothiazol) inhibitors but not complex I blockers. A saponin concentration of 30 μg/mL has been shown to efficiently permeabilize cell membrane and abolish glucose metabolism without promoting any significant alteration of the mitochondrial metabolism of substrates such as malate and succinate [67]. Validation of the assay in the presence of succinate confirmed a lack of activity of the complex I inhibitors rotenone and pyridaben regardless of the presence or absence of the EMT phenotype. When compared to HMLER parental cells, HMLER-EMT mitochondria were slightly more resistant to the highest concentrations of the complex II inhibitors malonate and carboxin and highly refractory to complex III blockade by antimycin A and myxothiazol (Figure 8C).

4. Discussion

The coupled cell fate decision-making processes of metabolism and EMT can be viewed as a key contributor to cancer therapy resistance, tumor immune evasion, and metastasis [68,69]. Our present analysis reveals significant differences in bioenergetic/1C metabolic signatures, utilization of preferred mitochondrial substrates, and sensitivity to mitochondrial drugs when EMT is executed in non-tumorigenic and tumorigenic backgrounds.

We first explored whether the use of central cytosolic/mitochondrial metabolic nodes differ between human breast epithelial cells engineered to acquire a mesenchymal phenotype in the absence or presence of the H-Ras^{V12} oncogene—a well-recognized driver of the cancer metabolic landscape [70,71]. Targeted analysis revealed that "upper" and "lower" glycolysis appear to work at different rates upon EMT activation in non-tumorigenic and H-Ras^{V12}-driven tumorigenic backgrounds. Indeed, 6-carbon molecules in the "upper" chain of the glycolytic–gluconeogenic reaction pathway, which connects glucose to G3P, were those most affected by EMT activation in a non-tumorigenic background. Because the concentration of fructose-1,6-bisphosphate mirrors glycolytic flux [72], our data support a scenario wherein the metabolic reprogramming accompanying EMT in a non-tumorigenic background likely involves changes in upper glycolytic enzymes controlling both glycolytic flux and metabolite levels. Conversely, 3-carbon molecules in the "lower" reaction chain in the same glycolytic pathway—also known as the "trunk pathway" connecting G3P to pyruvate—were the most significantly affected upon EMT activation in a tumorigenic background. Because enzyme steps in lower glycolysis do not control pathway flux but carry a higher flux than any biochemically-possible alternative [73], the massive accumulation of phosphoenolpyruvate in tumorigenic EMT cells might reflect their ability to decouple ATP production from phosphoenolpyruvate-mediated phosphotransfer [74], which can act through feedback mechanisms to inhibit glycolysis, thereby allowing for the high rate of glycolysis to support anabolic metabolism.

Examination of the homocysteine–methionine 1C cycle, a metabolic sensor system controlling methylation-regulated pathological signaling [75–77], revealed differential changes upon EMT activation in non-tumorigenic and tumorigenic backgrounds. The demethylation pathway generates the universal methyl group donor SAM and the methylation inhibitor SAH, whereas the remethylation pathway converts homocysteine back into methionine by receiving a methyl group from the folate cycle or from choline/betaine metabolism via methionine synthase or via betaine–homocysteine methyltransferase, respectively. Homocysteine is the sulfur-containing precursor that is ultimately channeled to the transsulfuration pathway via conversion to another sulfur-containing amino acid, cysteine, through cystathionine. Accordingly, the evident accumulation of homocysteine in non-tumorigenic HMLE-EMT cells should result from a decrease in its utilization, from altered remethylation to methionine and/or impaired transsulfuration activity [76,77]. The impairment in remethylation and transsulfuration pathways that accompanies non-tumorigenic EMT was characterized not only by the accumulation of homocysteine, but also by the depletion of SAM, cystathionine, and cysteine. Intriguingly, a completely different functioning of the homocysteine–methionine 1C cycle appears to occur when EMT is activated in a H-Ras^{V12}-driven oncogenic background. The observed increase in SAM, SAH, and cystathionine in HLMER-EMT cells strongly suggests an augmented transmethylation activity of SAM, whose elevation is known to increase the catalytic activity of cystathionine-β-synthase—the first and rate-limiting enzyme in the transsulfuration pathway [78]. The differential activation and maintenance of methylogenesis and SAM:homocysteine ratios might underlie dynamic and reversible changes in the DNA methylome of EMT cells, an epigenetically conserved mechanism contributing to cellular transformation, tumoral progression, and therapy resistance [79–81]. Because the transsulfuration pathway is a highly plastic emergency response mechanism for maintaining cysteine pools and redox homeostasis in harsh tumor microenvironments, it is tempting to speculate that its functioning may enable tumorigenic EMT cells to circumvent nutrient scarcity and high oxidative stress, and to evade drug-induced cell death [76,77,82]. Nonetheless, we acknowledge that one major limitation of the steady-state metabolomic approach employed here is that it does not allow us to discern whether the observed changes in metabolites are causally associated with changes in production or utilization. Metabolic flux experiments utilizing ^{13}C-labeled carbon, glutamine, serine, and methionine tracers will be needed as a next step to elucidate the nature of the observed changes within the glycolytic pathway and the methionine–homocysteine 1C cycle in non-tumorigenic and tumorigenic EMT cells.

We next performed functional mitochondrial phenotyping to test epithelial and EMT-activated cells for their ability to utilize bioenergetic substrates. We observed that lactate could support mitochondrial energy production in non-tumorigenic and tumorigenic EMT cells but not in their epithelial counterparts. For many years, lactate had been seen as a metabolic waste product of glycolytic metabolism; however, an ever-growing body of evidence has revealed novel roles of lactate in the tumor microenvironment, either as a signaling molecule or as a metabolic fuel [83–86]. In the latter regard, tumorigenic EMT cells were notably capable of utilizing not only lactate as a mitochondrial fuel but also the glycolysis end-product pyruvate when simultaneously provided with an additional exogenous substrate such as malic acid. Indeed, not only were high-energy glycolysis end-products utilized at significantly higher rates in EMT cells than in non-EMT cells, but the same was true for the mitochondrial β-fatty acid oxidation (FAO) substrate palmitoyl–carnitine. Mitochondrial FAO has recently been described as a druggable metabolic "gateway" that is activated for EMT cell-state transitions to occur [87]. Previous findings using intact cells revealed that EMT is accompanied by a metabolic infrastructure that enables the scavenging and catabolization of high-energy nutrients such as pyruvate and lactate and the ketone body (and mitochondrial β-oxidation substrate) β-hydroxybutyrate, supporting mitochondrial energy production [88]. We confirm that the mitochondrial phenotype of the EMT phenomenon might constitute an efficient adaptive strategy through which lactate and pyruvate can effectively substitute for glucose as efficient mitochondrial substrates, thereby providing a bioenergetic advantage in hostile microenvironmental conditions involving nutrient starvation. Although it is well established that tumor cells can take-up and oxidize lactate as a fuel under metabolically stressful circumstances when glucose becomes limited [89,90], there is controversy as to whether lactate must first be converted to glucose via gluconeogenesis. The Biolog MitoPlate S-1™ assay directly measures electron flow into and through the ETC from various mitochondrial substrates that produce NADH and $FADH_2$ under conditions of saponin permeabilization. Notably, saponin permeabilizes only the plasma membrane, leaving the intracellular membranes of the mitochondria intact while equilibrating the intracellular spaces with incubation medium [67,91]. Our findings, therefore, support the notion that lactate could be imported and converted into pyruvate inside mitochondria to directly feed the TCA cycle in EMT cells.

Finally, we used a modified version of the MitoPlate I-1™ assay to carry out cytotoxic screenings and test the notion that mitochondria-centered metabolic reprogramming is necessary for the survival of EMT cells. With the exception of a slightly augmented sensitivity to meclizine, an antiemetic that indirectly attenuates mitochondrial respiration by targeting cytosolic phosphoethanolamine metabolism [92,93], EMT activation in a non-tumorigenic background had no phenotypic (cell viability) consequences in terms of altered responsiveness to mitochondrial poisons. By contrast, tumorigenic EMT cells showed enhanced sensitivity to several agents, including gossypol, a naturally occurring mitochondrial aldehyde dehydrogenase inhibitor extracted from a cotton plant [94,95], the phenolic lignan NDGA, which promotes mitochondrial depolarization by targeting glutathione oxidation [96–99], and the antipsychotic trifluoperazine, an inhibitor of mitochondrial permeability transition [100]. Intriguingly, we found an unanticipated resistance to the mitochondrial complex III inhibitors antimycin A and myxothiazol upon EMT activation in a tumorigenic background. Mitochondrial complex I and II donate electrons to ubiquinone, resulting in the generation of ubiquinol and the regeneration of the NAD^+ and FAD cofactors, whereas complex III oxidizes ubiquinol back to ubiquinone. This raises the question of how tumorigenic EMT phenomena circumvent the cytotoxic effects of blockade of mitochondrial ubiquinol oxidation imposed by complex III inhibitors. Because mitochondrial thioredoxin reductase (TrxR2) can reduce cytochrome c to promote resistance to complex III inhibition upon both antimycin A and myxothiazol treatment [101], it is possible that the complex III-bypassing function of TrxR2 might play a cytoprotective role in tumorigenic EMT cells. However, it has recently been reported that the essential function of mitochondrial complex III for tumor growth is ubiquinol oxidation and not its ability to proton pump or donate electrons to the downstream electron carrier cytochrome c [102]. In this line, we found that tumorigenic EMT cells show enhanced utilization of succinate, which might be consistent with an enhanced complex II activity and an over-reduction of the ubiquinone pool, thereby driving electrons backwards into complex I in a process known as reverse electron transport (RET). In the latter regard, it should be noted that a significant alteration in the electron flow intensity from succinate to mitochondrial complex II and III was indirectly confirmed in saponin-permeabilized tumorigenic EMT cells, in which the mitochondria functioning exhibited partial resistance to respiratory complex II inhibitors and a highly significant refractoriness to complex III inhibitors. Whether succinate-energized mitochondria enabling an enhanced $NADH/NAD^+$ cycling, the activation of RET, and/or changes to the structure and organization of the ETC can explain the augmented resistance to complex III inhibition in tumorigenic EMT cells requires further study [103]. Because altered sensitivity to ionophores perturbing ion homeostasis affects not only mitochondrial functions but also other cellular processes ranging from vacuolar function, through translation to stress responses [104], the acquired resistance of tumorigenic EMT cells to valinomycin is likely pleiotropic and multi-faceted.

5. Conclusions

Metabolic rewiring, mitochondria functioning, and EMT cooperate to regulate cell fate in non-cancer scenarios such as induced pluripotency [105]. The close cooperation between EMT induction and an active form of RAS is sufficient to trigger malignant transformation of mammary epithelial cells including the acquisition of stem cell-like traits [106,107]. The interdependence of metabolism and EMT also suggests that repurposed metabolic inhibitors could be considered as novel therapeutic interventions for blocking EMT-associated metabolic traits that can trigger cancer recurrence [108]. Our present description of a distinctive landscape of metabolic traits in non-tumorigenic and tumorigenic EMT suggests not only context-specific supportive bioenergetic roles, but likely also instructive roles in determining and maintaining cell fate decisions. Moreover, our findings strongly opine that yet undefined links between metabolism and EMT could compromise the efficacy of metabolic therapies in breast cancer. Accordingly, mitochondrial phenotypes should be carefully evaluated when aiming to use mitochondria-targeting drugs to target EMT-driven biological aggressiveness and therapeutic resistance in breast cancer.

Supplementary Materials: The following supporting information can be downloaded at: https://www.mdpi.com/article/10.3390//cancers14246214/s1, Figure S1: Correlation of the metabolomic data. Table S1: Concentration of bioenergetic metabolites in HMLE/HMLE-EMT and HMLER/HMLER-EMT cells; Table S2: Concentration of homocysteine–methionine 1C metabolites in HMLE/HMLE-EMT and HMLER/HMLER-EMT cells.

Author Contributions: Conceptualization, E.C. and J.A.M.; methodology, S.F.-A., E.C., R.L. and J.A.M.; formal analysis, S.F.-A., E.C., S.V., R.L., J.J. and J.A.M.; investigation, E.C., S.F.-A., S.V., R.L., J.J. and J.A.M.; validation, E.C., S.F.-A. and S.V.; data curation, E.C., S.F.-A., S.V., R.L. and J.A.M.; writing—original draft preparation, E.C. and J.A.M.; writing—review and editing, J.A.M.; visualization, E.C., S.F.-A. and J.A.M.; supervision, S.F.-A., E.C., J.J. and J.A.M.; project administration, E.C.; funding acquisition, E.C. and J.A.M. All authors have read and agreed to the published version of the manuscript.

Funding: Work in the Menendez laboratory is supported by the Spanish Ministry of Science and Innovation (Grant PID2019-10455GB-I00, Plan Nacional de I+D+I, founded by the European Regional Development Fund, Spain). Elisabet Cuyàs holds a "Miguel Servet" research contract (CP20/00003) from the Instituto de Salud Carlos III (Spain) and is supported by the Spanish Ministry of Science and Innovation (Grant PI22/00297, Proyectos de I+D+I en Salud, Acción Estratégica en Salud 2021–2023, founded by the European Regional Development Fund, Spain).

Institutional Review Board Statement: Not applicable.

Informed Consent Statement: Not applicable.

Data Availability Statement: All data generated or analyzed during this study are included in this published article.

Acknowledgments: We are greatly indebted to Robert A. Weinberg (Whitehead Institute for Biomedical Research, Cambridge, MA, USA) for providing the HMLE^{shControl}, HMLE^{shECad}, HMLER^{shCntrol}, and HMLER^{shEcad} cells used in this work. The authors would like to thank Kenneth McCreath for detailed editing of this manuscript.

Conflicts of Interest: The authors declare that the research was conducted in the absence of any commercial or financial relationships that could be construed as a potential conflict of interest.

References

1. Thiery, J.P. Epithelial-mesenchymal transitions in tumour progression. *Nat. Rev. Cancer* **2002**, *2*, 442–454. [CrossRef] [PubMed]
2. Huber, M.A.; Kraut, N.; Beug, H. Molecular requirements for epithelial-mesenchymal transition during tumor progression. *Curr. Opin. Cell Biol.* **2005**, *17*, 548–558. [CrossRef] [PubMed]

3. Polyak, K.; Weinberg, R.A. Transitions between epithelial and mesenchymal states: Acquisition of malignant and stem cell traits. *Nat. Rev. Cancer* **2009**, *9*, 265–273. [CrossRef] [PubMed]
4. Ye, X.; Weinberg, R.A. Epithelial-Mesenchymal Plasticity: A Central Regulator of Cancer Progression. *Trends Cell Biol.* **2015**, *25*, 675–686. [CrossRef] [PubMed]
5. Shibue, T.; Weinberg, R.A. EMT, CSCs, and drug resistance: The mechanistic link and clinical implications. *Nat. Rev. Clin. Oncol.* **2017**, *14*, 611–629. [CrossRef] [PubMed]
6. Brabletz, T.; Kalluri, R.; Nieto, M.A.; Weinberg, R.A. EMT in cancer. *Nat. Rev. Cancer* **2018**, *18*, 128–134. [CrossRef]
7. Dongre, A.; Weinberg, R.A. New insights into the mechanisms of epithelial-mesenchymal transition and implications for cancer. *Nat. Rev. Mol. Cell Biol.* **2019**, *20*, 69–84. [CrossRef]
8. Fischer, K.R.; Durrans, A.; Lee, S.; Sheng, J.; Li, F.; Wong, S.T.; Choi, H.; El Rayes, T.; Ryu, S.; Troeger, J.; et al. Epithelial-to-mesenchymal transition is not required for lung metastasis but contributes to chemoresistance. *Nature* **2015**, *527*, 472–476. [CrossRef]
9. Zheng, X.; Carstens, J.L.; Kim, J.; Scheible, M.; Kaye, J.; Sugimoto, H.; Wu, C.C.; LeBleu, V.S.; Kalluri, R. Epithelial-to-mesenchymal transition is dispensable for metastasis but induces chemoresistance in pancreatic cancer. *Nature* **2015**, *527*, 525–530. [CrossRef]
10. Neelakantan, D.; Zhou, H.; Oliphant, M.U.J.; Zhang, X.; Simon, L.M.; Henke, D.M.; Shaw, C.A.; Wu, M.F.; Hilsenbeck, S.G.; White, L.D.; et al. EMT cells increase breast cancer metastasis via paracrine GLI activation in neighbouring tumour cells. *Nat. Commun.* **2017**, *8*, 15773. [CrossRef]
11. Li, W.; Kang, Y. Probing the Fifty Shades of EMT in Metastasis. *Trends Cancer* **2016**, *2*, 65–67. [CrossRef] [PubMed]
12. Jolly, M.K.; Ware, K.E.; Gilja, S.; Somarelli, J.A.; Levine, H. EMT and MET: Necessary or permissive for metastasis? *Mol. Oncol.* **2017**, *11*, 755–769. [CrossRef] [PubMed]
13. Aiello, N.M.; Kang, Y. Context-dependent EMT programs in cancer metastasis. *J. Exp. Med.* **2019**, *216*, 1016–1026. [CrossRef] [PubMed]
14. Jolly, M.K.; Somarelli, J.A.; Sheth, M.; Biddle, A.; Tripathi, S.C.; Armstrong, A.J.; Hanash, S.M.; Bapat, S.A.; Rangarajan, A.; Levine, H. Hybrid epithelial/mesenchymal phenotypes promote metastasis and therapy resistance across carcinomas. *Pharmacol. Ther.* **2019**, *194*, 161–184. [CrossRef]
15. Moody, S.E.; Perez, D.; Pan, T.C.; Sarkisian, C.J.; Portocarrero, C.P.; Sterner, C.J.; Notorfrancesco, K.L.; Cardiff, R.D.; Chodosh, L.A. The transcriptional repressor Snail promotes mammary tumor recurrence. *Cancer Cell* **2005**, *8*, 197–209. [CrossRef]
16. Creighton, C.J.; Li, X.; Landis, M.; Dixon, J.M.; Neumeister, V.M.; Sjolund, A.; Rimm, D.L.; Wong, H.; Rodriguez, A.; Herschkowitz, J.I.; et al. Residual breast cancers after conventional therapy display mesenchymal as well as tumor-initiating features. *Proc. Natl. Acad. Sci. USA* **2009**, *106*, 13820–13825. [CrossRef]
17. Li, X.; Lewis, M.T.; Huang, J.; Gutierrez, C.; Osborne, C.K.; Wu, M.F.; Hilsenbeck, S.G.; Pavlick, A.; Zhang, X.; Chamness, G.C.; et al. Intrinsic resistance of tumorigenic breast cancer cells to chemotherapy. *J. Natl. Cancer Inst.* **2008**, *100*, 672–679. [CrossRef]
18. Terry, S.; Savagner, P.; Ortiz-Cuaran, S.; Mahjoubi, L.; Saintigny, P.; Thiery, J.P.; Chouaib, S. New insights into the role of EMT in tumor immune escape. *Mol. Oncol.* **2017**, *11*, 824–846. [CrossRef]
19. Kallergi, G.; Papadaki, M.A.; Politaki, E.; Mavroudis, D.; Georgoulias, V.; Agelaki, S. Epithelial to mesenchymal transition markers expressed in circulating tumour cells of early and metastatic breast cancer patients. *Breast Cancer Res.* **2011**, *13*, R59. [CrossRef]
20. Bonnomet, A.; Brysse, A.; Tachsidis, A.; Waltham, M.; Thompson, E.W.; Polette, M.; Gilles, C. Epithelial-to-mesenchymal transitions and circulating tumor cells. *J. Mammary Gland Biol. Neoplasia* **2010**, *15*, 261–273. [CrossRef]
21. Yu, M.; Bardia, A.; Wittner, B.S.; Stott, S.L.; Smas, M.E.; Ting, D.T.; Isakoff, S.J.; Ciciliano, J.C.; Wells, M.N.; Shah, A.M.; et al. Circulating breast tumor cells exhibit dynamic changes in epithelial and mesenchymal composition. *Science* **2013**, *339*, 580–584. [CrossRef] [PubMed]
22. Huang, Y.; Hong, W.; Wei, X. The molecular mechanisms and therapeutic strategies of EMT in tumor progression and metastasis. *J. Hematol. Oncol.* **2022**, *15*, 129. [CrossRef] [PubMed]
23. Xu, Z.; Zhang, Y.; Dai, H.; Han, B. Epithelial-Mesenchymal Transition-Mediated Tumor Therapeutic Resistance. *Molecules* **2022**, *27*, 4750. [CrossRef] [PubMed]
24. Pattabiraman, D.R.; Weinberg, R.A. Tackling the cancer stem cells—What challenges do they pose? *Nat. Rev. Drug Discov.* **2014**, *13*, 497–512. [CrossRef] [PubMed]
25. Marcucci, F.; Stassi, G.; De Maria, R. Epithelial-mesenchymal transition: A new target in anticancer drug discovery. *Nat. Rev. Drug Discov.* **2016**, *15*, 311–325. [CrossRef]
26. Lambert, A.W.; Weinberg, R.A. Linking EMT programmes to normal and neoplastic epithelial stem cells. *Nat. Rev. Cancer* **2021**, *21*, 325–338. [CrossRef]
27. Williams, E.D.; Gao, D.; Redfern, A.; Thompson, E.W. Controversies around epithelial-mesenchymal plasticity in cancer metastasis. *Nat. Rev. Cancer* **2019**, *19*, 716–732. [CrossRef]
28. Grassian, A.R.; Lin, F.; Barrett, R.; Liu, Y.; Jiang, W.; Korpal, M.; Astley, H.; Gitterman, D.; Henley, T.; Howes, R.; et al. Isocitrate dehydrogenase (IDH) mutations promote a reversible ZEB1/microRNA (miR)-200-dependent epithelial-mesenchymal transition (EMT). *J. Biol. Chem.* **2012**, *287*, 42180–42194. [CrossRef]
29. Cuyàs, E.; Corominas-Faja, B.; Menendez, J.A. The nutritional phenome of EMT-induced cancer stem-like cells. *Oncotarget* **2014**, *5*, 3970–3982. [CrossRef]

30. Aspuria, P.P.; Lunt, S.Y.; Väremo, L.; Vergnes, L.; Gozo, M.; Beach, J.A.; Salumbides, B.; Reue, K.; Wiedemeyer, W.R.; Nielsen, J.; et al. Succinate dehydrogenase inhibition leads to epithelial-mesenchymal transition and reprogrammed carbon metabolism. *Cancer Metab.* **2014**, *2*, 21. [CrossRef]
31. Bhowmik, S.K.; Ramirez-Peña, E.; Arnold, J.M.; Putluri, V.; Sphyris, N.; Michailidis, G.; Putluri, N.; Ambs, S.; Sreekumar, A.; Mani, S.A. EMT-induced metabolite signature identifies poor clinical outcome. *Oncotarget* **2015**, *6*, 42651–42660. [CrossRef] [PubMed]
32. Sciacovelli, M.; Gonçalves, E.; Johnson, T.I.; Zecchini, V.R.; da Costa, A.S.; Gaude, E.; Drubbel, A.V.; Theobald, S.J.; Abbo, S.R.; Tran, M.G.; et al. Fumarate is an epigenetic modifier that elicits epithelial-to-mesenchymal transition. *Nature* **2016**, *537*, 544–547. [CrossRef] [PubMed]
33. Colvin, H.; Nishida, N.; Konno, M.; Haraguchi, N.; Takahashi, H.; Nishimura, J.; Hata, T.; Kawamoto, K.; Asai, A.; Tsunekuni, K.; et al. Oncometabolite D-2-Hydroxyglurate Directly Induces Epithelial-Mesenchymal Transition and is Associated with Distant Metastasis in Colorectal Cancer. *Sci. Rep.* **2016**, *6*, 36289. [CrossRef] [PubMed]
34. Sciacovelli, M.; Frezza, C. Metabolic reprogramming and epithelial-to-mesenchymal transition in cancer. *FEBS J.* **2017**, *284*, 3132–3144. [CrossRef]
35. Guerra, F.; Guaragnella, N.; Arbini, A.A.; Bucci, C.; Giannattasio, S.; Moro, L. Mitochondrial Dysfunction: A Novel Potential Driver of Epithelial-to-Mesenchymal Transition in Cancer. *Front. Oncol.* **2017**, *7*, 295. [CrossRef]
36. Morandi, A.; Taddei, M.L.; Chiarugi, P.; Giannoni, E. Targeting the Metabolic Reprogramming That Controls Epithelial-to-Mesenchymal Transition in Aggressive Tumors. *Front. Oncol.* **2017**, *7*, 40. [CrossRef]
37. Bhattacharya, D.; Scimè, A. Metabolic Regulation of Epithelial to Mesenchymal Transition: Implications for Endocrine Cancer. *Front. Endocrinol.* **2019**, *10*, 773. [CrossRef]
38. Kang, H.; Kim, H.; Lee, S.; Youn, H.; Youn, B. Role of Metabolic Reprogramming in Epithelial–Mesenchymal Transition (EMT). *Int. J. Mol. Sci.* **2019**, *20*, E2042. [CrossRef]
39. Ramirez-Peña, E.; Arnold, J.; Shivakumar, V.; Joseph, R.; Vidhya Vijay, G.; den Hollander, P.; Bhangre, N.; Allegakoen, P.; Prasad, R.; Conley, Z.; et al. The Epithelial to Mesenchymal Transition Promotes Glutamine Independence by Suppressing *GLS2* Expression. *Cancers* **2019**, *11*, E1610. [CrossRef]
40. Røsland, G.V.; Dyrstad, S.E.; Tusubira, D.; Helwa, R.; Tan, T.Z.; Lotsberg, M.L.; Pettersen, I.K.N.; Berg, A.; Kindt, C.; Hoel, F.; et al. Epithelial to mesenchymal transition (EMT) is associated with attenuation of succinate dehydrogenase (SDH) in breast cancer through reduced expression of *SDHC*. *Cancer Metab.* **2019**, *7*, 6. [CrossRef]
41. Dong, C.; Yuan, T.; Wu, Y.; Wang, Y.; Fan, T.W.; Miriyala, S.; Lin, Y.; Yao, J.; Shi, J.; Kang, T.; et al. Loss of FBP1 by Snail-mediated repression provides metabolic advantages in basal-like breast cancer. *Cancer Cell* **2013**, *23*, 316–331. [CrossRef] [PubMed]
42. Kim, N.H.; Cha, Y.H.; Lee, J.; Lee, S.H.; Yang, J.H.; Yun, J.S.; Cho, E.S.; Zhang, X.; Nam, M.; Kim, N.; et al. Snail reprograms glucose metabolism by repressing phosphofructokinase PFKP allowing cancer cell survival under metabolic stress. *Nat. Commun.* **2017**, *8*, 14374. [CrossRef] [PubMed]
43. Shaul, Y.D.; Freinkman, E.; Comb, W.C.; Cantor, J.R.; Tam, W.L.; Thiru, P.; Kim, D.; Kanarek, N.; Pacold, M.E.; Chen, W.W.; et al. Dihydropyrimidine accumulation is required for the epithelial-mesenchymal transition. *Cell* **2014**, *158*, 1094–1109. [CrossRef] [PubMed]
44. Chakrabarty, R.P.; Chandel, N.S. Mitochondria as Signaling Organelles Control Mammalian Stem Cell Fate. *Cell Stem Cell* **2021**, *28*, 394–408. [CrossRef]
45. Lunetti, P.; Di Giacomo, M.; Vergara, D.; De Domenico, S.; Maffia, M.; Zara, V.; Capobianco, L.; Ferramosca, A. Metabolic reprogramming in breast cancer results in distinct mitochondrial bioenergetics between luminal and basal subtypes. *FEBS J.* **2019**, *286*, 688–709. [CrossRef]
46. Hua, W.; Ten Dijke, P.; Kostidis, S.; Giera, M.; Hornsveld, M. TGFβ-induced metabolic reprogramming during epithelial-to-mesenchymal transition in cancer. *Cell. Mol. Life Sci.* **2019**, *77*, 2103–2123. [CrossRef]
47. Wu, M.J.; Chen, Y.S.; Kim, M.R.; Chang, C.C.; Gampala, S.; Zhang, Y.; Wang, Y.; Chang, C.Y.; Yang, J.Y.; Chang, C.J. Epithelial-Mesenchymal Transition Directs Stem Cell Polarity via Regulation of Mitofusin. *Cell Metab.* **2019**, *29*, 993–1002.e6. [CrossRef]
48. Peiris-Pagès, M.; Bonuccelli, G.; Sotgia, F.; Lisanti, M.P. Mitochondrial fission as a driver of stemness in tumor cells: mDIVI1 inhibits mitochondrial function, cell migration and cancer stem cell (CSC) signalling. *Oncotarget* **2018**, *9*, 13254–13275. [CrossRef]
49. Cuyàs, E.; Verdura, S.; Folguera-Blasco, N.; Bastidas-Velez, C.; Martin, Á.G.; Alarcón, T.; Menendez, J.A. Mitostemness. *Cell Cycle* **2018**, *17*, 918–926. [CrossRef]
50. Kingnate, C.; Charoenkwan, K.; Kumfu, S.; Chattipakorn, N.; Chattipakorn, S.C. Possible Roles of Mitochondrial Dynamics and the Effects of Pharmacological Interventions in Chemoresistant Ovarian Cancer. *EBioMedicine* **2018**, *34*, 256–266. [CrossRef]
51. Riera-Borrull, M.; Rodríguez-Gallego, E.; Hernández-Aguilera, A.; Luciano, F.; Ras, R.; Cuyàs, E.; Camps, J.; Segura-Carretero, A.; Menendez, J.A.; Joven, J.; et al. Exploring the Process of Energy Generation in Pathophysiology by Targeted Metabolomics: Performance of a Simple and Quantitative Method. *J. Am. Soc. Mass Spectrom.* **2016**, *27*, 168–177. [CrossRef] [PubMed]
52. Cuyàs, E.; Fernández-Arroyo, S.; Alarcón, T.; Lupu, R.; Joven, J.; Menendez, J.A. Germline BRCA1 mutation reprograms breast epithelial cell metabolism towards mitochondrial-dependent biosynthesis: Evidence for metformin-based "starvation" strategies in BRCA1 carriers. *Oncotarget* **2016**, *7*, 52974–52992. [CrossRef] [PubMed]
53. Cuyàs, E.; Fernández-Arroyo, S.; Corominas-Faja, B.; Rodríguez-Gallego, E.; Bosch-Barrera, J.; Martin-Castillo, B.; De Llorens, R.; Joven, J.; Menendez, J.A. Oncometabolic mutation IDH1 R132H confers a metformin-hypersensitive phenotype. *Oncotarget* **2015**, *6*, 12279–12296. [CrossRef] [PubMed]

54. Vazquez-Martin, A.; Van den Haute, C.; Cufí, S.; Corominas-Faja, B.; Cuyàs, E.; Lopez-Bonet, E.; Rodriguez-Gallego, E.; Fernández-Arroyo, S.; Joven, J.; Baekelandt, V.; et al. Mitophagy-driven mitochondrial rejuvenation regulates stem cell fate. *Aging* **2016**, *8*, 1330–1352. [CrossRef]
55. Fernández-Arroyo, S.; Cuyàs, E.; Bosch-Barrera, J.; Alarcón, T.; Joven, J.; Menendez, J.A. Activation of the methylation cycle in cells reprogrammed into a stem cell-like state. *Oncoscience* **2016**, *2*, 958–967. [CrossRef]
56. Riera-Borrull, M.; García-Heredia, A.; Fernández-Arroyo, S.; Hernández-Aguilera, A.; Cabré, N.; Cuyàs, E.; Luciano-Mateo, F.; Camps, J.; Menendez, J.A.; Joven, J. Metformin Potentiates the Benefits of Dietary Restraint: A Metabolomic Study. *Int. J. Mol. Sci.* **2017**, *18*, 2263. [CrossRef]
57. Cuyàs, E.; Fernández-Arroyo, S.; Buxó, M.; Pernas, S.; Dorca, J.; Álvarez, I.; Martínez, S.; Pérez-Garcia, J.M.; Batista-López, N.; Rodríguez-Sánchez, C.A.; et al. Metformin induces a fasting- and antifolate-mimicking modification of systemic host metabolism in breast cancer patients. *Aging* **2019**, *11*, 2874–2888. [CrossRef]
58. Chong, J.; Wishart, D.S.; Xia, J. Using MetaboAnalyst 4.0 for Comprehensive and Integrative Metabolomics Data Analysis. *Curr. Protoc. Bioinform.* **2019**, *68*, e86. [CrossRef]
59. Mani, S.A.; Guo, W.; Liao, M.J.; Eaton, E.N.; Ayyanan, A.; Zhou, A.Y.; Brooks, M.; Reinhard, F.; Zhang, C.C.; Shipitsin, M.; et al. The epithelial-mesenchymal transition generates cells with properties of stem cells. *Cell* **2008**, *133*, 704–715. [CrossRef]
60. Gupta, P.B.; Onder, T.T.; Jiang, G.; Tao, K.; Kuperwasser, C.; Weinberg, R.A.; Lander, E.S. Identification of selective inhibitors of cancer stem cells by high-throughput screening. *Cell* **2009**, *138*, 645–659. [CrossRef]
61. Elenbaas, B.; Spirio, L.; Koerner, F.; Fleming, M.D.; Zimonjic, D.B.; Donaher, J.L.; Popescu, N.C.; Hahn, W.C.; Weinberg, R.A. Human breast cancer cells generated by oncogenic transformation of primary mammary epithelial cells. *Genes Dev.* **2001**, *15*, 50–65. [CrossRef] [PubMed]
62. Liu, S.; Cong, Y.; Wang, D.; Sun, Y.; Deng, L.; Liu, Y.; Martin-Trevino, R.; Shang, L.; McDermott, S.P.; Landis, M.D.; et al. Breast cancer stem cells transition between epithelial and mesenchymal states reflective of their normal counterparts. *Stem Cell Rep.* **2013**, *2*, 78–91. [CrossRef] [PubMed]
63. Martin-Castillo, B.; Lopez-Bonet, E.; Cuyàs, E.; Viñas, G.; Pernas, S.; Dorca, J.; Menendez, J.A. Cancer stem cell-driven efficacy of trastuzumab (Herceptin): Towards a reclassification of clinically HER2-positive breast carcinomas. *Oncotarget* **2015**, *6*, 32317–32338. [CrossRef]
64. Lim, Y.Y.; Wright, J.A.; Attema, J.L.; Gregory, P.A.; Bert, A.G.; Smith, E.; Thomas, D.; Lopez, A.F.; Drew, P.A.; Khew-Goodall, Y.; et al. Epigenetic modulation of the miR-200 family is associated with transition to a breast cancer stem-cell-like state. *J. Cell Sci.* **2013**, *126*, 2256–2266. [CrossRef]
65. Dontu, G.; Abdallah, W.M.; Foley, J.M.; Jackson, K.W.; Clarke, M.F.; Kawamura, M.J.; Wicha, M.S. In vitro propagation and transcriptional profiling of human mammary stem/progenitor cells. *Genes Dev.* **2003**, *17*, 1253–1270. [CrossRef] [PubMed]
66. Manuel Iglesias, J.; Beloqui, I.; Garcia-Garcia, F.; Leis, O.; Vazquez-Martin, A.; Eguiara, A.; Cufi, S.; Pavon, A.; Menendez, J.A.; Dopazo, J.; et al. Mammosphere formation in breast carcinoma cell lines depends upon expression of E-cadherin. *PLoS ONE* **2013**, *8*, e77281. [CrossRef]
67. Lei, X.H.; Bochner, B.R. Optimization of cell permeabilization in electron flow based mitochondrial function assays. *Free Radic. Biol. Med.* **2021**, *177*, 48–57. [CrossRef]
68. Fedele, M.; Sgarra, R.; Battista, S.; Cerchia, L.; Manfioletti, G. The Epithelial-Mesenchymal Transition at the Crossroads between Metabolism and Tumor Progression. *Int. J. Mol. Sci.* **2022**, *23*, 800. [CrossRef]
69. Jia, D.; Park, J.H.; Kaur, H.; Jung, K.H.; Yang, S.; Tripathi, S.; Galbraith, M.; Deng, Y.; Jolly, M.K.; Kaipparettu, B.A.; et al. Towards decoding the coupled decision-making of metabolism and epithelial-to-mesenchymal transition in cancer. *Br. J. Cancer* **2021**, *124*, 1902–1911. [CrossRef]
70. Kimmelman, A.C. Metabolic Dependencies in RAS-Driven Cancers. *Clin. Cancer Res.* **2015**, *21*, 1828–1834. [CrossRef]
71. Mukhopadhyay, S.; Vander Heiden, M.G.; McCormick, F. The Metabolic Landscape of RAS-Driven Cancers from biology to therapy. *Nat. Cancer* **2021**, *2*, 271–283. [CrossRef] [PubMed]
72. Tanner, L.B.; Goglia, A.G.; Wei, M.H.; Sehgal, T.; Parsons, L.R.; Park, J.O.; White, E.; Toettcher, J.E.; Rabinowitz, J.D. Four Key Steps Control Glycolytic Flux in Mammalian Cells. *Cell Syst.* **2018**, *7*, 49–62.e8. [CrossRef]
73. Court, S.J.; Waclaw, B.; Allen, R.J. Lower glycolysis carries a higher flux than any biochemically possible alternative. *Nat. Commun.* **2015**, *6*, 8427. [CrossRef] [PubMed]
74. Vander Heiden, M.G.; Locasale, J.W.; Swanson, K.D.; Sharfi, H.; Heffron, G.J.; Amador-Noguez, D.; Christofk, H.R.; Wagner, G.; Rabinowitz, J.D.; Asara, J.M.; et al. Evidence for an alternative glycolytic pathway in rapidly proliferating cells. *Science* **2010**, *329*, 1492–1499. [CrossRef] [PubMed]
75. Shen, W.; Gao, C.; Cueto, R.; Liu, L.; Fu, H.; Shao, Y.; Yang, W.Y.; Fang, P.; Choi, E.T.; Wu, Q.; et al. Homocysteine-methionine cycle is a metabolic sensor system controlling methylation-regulated pathological signaling. *Redox Biol.* **2020**, *28*, 101322. [CrossRef]
76. Sbodio, J.I.; Snyder, S.H.; Paul, B.D. Regulators of the transsulfuration pathway. *Br. J. Pharmacol.* **2019**, *176*, 583–593. [CrossRef]
77. Zhang, H.F.; Klein Geltink, R.I.; Parker, S.J.; Sorensen, P.H. Transsulfuration, minor player or crucial for cysteine homeostasis in cancer. *Trends Cell Biol.* **2022**, *32*, 800–814. [CrossRef]
78. Prudova, A.; Bauman, Z.; Braun, A.; Vitvitsky, V.; Lu, S.C.; Banerjee, R. S-adenosylmethionine stabilizes cystathionine beta-synthase and modulates redox capacity. *Proc. Natl. Acad. Sci. USA* **2006**, *103*, 6489–6494. [CrossRef]

79. Carmona, F.J.; Davalos, V.; Vidal, E.; Gomez, A.; Heyn, H.; Hashimoto, Y.; Vizoso, M.; Martinez-Cardus, A.; Sayols, S.; Ferreira, H.J.; et al. A comprehensive DNA methylation profile of epithelial-to-mesenchymal transition. *Cancer Res.* **2014**, *74*, 5608–5619. [CrossRef]
80. Wang, Y.; Dong, C.; Zhou, B.P. Metabolic reprogram associated with epithelial-mesenchymal transition in tumor progression and metastasis. *Genes Dis.* **2019**, *7*, 172–184. [CrossRef]
81. Lai, X.; Li, Q.; Wu, F.; Lin, J.; Chen, J.; Zheng, H.; Guo, L. Epithelial-Mesenchymal Transition and Metabolic Switching in Cancer: Lessons from Somatic Cell Reprogramming. *Front. Cell Dev. Biol.* **2020**, *8*, 760. [CrossRef] [PubMed]
82. Lien, E.C.; Ghisolfi, L.; Geck, R.C.; Asara, J.M.; Toker, A. Oncogenic PI3K promotes methionine dependency in breast cancer cells through the cystine-glutamate antiporter xCT. *Sci. Signal.* **2017**, *10*, eaao6604. [CrossRef] [PubMed]
83. Baltazar, F.; Afonso, J.; Costa, M.; Granja, S. Lactate Beyond a Waste Metabolite: Metabolic Affairs and Signaling in Malignancy. *Front. Oncol.* **2020**, *10*, 231. [CrossRef]
84. de la Cruz-López, K.G.; Castro-Muñoz, L.J.; Reyes-Hernández, D.O.; García-Carrancá, A.; Manzo-Merino, J. Lactate in the Regulation of Tumor Microenvironment and Therapeutic Approaches. *Front. Oncol.* **2019**, *9*, 1143. [CrossRef]
85. Louie, M.C.; Ton, J.; Brady, M.L.; Le, D.T.; Mar, J.N.; Lerner, C.A.; Gerencser, A.A.; Mookerjee, S.A. Total Cellular ATP Production Changes with Primary Substrate in MCF7 Breast Cancer Cells. *Front. Oncol.* **2020**, *10*, 1703. [CrossRef]
86. Martínez-Reyes, I.; Chandel, N.S. Waste Not, Want Not: Lactate Oxidation Fuels the TCA Cycle. *Cell Metab.* **2017**, *26*, 803–804. [CrossRef]
87. Loo, S.Y.; Toh, L.P.; Xie, W.H.; Pathak, E.; Tan, W.; Ma, S.; Lee, M.Y.; Shatishwaran, S.; Yeo, J.Z.Z.; Yuan, J.; et al. Fatty acid oxidation is a druggable gateway regulating cellular plasticity for driving metastasis in breast cancer. *Sci. Adv.* **2021**, *7*, eabh2443. [CrossRef]
88. Soukupova, J.; Malfettone, A.; Bertran, E.; Hernández-Alvarez, M.I.; Peñuelas-Haro, I.; Dituri, F.; Giannelli, G.; Zorzano, A.; Fabregat, I. Epithelial-Mesenchymal Transition (EMT) Induced by TGF-β in Hepatocellular Carcinoma Cells Reprograms Lipid Metabolism. *Int. J. Mol. Sci.* **2021**, *22*, 5543. [CrossRef]
89. Faubert, B.; Li, K.Y.; Cai, L.; Hensley, C.T.; Kim, J.; Zacharias, L.G.; Yang, C.; Do, Q.N.; Doucette, S.; Burguete, D.; et al. Lactate Metabolism in Human Lung Tumors. *Cell* **2017**, *171*, 358–371.e9. [CrossRef]
90. Hui, S.; Ghergurovich, J.M.; Morscher, R.J.; Jang, C.; Teng, X.; Lu, W.; Esparza, L.A.; Reya, T.; Zhan, L.; Guo, J.Y.; et al. Glucose feeds the TCA cycle via circulating lactate. *Nature* **2017**, *551*, 115–118. [CrossRef]
91. Kuznetsov, A.V.; Javadov, S.; Margreiter, R.; Hagenbuchner, J.; Ausserlechner, M.J. Analysis of Mitochondrial Function, Structure, and Intracellular Organization In Situ in Cardiomyocytes and Skeletal Muscles. *Int. J. Mol. Sci.* **2022**, *23*, 2252. [CrossRef] [PubMed]
92. Gohil, V.M.; Sheth, S.A.; Nilsson, R.; Wojtovich, A.P.; Lee, J.H.; Perocchi, F.; Chen, W.; Clish, C.B.; Ayata, C.; Brookes, P.S.; et al. Nutrient-sensitized screening for drugs that shift energy metabolism from mitochondrial respiration to glycolysis. *Nat. Biotechnol.* **2010**, *28*, 249–255. [CrossRef]
93. Gohil, V.M.; Zhu, L.; Baker, C.D.; Cracan, V.; Yaseen, A.; Jain, M.; Clish, C.B.; Brookes, P.S.; Bakovic, M.; Mootha, V.K. Meclizine inhibits mitochondrial respiration through direct targeting of cytosolic phosphoethanolamine metabolism. *J. Biol. Chem.* **2013**, *288*, 35387–35395. [CrossRef]
94. Kang, J.H.; Lee, S.H.; Lee, J.S.; Nam, B.; Seong, T.W.; Son, J.; Jang, H.; Hong, K.M.; Lee, C.; Kim, S.Y. Aldehyde dehydrogenase inhibition combined with phenformin treatment reversed NSCLC through ATP depletion. *Oncotarget* **2016**, *7*, 49397–49410. [CrossRef]
95. Park, J.; Shim, J.K.; Kang, J.H.; Choi, J.; Chang, J.H.; Kim, S.Y.; Kang, S.G. Regulation of bioenergetics through dual inhibition of aldehyde dehydrogenase and mitochondrial complex I suppresses glioblastoma tumorspheres. *Neuro Oncol.* **2018**, *20*, 954–965. [CrossRef] [PubMed]
96. Pavani, M.; Fones, E.; Oksenberg, D.; Garcia, M.; Hernandez, C.; Cordano, G.; Muñoz, S.; Mancilla, J.; Guerrero, A.; Ferreira, J. Inhibition of tumoral cell respiration and growth by nordihydroguaiaretic acid. *Biochem. Pharmacol.* **1994**, *48*, 1935–1942. [CrossRef]
97. Hernández-Damián, J.; Andérica-Romero, A.C.; Pedraza-Chaverri, J. Paradoxical cellular effects and biological role of the multifaceted compound nordihydroguaiaretic acid. *Arch. Pharm.* **2014**, *347*, 685–697. [CrossRef] [PubMed]
98. Biswal, S.S.; Datta, K.; Shaw, S.D.; Feng, X.; Robertson, J.D.; Kehrer, J.P. Glutathione oxidation and mitochondrial depolarization as mechanisms of nordihydroguaiaretic acid-induced apoptosis in lipoxygenase-deficient FL5.12 cells. *Toxicol. Sci.* **2000**, *53*, 77–83. [CrossRef]
99. Manda, G.; Rojo, A.I.; Martínez-Klimova, E.; Pedraza-Chaverri, J.; Cuadrado, A. Nordihydroguaiaretic Acid: From Herbal Medicine to Clinical Development for Cancer and Chronic Diseases. *Front. Pharmacol.* **2020**, *11*, 151. [CrossRef]
100. Huang, C.; Lan, W.; Fraunhoffer, N.; Meilerman, A.; Iovanna, J.; Santofimia-Castaño, P. Dissecting the Anticancer Mechanism of Trifluoperazine on Pancreatic Ductal Adenocarcinoma. *Cancers* **2019**, *11*, 1869. [CrossRef]
101. Nalvarte, I.; Damdimopoulos, A.E.; Spyrou, G. Human mitochondrial thioredoxin reductase reduces cytochrome c and confers resistance to complex III inhibition. *Free Radic. Biol. Med.* **2004**, *36*, 1270–1278. [CrossRef]
102. Martínez-Reyes, I.; Cardona, L.R.; Kong, H.; Vasan, K.; McElroy, G.S.; Werner, M.; Kihshen, H.; Reczek, C.R.; Weinberg, S.E.; Gao, P.; et al. Mitochondrial ubiquinol oxidation is necessary for tumour growth. *Nature* **2020**, *585*, 288–292. [CrossRef] [PubMed]

103. Raimondi, V.; Ciccarese, F.; Ciminale, V. Oncogenic pathways and the electron transport chain: A dangeROS liaison. *Br. J. Cancer* **2020**, *122*, 168–181. [CrossRef] [PubMed]
104. Jakubkova, M.; Dzugasova, V.; Truban, D.; Abelovska, L.; Bhatia-Kissova, I.; Valachovic, M.; Klobucnikova, V.; Zeiselova, L.; Griac, P.; Nosek, J.; et al. Identification of Yeast Mutants Exhibiting Altered Sensitivity to Valinomycin and Nigericin Demonstrate Pleiotropic Effects of Ionophores on Cellular Processes. *PLoS ONE* **2016**, *11*, e0164175. [CrossRef] [PubMed]
105. Sun, H.; Yang, X.; Liang, L.; Zhang, M.; Li, Y.; Chen, J.; Wang, F.; Yang, T.; Meng, F.; Lai, X.; et al. Metabolic switch and epithelial-mesenchymal transition cooperate to regulate pluripotency. *EMBO J.* **2020**, *39*, e102961. [CrossRef]
106. Morel, A.P.; Lièvre, M.; Thomas, C.; Hinkal, G.; Ansieau, S.; Puisieux, A. Generation of breast cancer stem cells through epithelial-mesenchymal transition. *PLoS ONE* **2008**, *3*, e2888. [CrossRef]
107. Morel, A.P.; Hinkal, G.W.; Thomas, C.; Fauvet, F.; Courtois-Cox, S.; Wierinckx, A.; Devouassoux-Shisheboran, M.; Treilleux, I.; Tissier, A.; Gras, B.; et al. EMT inducers catalyze malignant transformation of mammary epithelial cells and drive tumorigenesis towards claudin-low tumors in transgenic mice. *PLoS Genet.* **2012**, *8*, e1002723. [CrossRef]
108. Ramesh, V.; Brabletz, T.; Ceppi, P. Targeting EMT in Cancer with Repurposed Metabolic Inhibitors. *Trends Cancer* **2020**, *6*, 942–950. [CrossRef]

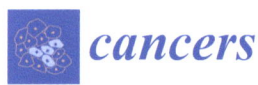 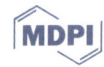

Article

Hypoxia-Inducible Factor-1 Alpha Expression Is Predictive of Pathological Complete Response in Patients with Breast Cancer Receiving Neoadjuvant Chemotherapy

César L. Ramírez-Tortosa [1], Rubén Alonso-Calderón [2], José María Gálvez-Navas [3,4,*], Cristina Pérez-Ramírez [3,4], José Luis Quiles [5], Pedro Sánchez-Rovira [2], Alberto Jiménez-Morales [3,†] and MCarmen Ramírez-Tortosa [4,†]

[1] Pathological Anatomy Service, University Hospital San Cecilio, Parque Tecnológico de la Salud (PTS), Avda. del Conocimiento, 18016 Granada, Spain
[2] Medical Oncology Service, Complejo Hospitalario de Jaén, Avda. del Ejército Español 10, 23007 Jaén, Spain
[3] Pharmacogenetics Unit, Pharmacy Service, University Hospital Virgen de las Nieves, Avda. de las Fuerzas Armadas 2, 18004 Granada, Spain
[4] Department of Biochemistry and Molecular Biology II, Faculty of Pharmacy, Campus Universitario de Cartuja, Universidad de Granada, 18011 Granada, Spain
[5] Department of Physiology, Faculty of Pharmacy, Campus Universitario de Cartuja, University of Granada, 18011 Granada, Spain
* Correspondence: jmgalna7@gmail.com
† These authors contributed equally to this work.

Simple Summary: Standard neoadjuvant chemotherapy, based on taxanes and anthracyclines, makes conservative treatment of breast cancer possible and it allows for the evaluation of the tumor response in terms of achieving pathological complete response. Whereas hypoxia participates in carcinogenesis, resulting in less differenced tumor cells and poorer prognosis, HIF-1α could be predictive of the tumor response to treatment. Nonetheless, very few studies have evaluated the predictive value of HIF-1α in breast cancer in patients receiving neoadjuvant chemotherapy.

Abstract: To demonstrate the value of hypoxia-inducible factor-1α (HIF-1α) in predicting response in patients with breast cancer receiving standard neoadjuvant chemotherapy (NAC). Methods: Ninety-five women enrolled in two prospective studies underwent biopsies for the histopathological diagnosis of breast carcinoma before receiving NAC, based on anthracyclines and taxanes. For expression of HIF-1α, EGFR, pAKT and pMAPK, tumor samples were analyzed by immunohistochemistry in tissues microarrays. Standard statistical methods (Pearson chi-square test, Fisher exact test, Kruskal–Wallis test, Mann–Whitney test and Kaplan–Meier method) were used to study the association of HIF-1α with tumor response, survival and other clinicopathologic variables/biomarkers. Results: HIF-1α expression was positive in 35 (39.7%) cases and was significantly associated to complete pathological response (pCR) ($p = 0.014$). HIF-1α expression was correlated positively with tumor grade ($p = 0.015$) and Ki-67 expression ($p = 0.001$) and negativity with progesterone receptors (PR) ($p = 0.04$) and luminal A phenotype expression ($p = 0.005$). No correlation was found between HIF-1α expression and EGFR, pAKT and pMAPK. In terms of survival, HIF-1α expression was associated with a significantly shorter disease-free survival ($p = 0.013$), being identified as an independent prognostic factor in multivariate analysis. Conclusions: Overexpression of HIF-1α is a predictor of pCR and shorter DFS; it would be valuable to confirm these results in prospective studies.

Keywords: hypoxia-inducible factor 1; breast cancer; neoadjuvant chemotherapy; prognostic factor; pathological complete response

Citation: Ramírez-Tortosa, C.L.; Alonso-Calderón, R.; Gálvez-Navas, J.M.; Pérez-Ramírez, C.; Quiles, J.L.; Sánchez-Rovira, P.; Jiménez-Morales, A.; Ramírez-Tortosa, M. Hypoxia-Inducible Factor-1 Alpha Expression Is Predictive of Pathological Complete Response in Patients with Breast Cancer Receiving Neoadjuvant Chemotherapy. *Cancers* **2022**, *14*, 5393. https://doi.org/10.3390/cancers14215393

Academic Editor: Paola Tucci

Received: 26 September 2022
Accepted: 31 October 2022
Published: 2 November 2022

Publisher's Note: MDPI stays neutral with regard to jurisdictional claims in published maps and institutional affiliations.

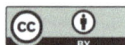

Copyright: © 2022 by the authors. Licensee MDPI, Basel, Switzerland. This article is an open access article distributed under the terms and conditions of the Creative Commons Attribution (CC BY) license (https://creativecommons.org/licenses/by/4.0/).

1. Introduction

Standard neoadjuvant chemotherapy (NAC), based on a schedule of anthracyclines and taxanes, is the treatment of choice for locally advanced breast tumors and inflammatory carcinomas [1]. The administration of NAC not only makes conservative treatment possible, but also precision medicine according to its efficacy [1] and the evaluation of the pathologic response of the tumor in terms of achieving pathologic complete response (pCR) with rates ranging from 3% to 48% and a partial response with a rate of 61.2% [2,3]. It has been shown that pCR is a prognostic factor for disease-free survival (DFS) and overall survival (OS) [4,5], probably because it reflects the eradication of micrometastatic disease [5]. For this reason, predictive markers of response identification have been a topic of study for a long time; estrogen (ER) and progesterone receptors (PR) and human epidermal growth receptor 2 (HER2) status are the best known of these markers.

Multiple factors affect cancer development [6,7]. When a situation of hypoxia develops in the tumor microenvironment during the process of neoplastic progression, cells with more aggressive tumor phenotypes, higher mutation rates and increased metastatic potential are selected [8]. The HIF-1α (hypoxia-inducible factor 1α) transcription factor seems to be the key molecular complex in the cellular response to hypoxia [8,9]. Furthermore, the synthesis of HIF-1α can be regulated for other mechanisms, independent of tissue oxygenation, across activation of the phosphatidylinositol 3-kinase (PI3K/AKT) and mitogen-activated protein kinase (Ras/Raf/MAPK) pathways [10,11]. These pathways can be activated by receptors with tyrosine kinase activity, such as the epidermal growth factor receptor (EGFR) [12].

Several studies have examined the role of HIF-1α as a prognosis factor in breast cancer and have associated HIF-1α overexpression with shorter DFS and OS [13]. However, little is known about the predictive value of HIF-1α response in breast cancer. To date, few published papers have demonstrated the relation between HIF-1α overexpression and pCR after treatment with NAC based on anthracyclines and taxanes. The objectives of our study were to demonstrate the value of HIF-1α in predicting response in patients diagnosed with breast cancer and given an NAC schedule of anthracyclines and taxanes, to study the relation between HIF-1α overexpression and other clinicopathologic variables of well-established predictive value and, finally, to study the intracellular signaling pathways involved in HIF-1α regulation and to analyze the potential prognostic value of HIF-1α.

2. Materials and Methods

2.1. Patients and Treatment Management

The study included 95 patients diagnosed with stage II-III breast cancer who received neoadjuvant chemotherapy at Complejo Hospitalario de Jaén. All patients were participants in two prospective phase 2 studies. In study A, 73 patients received 3 cycles of epirubicin (90 mg/m^2) and cyclophosphamide (600 mg/m^2), followed by 6 cycles of paclitaxel (150 mg/m^2) and gemcitabine (2500 mg/m^2), with or without trastuzumab (2 mg/kg/week, with a loading dose of 4 mg/kg) in accordance with HER2 status [14]. In study B, 22 patients received 4 cycles of doxorubicin (60 mg/m^2) and cyclophosphamide (600 mg/m^2) followed by 4 cycles of docetaxel (100 mg/m^2) [15]. Previous axillar status to chemotherapy was firstly evaluated using sonography. Suspicious cases were confirmed by needle core biopsy. All women underwent surgery after cytostatic treatment. Modified radical mastectomy or conservative surgery was performed according to surgeons' criteria. Patients with cN0 were submitted to axillary intraoperative study through sentinel lymph node biopsy. Axillary lymphadenectomy was performed in cN+ patients. Patients who underwent conservative surgery also received radiotherapy. All patients with hormone-receptor-positive tumors were treated with hormonal therapy for 5 years. The median follow-up of patients was 7.4 years. The patients' characteristics are shown in Table 1.

Table 1. Clinicopathologic characteristics of patients.

Characteristics	Number of Cases (%)
Age at diagnosis (years)	
<40	19 (20%)
40–49	38 (40%)
50–59	18 (18.9%)
>60	20 (21.1%)
Mean	20 (21.1%)
Range	27–74
Pretreatment tumor size (cm)	
1–1.9	4 (4.2%)
2–2.9	22 (23.2%)
3–3.9	22 (23.2%)
4–4.9	17 (17.9%)
>4.9	23 (24.2%)
Not measurable	7 (7.4%)
Histological type	
Ductal infiltrating	72 (75.8%)
Lobular infiltrating	9 (9.5%)
Inflammatory	6 (6.3%)
Mucinous	6 (6.3%)
Mixed	2 (2.1%)
Histological grade	
1	20 (21%)
2	37 (39%)
3	34 (35.8%)
Not evaluable	4 (4.2%)
Clinical TNM at diagnosis	
T	
T1	6 (6.3%)
T2	62 (65.3%)
T3	16 (16.8%)
T4	8 (8.4%)
Tx	3 (3.2%)
N	
N0	34 (35.8%)
N1	46 (48.4%)
N2	15 (15.8%)
N3	0 (0%)
Nx	0 (0%)
M	
M0	95 (100%)
M1	0 (0%)
Clinical stage	
IIA	32 (33.7%)
IIB	31 (32.6%)
IIIA	21 (21.1%)
IIIB	8 (8.4%)
Not evaluable	3 (3.2%)
ER	
≥10%	69 (72.6%)
<10%	25 (26.3%)
Not evaluable	1 (1.1%)
Count ≥ 3	71 (74.7%)

Table 1. Cont.

Characteristics	Number of Cases (%)
Count < 3	23 (24.2%)
Not evaluable	1 (1.1%)
PR	
≥10%	54 (56.8%)
<10%	40 (42.1%)
Not evaluable	1 (1.1%)
Count ≥ 3	58 (61.1%)
Count < 3	36 (37.1%)
Not evaluable	1 (1.1%)
HER2	
Positive	20 (21.1%)
Negative	72 (75.8%)
Not evaluable	3 (3.1%)
Ki-67	
≥20%	38 (40%)
<20%	56 (58.9%)
Not evaluable	1 (1.1%)
Phenotype	
Basal	13 (13.7%)
HER2	20 (21%)
Luminal A	31 (32.6%)
Luminal B	28 (29.5%)
Not evaluable	3 (3.2%)
Type of surgery	
Conservative	38 (40%)
Not conservative	56 (58.9%)
Not evaluable	1 (1.1%)
Pathological response (M&P)	
Grade 1	8 (8.4%)
Grade 2	22 (23.1%)
Grade 3	28 (29.5%)
Grade 4	17 (17.9%)
Grade 5 (pCR)	20 (21.1%)

Abbreviations: ER, estrogen receptor; PR, progesterone receptor.

2.2. Histology and Response Pathological Evaluation

Histological examinations were performed on slides stained by hematoxylin–eosin from those that were paraffin embedded. Histological grade was determined according to the modified Bloom–Richardson classification [16]. pCR was defined as the absence of invasive carcinoma in the breast and lymph nodes according to the Miller–Payne criteria. Additionally, the single presence of carcinoma in situ was equally considered as pCR [17].

2.3. Tissue Microarray Construction

Hematoxylin-and-eosin-stained sections from core biopsies (pretreatment) and surgical specimens (post-treatment) were marked on individual paraffin blocks. Two tissue cores (1.5 mm in diameter) were obtained from each specimen. Additionally, other tissues, both non-neoplastic and neoplastic samples, were included as controls following the Kononen methodology [18]. A hematoxylin-and-eosin-stained section was reviewed to confirm the presence of morphologically representative areas of the original lesions.

2.4. Immunohistochemistry

The immunohistochemical analysis was blinded. The sections of tissue were deparaffinized with xylene and hydrated in gradient alcohols. After the deparaffinization of tissue sections, antigen retrieval was performed with the PTLink module (Dako, Glostrup, Denmark) using Dako pH Antigen Retrieval fluid (Dako) followed by several washes in water. They were then placed onto an Autostainer Plus Link (Dako, Demark) where the remainder of the immunohistochemical staining was performed using Envision FLEX (DAKO). Briefly, sections were first placed in washing buffer followed by blockade of endogenous peroxidase with 3% hydrogen peroxide for 5 min. Then, the primary antibody ER (rabbit monoclonal antibody, prediluted, clone SP1 Master Diagnostica), PR (rabbit monoclonal antibody, prediluted, clone Y85 Master Diagnostica), Ki-67 (rabbit monoclonal antibody, prediluted, clone SP6 Master Diagnostica), HIF-1α (mouse monoclonal antibody, diluted 1:50, Becton-Dickinson Biosciences, Palo Alto, CA, USA), pAKT (rabbit monoclonal antibody, diluted 1:25, clone 736E11 Cell Signaling Technology, Beverly, MA, USA) and pMAPK (rabbit monoclonal antibody, diluted 1:100 clone 20G11 Cell Signaling echnology) were applied for 30 (ER), 20 (PR), 30 (Ki-67), 120 (pAKT) and 60 (pMAPK) minutes at room temperature, except HIF-1α, which was applied overnight at 4 °C. Sections were then treated with immunodetection solution consisting of biotinylated secondary antibody for 30 min. Diluted 1:50 liquid 3,3'-diaminobenzidine (Dako) was used as a chromogenic agent and sections were counterstained in Meyer's hematoxylin. As a negative control, the primary antibody was replaced by a non-immune serum.

HER2 status was determined using the Dako HERceptest (Dako Denmark A/S, Glostrup, Denmark) as well as a fluorescence in situ hybridization test in biopsy specimens with a 2+ score via IHC analysis. EGFR expression was determined using the Dako EGFR pharma (Dako Denmark A/S, Glostrup, Denmark).

2.5. Evaluation of Immunohistochemical Staining

For ER and PR, two approaches were used. All red method scoring was used for assessing staining intensity and the percentage of positive cells. The total score is obtained by adding the staining score and intensity score. Any score between 0 and 2 is considered ER or PR negative; any score above 2 is considered ER or PR positive [19]. A case was considered positive when staining for ER and PR was found in 10% or more of tumor cells [20]. Tumors were considered to have high rates of proliferation according to the Ki-67 labeling index if 20% of cell nuclei stained positive for Ki-67 [21]. HER2-positive cases were defined as having membrane staining score of +3 or +2 with gene amplification by FISH [22].

HIF-1α was scored only according to the presence (1+) or absence (0) of nuclear expression: at least 5% of cells had to be stained to be considered positive [13,23]. However, pAKT and pMAPK were scored according to the presence (1+) or absence (0) of nuclear and/or cytoplasmic expression: the cutoff value was 10% [24]. For EGFR, all cells that exhibited some membrane staining were considered positive.

2.6. Statistical Analysis

Statistical analysis was carried out using SPSS version 27.0 software (SPSS Inc., Chicago, IL, USA) (SPSS IBM Statistics 27.0 for Windows). The Pearson chi-square test/Fisher exact test was used to study the association between pCR and HIF-1α with clinicopathologic variables. The association between protein expression and pCR was studied using non-parametric tests (Kruskal–Wallis/Mann–Whitney) and the Pearson chi-square test/Fisher exact test. Multivariate logistic regression was used to examine the predictors of pCR. The relation between the expressions of different proteins was studied using the Fisher exact test. Finally, survival was analyzed using the Kaplan–Meier method, with determination of significance using the long rank test. Multivariate analysis was carried out using Cox regression analysis. Data analysis is reported according to REMARK guidelines [25].

Probability (p) values of less than 0.05 were considered statistically significant.

3. Results

3.1. Relation between HIF-1α Expression and pCR

Out of 95 samples analyzed, HIF-1α expression was determined in 88 (92.6%). Of these, 35 (39.72%) were considered positive (Figure 1). The relation between HIF-1α and pCR was examined by studying the HIF-1α variable, both quantitatively as a percentage (%) and qualitatively as a dichotomy (≥5%). A statistically significant relation was found between HIF-1α expression and pCR: patients whose tumors overexpressed HIF-1α were more likely to achieve pCR (Table 2).

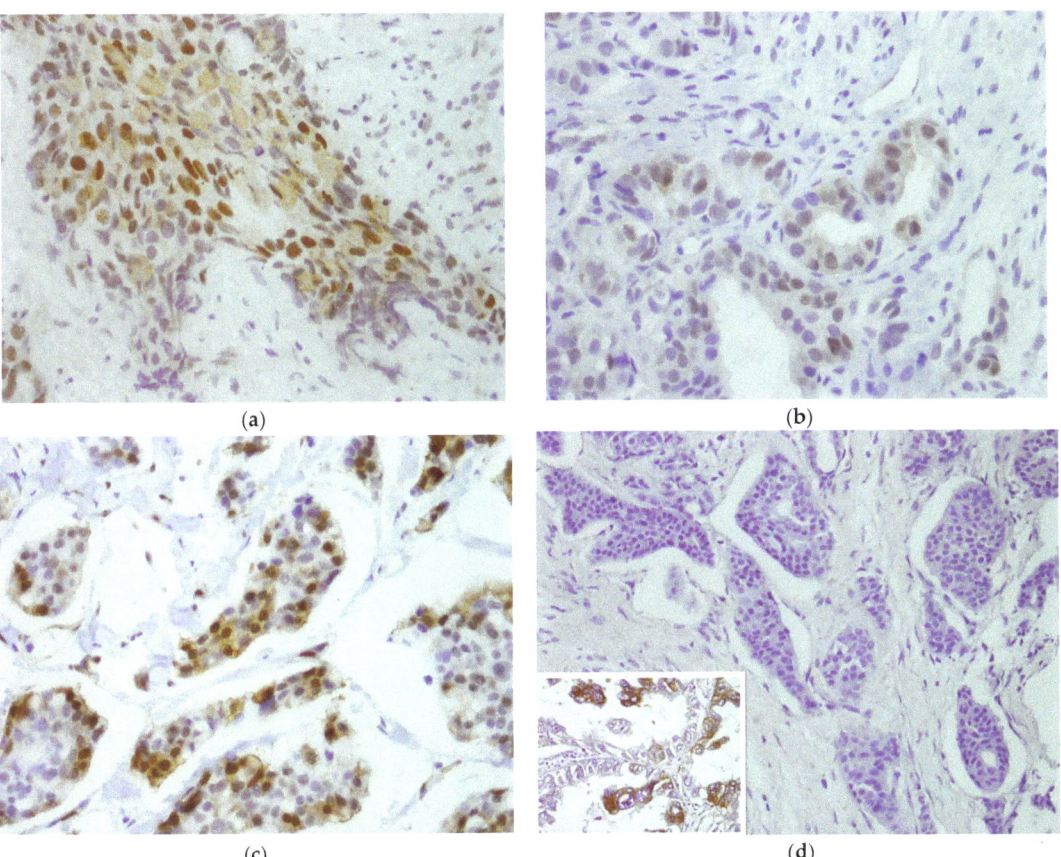

Figure 1. Evaluation of immunohistochemical staining. (**a**) For HIF-1α, moderate staining of nuclei and slight staining of some cytoplasmic areas, >5% in tumor cells. 40×. (**b**) For pAKT, mild-to-moderate nuclear and cytoplasmic staining, ≥10% in tumor cells. 40×. (**c**) For pMAPK, strong nuclear staining and mild-to-moderate cytoplasmic staining, >10% in tumor cells. 40×. (**d**) For EGFR, negative membrane staining. A staining positive control for EGFR of lung cancer was inserted in the image 40×.

Table 2. Relation between HIF-1α expression and pCR.

	Number of Cases (%)		p
	pCR	No pCR	
HIF-1α < 5%	6 (33.3%)	47 (67.1%)	*0.014* [a]
HIF-1α ≥ 5%	12 (66.7%)	23 (32.9%)	
HIF-1α%	18 (20.5%)	70 (79.5%)	*0.017* [b]
	x = 10.42; SD = 9.53	x = 5.05; SD = 7.52	

[a] Fisher exact test. [b] Mann–Whitney U test. Abbreviations: pCR, pathological complete response; x, mean; SD, standard deviation. Italic means the relation is significant.

3.2. Relation between HIF-1α Expression and Biological Markers

A positive relationship between HIF-1α expression and Grade (p = 0.015) and Ki-67 (p = 0.001) was identified. HIF-1α expression was negatively correlated with PR (p = 0.049) and Luminal A phenotype (p = 0.005) (Table 3).

Table 3. Relation between HIF-1α expression and clinicopathological variables.

Variable		HIF-1α < 5%	HIF-1α ≥ 5%	p
Grade 1		15 (83.3%)	3 (16.7%)	*0.015* [a]
Grade 2		22 (62.8%)	13 (37.2%)	
Grade 3		13 (41.9%)	18 (58.1%)	
Ki-67 < 20%		29 (80.6%)	7 (19.4%)	*0.001* [b]
Ki-67 ≥ 20%		23 (45.1%)	28 (54.9%)	
HER2 −		43 (63.2%)	25 (36.8%)	0.593 [b]
HER2 +		10 (55.6%)	8 (44.4%)	
ER < 10%		10 (43.5%)	13 (56.5%)	0.080 [b]
ER ≥ 10%		43 (67.2%)	21 (32.8%)	
ER count < 3		9 (42.9%)	12 (57.1%)	0.072 [b]
ER count ≥ 3		44 (66.7%)	22 (33.3%)	
PR < 10%		18 (48.6%)	19 (51.4%)	*0.049* [b]
PR ≥ 10%		35 (70%)	15 (30%)	
PR count < 3		16 (47.1%)	18 (52.9%)	*0.044* [b]
PR count ≥ 3		37 (69.8%)	16 (30.2%)	
Phenotype	Basal	5 (41.7%)	7 (58.3%)	
	HER2	10 (55.6%)	8 (44.4%)	
	Luminal A	26 (86.7%)	4 (13.3%)	*0.005* [b]
	Luminal B	12 (46.2%)	14 (53.8%)	

[a] Pearson chi-square. [b] Fisher exact test. Abbreviations: ER, estrogen receptor; PR, progesterone receptor. Italic means the relation is significant.

3.3. Relation between HIF-1α Expression and pATK, pMAK and EGFR

In 95 samples analyzed, pAKT expression was determined in 81 (85.3%) patients and it was considered positive in 57 (70.37%) (Figure 1). Using pMAPK, expression was determined in 74 (77.9%) patients and it was considered positive in 61 (82.43%) (Figure 1). For EGFR, expression was determined in 88 (92.6%) patients: of these, none were considered positive because there was no membrane staining of any tumor cells (Figure 1). No relation was found between the expression of these proteins and HIF-1α (Supplementary Table S1).

3.4. Predictive Factors of Response to Treatment—Multivariate Analysis

For the resulting model consisting of the variables Ki-67, HIF-1α and molecular phenotype, only basal phenotype was an independent predictive factor of pCR (p = 0.001) (Supplementary Table S2).

3.5. Sulvival Analysis—Prognostic Markers

In univariate analysis, the markers associated with shorter DFS were: HIF-1α positive (p = 0.013) (Figure 2), Ki-67 positive (p = 0.002), basal phenotype (p = 0.001), pAKT negative

(p = 0.009) and ER negative (p = 0.024, p = 0.010). As for OS, markers associated with decreased survival were HIF-1α positive (a trend that did not reach statistical significance, p = 0.08), Ki-67 positive (p = 0.022), basal phenotype (p = 0.007), pAKT negative (p = 0.007) and ER negative (p = 0.001).

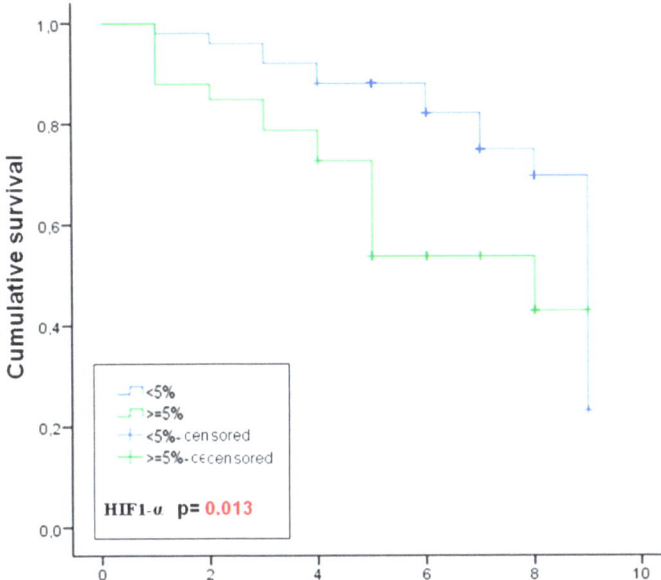

Figure 2. Kaplan–Meier curves of disease-free survival of patients stratified by HIF-1α expression.

In multivariate analysis with correlation of ER, grade, Ki-67, pCR, HIF-1α and pAKT, it was shown that pCR and the expression of Ki-67, HIF-1α and pAKT were independent predictors of DFS, while ER and pAKT were independent prognostic factors of OS (Table 4).

Table 4. Multivariate analysis (Cox regression) of prognostic factors for DFS and OS.

	DFS			OS		
	HR	95% CI	*p*-Value	HR	95% CI	*p*-Value
Grade 1 vs. 2 vs. 3	-	-	0.560	-	-	0.977
Ki-67 ≥ 20% vs. <20%	0.8	1.8–35.5	*0.006*	-	-	0.260
ER ≥ 10% vs. <10%	-	-	0.072	3.2	1.3–7.7	*0.008*
pCR vs. no pCR	0.2	0.0–0.6	*0.009*	-	-	0.06
HIF-1α ≥ 5% vs. <5%	2.5	1.0–6.2	*0.047*	-	-	0.295
pAKT ≥ 10% vs. <10%	2.4	1.0–5.9	*0.039*	2.4	1.0–5.7	*0.046*

Abbreviations: DFS, disease-free survival; ER, estrogen receptor; HR, Hazard ratio; OS, overall survival; Italic means the *p*-value is significant.

4. Discussion

To date, just a few studies have demonstrated the existence of statistically significant relations between the expression of HIF-1α and pCR in breast cancer after neoadjuvant chemotherapy based on anthracyclines and taxanes [26–28]. In our study, more than a third of patients were considered HIF-1α positive. These results concur with other findings reported in the literature from studies using the same cutoff point as in our study [13,23,29]. However, the rate of positivity in the studies that examined HIF-1α in breast cancer ranges from 1% to 80.2%, probably due to the use of different cutoff points and assessment systems [11].

Among the studies where the predictive value of HIF-1α in breast cancer is evaluated, very few have investigated the relation between the expression of HIF-1α and pCR or the predictive value of the molecule in breast cancer patients going under neoadjuvant chemotherapy based on anthracyclines and taxanes [26–31]. In the study published by Yamamoto et al. (2008), of all of the patients who achieved pCR, 100% were positive for HIF-1α, whereas only 66.7% of the other patients were. The difference did not reach statistical significance, probably because of the small study sample [29]. Another two studies conducted by Generali et al. analyzed the predictive value of HIF-1α. The first study is a phase 2 clinical trial where patients were randomized to receive neoadjuvant anthracycline-based chemotherapy versus anthracycline plus tamoxifen [30]. Overexpression of HIF-1α was associated with lower clinical response. However, no statistically significant relation was found between pCR and overexpression of HIF-1α, which makes the above findings questionable. Moreover, staining intensity was used to establish the cutoff point for HIF-1α (negative: 0, +1 vs. positive: +2). Of the five patients who achieved pCR, only one had no staining; the other four were classified as +1. In many other studies, including ours, the cutoff was the percentage of cells stained; therefore, weak staining, considered negative for HIF-1α in this study, could be considered positive by other authors, depending on the percentage of stained cells. The other study that evaluated the predictive value of HIF-1α was also a phase 2 trial, where patients were randomized to receive either letrozole or letrozole plus oral cyclophosphamide [31]. Overexpression of HIF-1α was associated with lower rates of clinical response, with no reference to the relation with pCR rate. In a recent meta-analysis, it was shown that pCR correlates with improved DFS and OS, pointing to the lack of prognostic value of the clinical responses [5]. In our study, pCR was an independent prognostic factor of longer DFS and almost significant for OS ($p = 0.06$).

Recent studies continue this evaluation. According to the study published by Tiezzi et al. (2013), an overall reduction in HIF-1α and HIF-2α expression was observed in patients after using NAC based on anthracycline and taxanes, but no association was observed between HIF-2α expression and its predictive value of pCR. However, the pCR rate in HIF-1α-negative patients was 5%, whereas in HIF-1α-positive patients, it was 21% ($p = 0.03$) [28]. These results are consistent with those in our study. Furthermore, in a cohort formed of 220 patients who received a treatment regime based on anthracyclines and taxanes, 68.2% were considered HIF-1α positive (150/220). Otherwise, in this case, HIF-1α-negative patients had a higher pCR rate rather than HIF-1α-positive patients ($p = 0.027$) [27]. In the most recent study, the expression of HIF-1α was identified in 104 tumor biopsies. Thus, more than a third of the patients were considered HIF-1α positive. The evaluation of the predictive value of HIF-1α showed significant association with resistance and favorable response to NAC based on anthracyclines and taxanes ($p < 0.001$). Specifically, patients with a lower expression of HIF-1α were in the favorable-response group while those in the resistance group had a higher expression of the molecule [26].

Other markers have more predictive value. In our study, we found that patients with negative hormone receptors, more undifferentiated tumors, a higher rate of proliferation and basal phenotype were significantly related to higher pCR rate. These results concur with those described in the literature [3,32,33].

An attempt was made to explain the paradoxical observation that some of the variables were predictive of both unfavorable prognosis and chemosensitivity. Some authors have related these discrepant findings with attaining pCR or not. That is to say that it seems clear that patients with a triple-negative phenotype who receive NAC and do not reach pCR, despite good clinical response, have a less prolonged survival. However, those who attain pCR apparently have an excellent prognosis [34,35].

On the other hand, we found a statistically significant relation between HIF-1α expression and hormone receptor negativity. It has been demonstrated that hypoxia decreases ER and PR levels in breast cancer, suggesting a relation between HIF-1α expression and resistance to hormonal therapy [36]. We also found a statistically significant positive relation between HIF-1α expression and the proliferation marker Ki-67. These results are consistent with the findings reported in the literature, as it has been suggested that the higher proliferation rate of tumor cells causes HIF-1α activation [37]. The expression of HIF1-α has also been linked with poorly differentiated tumors [37,38]. Our findings also support these statements; it is considered that hypoxia induces genetic alterations, promoting morphological changes in the cell itself and in its nucleus, resulting in more undifferentiated tumor cells [7,39].

The third objective of our study was to determine whether the activation of HIF-1α is independent of tissue oxygen concentration, so we studied the molecular pathways that might be involved. One of the membrane receptors related with HIF-1α activation in normoxic conditions is EGFR [12]. Jögi et al. found a significant relationship between the expression of EGFR and HIF-1α [40]. We did not find EGFR expression in any of the patients in the study, although the external controls were positive, suggesting that there may be other receptor tyrosine kinases capable of inducing the transcriptional activity or increasing HIF-1α stability under normoxic conditions but ROS dependent [41]. Some authors have elucidated a role for mitochondrial-generated ROS in tumoral HIF-1α stabilization [9,42]. On the basis of the foregoing, this pathway could be the reason why HIF-1α expression incremented in this study due to the increase in oxidative stress status in breast cancer patients who received neoadjuvant chemotherapy treatment, as described in previous investigations of our group [43].

Once the membrane receptor is stimulated, there are several intracellular signaling pathways that are associated with the synthesis of HIF-1α under normoxic conditions. These pathways include the PI3K/AKT/mTOR and RAS/RAF/MAPK pathways. We found overexpressed pAKT in 70% of cases, which is consistent with the results of other published studies [24,44]. The relation between the expression of HIF-1α and pAKT was examined by immunohistochemistry in breast cancer in a single study. Gort et al. [44] studied the overexpression of both proteins in 95 patients and concluded that low pAKT expression correlated significantly with low HIF-1α expression. We found no relation between the two molecules in our study. With respect to the RAS/RAF/MAPK pathway, we detected positivity in 83%, as reported in other published studies [45,46]. No significant association was found between overexpression of HIF-1α and pMAPK. Kronblad et al. [45] studied the expression of pMAPK and HIF-1α in 21 samples of ductal carcinoma in situ breast cancer, finding a positive relation between the expression of both molecules; the authors emphasized the overexpression of pMAPK in less-hypoxic areas. These results are consistent with the ones shown in the study conducted by Hsu et al. (2016) [46]. These findings and our results support activation of HIF-1α mediated by the hypoxic conditions existing in the tumor microenvironment.

As for the prognostic value of HIF-1α, in our study, we saw how overexpression of this protein was an independent prognostic factor for shorter DFS. Our results confirm those of other authors included in a meta-analysis of 5177 patients who used the same cutoff value as in our study [37].

Interestingly, in our study, we also found that pAKT overexpression was an independent prognostic factor of more prolonged DFS and OS. The largest study to analyze the prognostic value of pAKT was carried out by Yang et al. [47] with 1202 patients enrolled in the study of neoadjuvant NSABP B-28; patients who overexpressed pAKT had a longer DFS compared to patients who did not overexpress this protein.

5. Conclusions

It was shown that overexpression of HIF-1α is a predictor of pCR and shorter DFS in patients who received a neoadjuvant chemotherapy schedule based on anthracyclines and taxanes. In addition, HIF-1α is related to other variables with a more consolidated predictive and prognostic value. All these variables are associated with a more aggressive and hypoxic tumor microenvironment. We believe that it would be interesting to confirm these results in prospective studies, given the need for expanding the small panel of predictive markers in breast cancer.

Supplementary Materials: The following supporting information can be downloaded at: https://www.mdpi.com/article/10.3390/cancers14215393/s1, Table S1: Relation between HIF-1α expression and pAKT and pMAPK; Table S2: Logistic regression model as a predictive factor of response to treatment.

Author Contributions: C.L.R.-T. and P.S.-R. designed and conceived the experiments; C.L.R.-T., J.L.Q. and R.A.-C. performed the experiments, P.S.-R. and R.A.-C. collected samples; M.R.-T., C.L.R.-T. and J.M.G.-N. analyzed the data; J.M.G.-N. and C.P.-R. contributed materials and analysis tools; J.M.G.-N. prepared the original draft; J.L.Q., C.L.R.-T., M.R.-T. and P.S.-R. reviewed and edited the draft; C.P.-R., R.A.-C. and A.J.-M. reviewed the analysis and interpretation; A.J.-M. supervised funding acquisition. Every author participated in reviewing the manuscript and improving the intellectual content. All authors have read and agreed to the published version of the manuscript.

Funding: This research received no external funding.

Institutional Review Board Statement: The study was conducted in accordance with the Declaration of Helsinki and approved by the Ethics and Research Committee of the Complejo Hospitalario de Jaén, Spain (code: PI-0695-2012).

Informed Consent Statement: Informed consent was obtained from all subjects involved in the study.

Data Availability Statement: Not applicable.

Conflicts of Interest: The authors declare no conflict of interest.

Abbreviations

DFS: disease-free survival; EGFR: epidermal growth factor receptor; ER: estrogen receptor; HER2: human epidermal growth receptor 2; HIF-1α: hypoxia-inducible factor-1α; MAPK: mitogen activated protein kinase; M–P: Miller and Payne scale; NAC: neoadjuvant chemotherapy; OS: overall survival; pCR: pathologic complete response; PI3K: phosphatidylinositol 3-kinase; PR: progesterone receptors.

References

1. Shien, T.; Iwata, H. Adjuvant and neoadjuvant therapy for breast cancer. *Jpn. J. Clin. Oncol.* **2020**, *50*, 225–229. [CrossRef] [PubMed]
2. Shuai, Y.; Ma, L. Prognostic value of pathologic complete response and the alteration of breast cancer immunohistochemical biomarkers after neoadjuvant chemotherapy. *Pathol. Res. Pract.* **2019**, *215*, 29–33. [CrossRef] [PubMed]
3. Greenwell, K.; Hussain, L.; Lee, D.; Bramlage, M.; Bills, G.; Mehta, A.; Jackson, A.; Wexelman, B. Complete pathologic response rate to neoadjuvant chemotherapy increases with increasing HER2/CEP17 ratio in HER2 overexpressing breast cancer: Analysis of the National Cancer Database (NCDB). *Breast Cancer Res. Treat.* **2020**, *181*, 249–254. [CrossRef] [PubMed]
4. Al-Masri, M.; Aljalabneh, B.; Al-Najjar, H.; Al-Shamaileh, T. Effect of time to breast cancer surgery after neoadjuvant chemotherapy on survival outcomes. *Breast Cancer Res. Treat.* **2021**, *186*, 7–13. [CrossRef] [PubMed]
5. Cullinane, C.; Shrestha, A.; Al Maksoud, A.; Rothwell, J.; Evoy, D.; Geraghty, J.; McCartan, D.; McDermott, E.W.; Prichard, R. Optimal timing of surgery following breast cancer neoadjuvant chemotherapy: A systematic review and meta-analysis. *Eur. J. Surg. Oncol.* **2021**, *47*, 1507–1513. [CrossRef] [PubMed]
6. Gálvez-Navas, J.M.; Pérez-Ramírez, C.; Ramírez-Tortosa, M.C. [Secreted Frizzled-Related Protein 4 and breast cancer]. *Ars. Pharm.* **2021**, *62*, 438–450. [CrossRef]
7. Pineda-Lancheros, L.E.; Pérez-Ramírez, C.; Sánchez-Martín, A.; Gálvez-Navas, J.M.; Martínez-Martínez, F.; Ramírez-Tortosa, M.C.; Jiménez-Morales, A. Impact of Genetic Polymorphisms on the Metabolic Pathway of Vitamin D and Survival in Non-Small Cell Lung Cancer. *Nutrients* **2021**, *13*, 3783. [CrossRef] [PubMed]
8. Vaupel, P.; Multhoff, G. Hypoxia-/HIF-1alpha-Driven Factors of the Tumor Microenvironment Impeding Antitumor Immune Responses and Promoting Malignant Progression. *Adv. Exp. Med. Biol.* **2018**, *1072*, 171–175. [CrossRef]
9. Zhang, T.; Suo, C.; Zheng, C.; Zhang, H. Hypoxia and Metabolism in Metastasis. *Adv. Exp. Med. Biol.* **2019**, *1136*, 87–95. [CrossRef]
10. Zhang, Z.; Yao, L.; Yang, J.; Wang, Z.; Du, G. PI3K/Akt and HIF-1 signaling pathway in hypoxia-ischemia (Review). *Mol. Med. Rep.* **2018**, *18*, 3547–3554. [CrossRef]
11. Masoud, G.N.; Li, W. HIF-1α pathway: Role, regulation and intervention for cancer therapy. *Acta Pharm. Sin. B* **2015**, *5*, 378–389. [CrossRef] [PubMed]
12. Wee, P.; Wang, Z. Epidermal Growth Factor Receptor Cell Proliferation Signaling Pathways. *Cancers* **2017**, *9*, 52. [CrossRef] [PubMed]
13. Shamis, S.A.K.; McMillan, D.C.; Edwards, J. The relationship between hypoxia-inducible factor 1α (HIF-1α) and patient survival in breast cancer: Systematic review and meta-analysis. *Crit. Rev. Oncol. Hematol.* **2021**, *159*, 103231. [CrossRef] [PubMed]

14. Sanchez-Munoz, A.; Duenas-Garcia, R.; Jaen-Morago, A.; Carrasco, E.; Chacon, I.; Garcia-Tapiador, A.M.; Ortega-Granados, A.L.; Martínez-Ortega, E.; Ribelles, N.; Fernández-Navarro, M.; et al. Is it posible to increase pCR in the neoadjuvant treatment with dose-dense/sequential combination?: Results from a phase II Trial combining epirubicin and cyclophosphamide followed by paclitaxel and gemtamicine +/− trastuzumab in stage II and III breast cancer patients. *Am. J. Clin. Oncol.* **2010**, *33*, 432–437. [CrossRef]
15. Schneeweiss, A.; Lauschner, I.; Ruiz, A.; Guerrero, A.; Sanchez-Rovira, P.; Segui, M.A.; Goerke, K.; Wolf, M.; Manikhas, A.G.; Wacker, J.; et al. Doxorubicin/pemetrexed followed by docetaxel as neoadjuvant treatment for early-stage breast cancer: A randomized phase II trial. *Clin. Breast Cancer* **2007**, *7*, 555–558. [CrossRef]
16. Oluogun, W.A.; Adedokun, K.A.; Oyenike, M.A.; Adeyeba, O.A. Histological classification, grading, staging, and prognostic indexing of female breast cancer in an African population: A 10-years restrospective study. *Int. J. Health Sci.* **2019**, *13*, 3–9.
17. Ogston, K.N.; Miller, I.D.; Payne, S.; Hutcheon, A.H.; Sarkar, T.K.; Smith, I.; Schofield, A.; Heys, S.D. A new histological grading system to assess response of breast cancer to primary chemotherapy: Prognostic significance and sulrvival. *Breast* **2003**, *12*, 320–327. [CrossRef]
18. Konoken, J.; Bubendorf, L.; Kallioniemi, A.; Barlund, M.; Schraml, P.; Leighton, S.; Torhorst, J.; Mihatsch, M.J.; Sauter, G.; Kallioniemi, O.P. Tissue microarrays for high-throughput molecular profiling of tumor specimens. *Nat. Med.* **1998**, *4*, 844–847. [CrossRef]
19. Zhu, Q.; Ademuyiwa, F.O.; Young, C.; Appleton, C.; Covington, M.F.; Ma, C.; Sanati, S.; Hagemann, I.S.; Mostafa, A.; Uddin KM, S.; et al. Early Assessment Window for Predicting Breast Cancer Neoadjuvant Therapy using Biomarkers, Ultrasound, and Diffuse Optical Tomography. *Breast Cancer Res. Treat.* **2021**, *188*, 615–630. [CrossRef]
20. Avci, N.; Deligonul, A.; Tolunay, S.; Cubukcu, E.; Olmez, O.F.; Ulas, A. Neoadjuvant chemotherapy-induced changes in immunohistochemucal expression of estrogen receptor, progesterone receptor, HER2, and Ki-67 in patients with breast cancer. *J. BUON* **2015**, *20*, 45–49.
21. Sánchez-Muñoz, A.; Plata-Fernández, Y.M.; Fernández, M.; Jaén-Morago, A.; Fernández-Navarro, M.; de la Torre-Cabrera, C.; Ramírez-Tortosa, C.; Lomas-Garrido, M.; Llácer, C.; Navarro-Pérez, V.; et al. The role of immunohistochemistry in breast cancer patients treated with neoadjuvant chemotherapy: And old tool with an enduring prognostic value. *Clin. Breast Cancer* **2013**, *13*, 46–52. [CrossRef] [PubMed]
22. Wolff, A.C.; Hammond, M.E.H.; Allison, K.H.; Harvey, B.E.; Mangu, P.B.; Bartlett, J.M.S.; Bilous, M.; Ellis, I.O.; Fitzgibbons, P.; Hanna, W.; et al. Human epidermal growth factor receptor 2 testing in breast cancer: American Society of Clinical Oncology/College of American Pathologists clinical practice guideline focused update. *Arch. Pathol. Lab. Med.* **2018**, *142*, 1364–1382. [CrossRef] [PubMed]
23. Vermeulen, M.A.; van Deurzen, C.H.; Schroder, C.P.; Matens, J.W.; van Diest, P.J. Expression of hipoxia-induced proteins in ductal carcinoma in situ invasive cancer of the male breast. *J. Clin. Pathol.* **2020**, *73*, 204–208. [CrossRef] [PubMed]
24. Iyikesici, M.S.; Basaran, G.; Dane, F.; Ekenel, M.; Yumuk, P.F.; Cabuk, D.; Ekenel, M.; Yukum, P.F.; Cabuk, D.; Teomete, M.; et al. Associations between clinicopathological prognostic factors and pAkt, pMAPK and topoisomerase II expression in breast cancer. *Int. J. Clin. Exp. Med.* **2014**, *7*, 1459–1464. [PubMed]
25. Sauerbrei, W.; Taube, S.E.; McShane, L.M.; Cavenagh, M.M.; Altman, D.G. Reporting Recommendations for Tumor Market Prognostic Studies (REMARK): An Abridged Explanation and Elaboration. *J. Nat. Cancer Inst.* **2018**, *110*, 803–811. [CrossRef]
26. Zhang, J.; Zhang, S.; Gao, S.; Ma, Y.; Tan, X.; Kang, Y.; Ren, W. HIF-1α, TWIST-1 and ITGB-1, associated with Tumor Stiffness, as Novel Predictive Markers for the Pathological Response to Neoadjuvant Chemotherapy in Breast Cancer. *Cancer Manag. Res.* **2020**, *12*, 2209–2222. [CrossRef]
27. Nie, C.; Lv, H.; Bie, L.; Hou, H.; Chen, X. Hypoxia-inducible factor 1-alpha expression correlated with response to neoadjuvant chemotherapy in women with breast cancer. *Medicine* **2018**, *97*, e13551. [CrossRef]
28. Tiezzi, D.G.; Clagnan, W.S.; Mandarano, L.R.; de Sousa, C.B.; Marana, H.R.; Tiezzi, M.G.; de Andrade, J.M. Expression of aldehyde dehydrogenase after neoadjuvant chemotherapy is associated with expression of hypoxia-inducible factors 1 and 2 alpha and predicts prognosis in locally advanced breast cancer. *Clinics* **2013**, *68*, 592–598. [CrossRef]
29. Yamamoto, Y.; Ibusuki, M.; Okumura, Y.; Kawasoe, T.; Kai, K.; Iyama, K.; Iwase, H. Hypoxia-inducible factor 1 alpha is closely linked to an aggressive phenotype in breast cancer. *Breast Cancer Res Treat.* **2008**, *110*, 465–475. [CrossRef]
30. Generali, D.; Berruti, A.; Brizzi, M.P.; Campo, L.; Bonardi, S.; Wigfield, S.; Bersiga, A.; Allevi, G.; Milani, M.; Aguggini, S.; et al. Hypoxia-inducible factor-1 alpha expression predicts a poor response to primary chemoendocrine therapy and disease-free survival in primary human breast cancer. *Clin. Cancer Res.* **2006**, *12*, 4562–4568. [CrossRef]
31. Generali, D.; Buffa, F.M.; Berruti, A.; Brizzi, M.P.; Campo, L.; Bonardi, S.; Bersiga, A.; Allevi, G.; Milani, M.; Aguggini, S.; et al. Phosphorylated ER alpha, HIF-1 alpha, and MAPK signaling as predictors of primary endocrine treatment response and resistance in patients with breast cancer. *J. Clin. Oncol.* **2009**, *27*, 227–234. [CrossRef] [PubMed]
32. Sanchez-Rovira, P.; Anton, A.; Barnadas, A.; Velasco, A.; Lomas, M.; Rodriguez-Pinilla, M.; Ramírez, J.L.; Ramírez, C.; Ríos, M.J.; Castellá, E.; et al. Classical markers like ER and Ki-67, but also surviving and pERK, could be involved in the pathological response to gemcitabine, Adriamycin and paclitaxel (GAT) in locally advanced breast cancer patients: Results from the GEICAM/2002-01 phase II study. *Clin. Transl. Oncol.* **2012**, *14*, 430–436. [CrossRef] [PubMed]

33. Foldi, J.; Silber, A.; Reisenbichler, E.; Singh, K.; Fishbach, N.; Persico, J.; Adelson, K.; Katoch, A.; Horowitz, N.; Lannin, D.; et al. Neoadjuvant durvalumab plus weekly nab-paclitaxel and dose-dense doxorubicin/cyclophosphamide in triple-negative breast cancer. *Npj Breast Cancer* **2021**, *7*, 9. [CrossRef] [PubMed]
34. Wong, W.; Brogi, E.; Reis-Filho, J.S.; Plitas, G.; Robson, M.; Norton, L.; Morrow, M.; Wen, H.Y. Poor response to neoadjuvant chemotherapy in metaplastic breast carcinoma. *Npj Breast Cancer* **2021**, *7*, 96. [CrossRef]
35. Miglietta, F.; Dieci, M.V.; Griguolo, G.; Guarneri, V. Neoadjuvant approach as a platform for treatment personalization: Focus on HER2-positive and triple-negative breast cancer. *Cancer Treat. Rev.* **2021**, *98*, 102222. [CrossRef]
36. Campbell, E.J.; Dachs, G.U.; Morrin, H.R.; Davey, V.C.; Robinson, B.A.; Vissers, M.C.M. Activation of the hypoxia pathway in breast cancer tissue and patient survival are inversely associated with tumor ascorbate levels. *BCM Cancer* **2019**, *19*, 307. [CrossRef] [PubMed]
37. Zhao, Z.; Mu, H.; Li, Y.; Liu, Y.; Zou, J.; Zhu, Y. Clinicopathological and prognostic value of hipoxia-inducible factor-1α in breast cancer: A meta-analysis including 5177 patients. *Clin. Trans. Oncol.* **2020**, *22*, 1892–19086. [CrossRef]
38. Infantino, V.; Santarsiero, A.; Convertini, P.; Todisco, S.; Iacobazzi, V. Cancer Cell Metabolism in Hypoxia: Role of HIF-1 as Key Regulator and Therapeutic Target. *Int. J. Mol. Sci.* **2021**, *22*, 5703. [CrossRef]
39. Sajnani, K.; Islam, F.; Smith, R.A.; Gopalan, V.; King-Yin Lam, A. Genetic alterations in Krebs cycle and its impact on cancer pathogenesis. *Biochimie* **2017**, *135*, 164–172. [CrossRef]
40. Jögi, A.; Ehinger, A.; Hartman, L.; Alkner, S. Expression of HIF-1α is related to a poor prognosis and tamoxifen resistance in contralateral breast cancer. *PLoS ONE* **2019**, *14*, e0226150. [CrossRef]
41. Bullen, J.W.; Tchernyshyov, I.; Holewinski, R.J.; DeVine, L.; Wu, F.; Venkatraman, V.; Kass, D.L.; Cole, R.N.; Van Eyk, J.; Semenza, G.L. Protein kinase A-dependent phosphorylation stimulates the transcriptional activity of hypoxia-inducible factor 1. *Sci. Signal.* **2016**, *9*, ra56. [CrossRef] [PubMed]
42. Hielscher, A.; Gerecht, S. Hypoxia and free radicals: Role in tumor progression and the use of engineering-based platforms to address these relationships. *Free Radic. Biol. Med.* **2015**, *79*, 281–291. [CrossRef] [PubMed]
43. Vera-Ramírez, L.; Sanchez-Rovira, P.; Ramírez-Tortosa, M.C.; Ramírez-Tortosa, C.L.; Granados-Principal, S.; Fernández-Navarro, M.; Lorente, J.A.; Quiles, J.L. Does chemotherapy-induced oxidative stress improve the survival rates of breast cancer patients? *ARS* **2011**, *15*, 903–909. [CrossRef] [PubMed]
44. Gort, E.H.; Groot, A.J.; Derks van de Ven, T.L.; van der Groep, P.; Verlaan, I.; van Laar, T.; van Diest, P.J.; van der Wall, E.; Shvarts, A. Hypoxia-inducible factor-1 alpha expression requires PI 3-kinase activity and correlates with Akt1 phosphorylation in invasive breast carcinomas. *Oncogene* **2006**, *25*, 6123–6127. [CrossRef] [PubMed]
45. Kronblad, A.; Hedenfalk, I.; Nisson, E.; Pahlman, S.; Landberg, G. ERK1/2 inhibition increases antiestrogen treatment efficacy by interfering with hypoxia-induced downregulation of ER alpha: A combination therapy potentially targeting hypoxic and dormant tumor cells. *Oncogene* **2005**, *24*, 6835–6841. [CrossRef] [PubMed]
46. Hsu, C.-W.; Huang, R.; Khuc, T.; Shou, D.; Bullock, J.; Grooby, S.; Griffin, S.; Zou, C.; Little, A.; Astley, H.; et al. Identification of approved and investigational drugs that inhibit hypoxia-inducible factor-1 signalling. *Oncotarget* **2016**, *7*, 8172–8183. [CrossRef] [PubMed]
47. Yang, S.X.; Constantino, J.P.; Kim, C.; Mamounas, E.P.; Nguyen, D.; Jeong, J.H.; Wolmark, N.; Kidwell, K.; Paik, S.; Swain, S.M. Akt phosphorylation as Ser473 predicts benefits of paclitaxel chemotherapy in node-positive breast cancer. *J. Clin. Oncol.* **2010**, *28*, 2974–2981. [CrossRef] [PubMed]

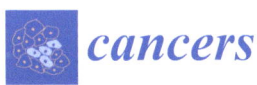

Article

Glycolysis-Related SLC2A1 Is a Potential Pan-Cancer Biomarker for Prognosis and Immunotherapy

Haosheng Zheng [1,†], Guojie Long [2,3,†], Yuzhen Zheng [1], Xingping Yang [1], Weijie Cai [1], Shiyun He [1], Xianyu Qin [1,*] and Hongying Liao [1,*]

[1] Department of Thoracic Surgery, Thoracic Cancer Center, The Sixth Affiliated Hospital, Sun Yat-sen University, Guangzhou 510655, China
[2] Guangdong Research Institute of Gastroenterology, The Sixth Affiliated Hospital, Sun Yat-sen University, Guangzhou 510655, China
[3] Department of Pancreatic Hepatobiliary Surgery, The Sixth Affiliated Hospital of Sun Yat-sen University, Guangzhou 510655, China
* Correspondence: qinxy27@mail.sysu.edu.cn (X.Q.); liaohy2@mail.sysu.edu.cn (H.L.); Tel.: +86-139-2884-5885 (H.L.)
† These authors contributed equally to this work.

Simple Summary: Enhanced glycolysis is a major feature of cancer glycometabolism, and SLC2A1 is one of the pivotal genes in cancer glycometabolism. Although SLC2A1 plays an important role in the growth of many cancers, pan-cancer analysis allows us to more comprehensively and systematically understand the function and role of SLC2A1 in cancers. In this study, we found that SLC2A1 was highly expressed in most cancers, and resulted in poor prognosis. M6A methylation might be one of the important factors for the high expression level of SLC2A1. SLC2A1 not only enhanced cancer glycolysis, but also affected the tumor microenvironment. Notably, SLC2A1 was significantly and positively correlated with the T-cell-exhaustion biomarkers PD-L1 and CTLA4. Collectively, SLC2A1 may provide new strategies for pan-cancer treatment, especially cancer immunotherapy.

Abstract: SLC2A1 plays a pivotal role in cancer glycometabolism. SLC2A1 has been proposed as a putative driver gene in various cancers. However, a pan-cancer analysis of SLC2A1 has not yet been performed. In this study, we explored the expression and prognosis of SLC2A1 in pan-cancer across multiple databases. We conducted genetic alteration, epigenetic, and functional enrichment analyses of SLC2A. We calculated the correlation between SLC2A1 and tumor microenvironment using the TCGA pan-cancer dataset. We observed high expression levels of SLC2A1 with poor prognosis in most cancers. The overall genetic alteration frequency of SLC2A1 was 1.8% in pan-cancer, and the SLC2A1 promoter was hypomethylation in several cancers. Most m6A-methylation-related genes positively correlated with the expression of SLC2A1 in 33 TCGA cancers. Moreover, SLC2A1 was mainly related to the functions including epithelial–mesenchymal transition, glycolysis, hypoxia, cell-cycle regulation, and DNA repair. Finally, SLC2A1 positively associated with neutrophils and cancer-associated fibroblasts in the tumor microenvironment of most cancers and significantly correlated with TMB and MSI in various cancers. Notably, SLC2A1 was remarkably positively correlated with PD-L1 and CTLA4 in most cancers. SLC2A1 might serve as an attractive pan-cancer biomarker for providing new insights into cancer therapeutics.

Keywords: SLC2A1; pan-cancer; glycometabolism; immune infiltration; biomarker; prognosis

Citation: Zheng, H.; Long, G.; Zheng, Y.; Yang, X.; Cai, W.; He, S.; Qin, X.; Liao, H. Glycolysis-Related SLC2A1 Is a Potential Pan-Cancer Biomarker for Prognosis and Immunotherapy. *Cancers* 2022, 14, 5344. https://doi.org/10.3390/cancers14215344

Academic Editor: Paola Tucci

Received: 29 September 2022
Accepted: 27 October 2022
Published: 29 October 2022
Corrected: 18 January 2023

Publisher's Note: MDPI stays neutral with regard to jurisdictional claims in published maps and institutional affiliations.

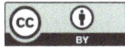

Copyright: © 2022 by the authors. Licensee MDPI, Basel, Switzerland. This article is an open access article distributed under the terms and conditions of the Creative Commons Attribution (CC BY) license (https:// creativecommons.org/licenses/by/ 4.0/).

1. Introduction

Cancer is one of the leading causes of death in humans. Although much progress has been made in the treatment of cancer, the overall therapeutic effect is unsatisfactory. Newly diagnosed cases are also increasing, placing a huge burden on society [1]. In recent years, cancer immunotherapy has considerably progressed, providing a powerful tool for cancer treatment and improving the prognosis of cancer patients [2]. In 2017, the U.S. FDA approved pembrolizumab for solid tumors with high microsatellite instability or mismatch repair gene defects (MSI-H/dMMR). Pembrolizumab has also become the first antitumor immune drug based on pan-cancer biomarkers without paying attention to the cancer type [3]. Pan-cancer analysis can help us understand the commonalities among different cancer types and provide new ideas for the treatment of pan-cancer [4].

Glucose is one of the basic metabolites needed by animal and plant cells. Cancer cells require a large amount of energy from the body for malignant proliferation [5]. Aberrant energy metabolism is an important feature of cancer cells. Even with ample oxygen supply, most tumor cells prefer enhanced glycolysis instead of oxidative phosphorylation to produce ATP [6]. Metabolite reprogramming provides energy and biological materials, providing a growth advantage to tumor cells under hypoxia [7]. Therefore, cancer metabolic reprogramming is an important direction in the search for novel pan-cancer biomarkers

Solute carrier family 2 member 1 (SLC2A1) is known as glucose transporter 1 (GLUT1) [8]. SLC2A1 plays a crucial role in the process of cell glycometabolism, whether in cancer or normal cells [9]. SLC2A1 is highly expressed in many kinds of cancer, and the overexpression of SLC2A1 can promote the growth and metastasis of cancers, such as liver, lung, endometrial, oral, breast, and gastric cancers [10–15]. Although the overexpression of SLC2A1 can further enhance glycolysis and cell proliferation in various cancers, a comprehensive pan-cancer analysis on SLC2A1 is lacking.

In this study, data from public databases and our own data convincingly showed that the expression of SLC2A1 was significantly increased in pan-cancer and conferred a poor prognosis. We explored the potential mechanism of SLC2A1 in pan-cancer through bioinformatics analysis. We further examined the association between SLC2A1 and the immune cell infiltration score, immune checkpoints, TMB, and MSI. Our results comprehensively revealed the potential mechanism of SLC2A1 in pan-cancer, and they highlight the impact of SLC2A1 on the tumor microenvironment (TME) and cancer immunotherapy.

2. Materials and Methods

2.1. Data Collection

We downloaded transcriptome data and clinical information from the University of California Santa Cruz (UCSC) Xena browser (https://xena.ucsc.edu/, accessed on 14 July 2022) and the Genotype-Tissue Expression (GTEx) database (https://www.gtexportal.org/home/-index.html, accessed on 14 July 2022), which included 15,776 samples of 33 cancer types and normal tissues. The abbreviations of all cancer types are shown in Table S1. Using the R package of "rma", we transformed the whole data by log2 (TPM +1), which we then filtered to remove missing and duplicated results. In addition, we searched 20 relative datasets from the Gene Expression Omnibus (GEO) database (https://www.ncbi.nlm.nih.gov/geo/, accessed on 14 July 2022) for validation. These datasets were GSE2088, GSE13507, GSE10927, GSE39001, GSE26566, GSE18520, GSE53757, GSE62452, GSE87211, GSE15605, GSE33630, GSE3218, GSE17025, GSE47861, GSE68468, GSE53625, GSE13601, GSE57927, GSE75037, and GSE26899. Detailed information on the GEO datasets is shown in Table S2.

We collected 90 pairs of samples (30 LUAD, 30 ESCA, and 30 COAD) from the Sixth Affiliated Hospital of Sun Yat-Sen University. Each sample contained paired tumors and adjacent normal tissues. The study was approved by the Ethics Committees of the Sixth Affiliated Hospital of Sun Yat-Sen University.

Finally, we used RT-qPCR method to validate the differential expression of SLC2A1 in LUAD and ESCA between cancer tissues and paired normal tissues. Using TRIzol reagent (Invitrogen, USA), we extracted the total RNA from the frozen tissues, which we then reverse-transcribed into cDNA with a PrimeScript RT reagent Kit with gDNA Eraser (TaKaRa). Next, we confirmed the expression of SLC2A1 with TB Green® Premix Ex Taq (TaKaRa), following the manufacturer's protocol, which we calculated using the $2-\Delta\Delta CT$ method. We used GAPDH as the endogenous control. The primers used in this study were as follows: SLC2A1 forward 5'-CTGCAACGGCTTAGACTTCGAC-3' and reverse 5'-TCTCTGGGTAACAGGGATCAAACA-3'; GAPDH forward 5'- GCTCTCTGCTCCTCC-TGTTC-3' and reverse 5'- ACGACCAAATCCGTTGACTC-3'.

2.2. Expression of SLC2A1 in Pan-Cancer

We extracted the expression data of SLC2A1 for each sample. We excluded cancer types with less than 3 samples. We used R software to calculate the expression differences between normal and tumor samples for each tumor by using Wilcoxon rank-sum and signed-rank tests. Moreover, we used the downloaded data to analyze the relationship between SLC2A1 level and clinicopathological parameters. We explored the protein level of SLC2A1 between human cancer and normal tissues by using the Human Protein Atlas (HPA: https://www.proteinatlas.org/) database. A previous study [16] from the Clinical Proteomic Tumor Analysis Consortium (CPTAC) identified 11 pan-cancer proteome-based subtypes (s1 to s11) using mass-spectrometry-based proteomic data from a compendium dataset of 2002 primary tumors compiled from 17 studies and 14 cancer types. The functions of proteome-based subtypes (s1 to s11) are described in detail in Table S3. The UALCAN database (http://ualcan.path.uab.edu, accessed on 14 July 2022) provides a pan-cancer protein expression analysis option based on the data from CPTAC. Therefore, we used the UALCAN database to perform pan-cancer protein expression analysis of SLC2A1.

2.3. Diagnostic Value of SLC2A1 in Pan-Cancer

To explore whether the mRNA levels of SLC2A1 exhibit diagnostic efficiency for distinguishing cancer from normal lung tissues, we performed receiver operating characteristic (ROC) curve analysis for the TCGA-GTEx pan-cancer dataset. The pROC package was used to plot ROC curves and calculate the areas under the curves (AUCs) values in R.

2.4. Prognostic Analysis of SLC2A1

We used the Kaplan–Meier (log-rank) method and univariate Cox regression to evaluate the overall survival (OS) of the patients from the TCGA pan-cancer cohort. We also assessed the progression-free interval (PFI), disease-specific survival (DSS), and the disease-free interval (DFI) of the patients from the TCGA pan-cancer cohort with univariate Cox regression analysis. We determined the optimal cut-off value using the R package 'survival'.

2.5. Genetic Alteration Analysis of SLC2A1

cBioPortal (http://cbioportal.org, accessed on 14 July 2022) is an open-access resource for exploring, visualizing, and analyzing multidimensional cancer genome data. It currently contained 225 cancer studies. We used cBioPortal to analyze the SLC2A1 gene genetic alterations in TCGA pan-cancer samples.

2.6. Epigenetic Analysis of SLC2A1

UALCAN database is a comprehensive, user-friendly, and interactive web resource for analyzing cancer OMICS data. We used UALCAN to evaluate promoter methylation of SLC2A1 in pan-cancer.

We collected 21 genes related to RNA m6A methylation from previous studies [17]. We extracted the SLC2A1 gene expression and 21 RNA m6A-methylation-related genes' expression data from each sample in the TCGA pan-cancer dataset. Then, we analyzed the correlation between SLC2A1 and RNA m6A-methylation-related genes in pan-cancer, and the results are presented in a heatmap.

2.7. Functional Enrichment Analysis of SLC2A1

We selected the TCGA LUAD cohort as an example to explore the underlying mechanisms of SLC2A1. Based on the median expression of SLC2A1, we divided the patients into high and low groups. After that, we conducted Gene Ontology (GO), Kyoto Encyclopedia of Genes and Genomes (KEGG), and Gene Set Enrichment Analysis

(GSEA) (www.gsea-msigdb.org/gsea/index.jsp, accessed on 14 July 2022). First, we used the "limma" package in R to screen differential expression genes (DEGs) between these two groups. We set FDR<0.05 and |log2FC| ≥ 1 as the threshold values for DEG identification. After that, the enrichGO and enrichKEGG functions of the ClusterProfiler package in Bioconductor were used to perform GO/KEGG analysis on SLC2A1-related DEGs, choosing p.adj < 0.05, q-value < 0.05, and count ≥2 as cut-off values. Second, we performed GSEA based on the HALLMARK and REACTOME gene sets. Under the condition of FDR (q-value) < 0.25 and p < 0.05, the results were considered statistically significant. In addition, we used the single-cell database CancerSEA (http://biocc.hrbmu.edu.cn/CancerSEA/, accessed on 14 July 2022) to study the potential functions of SLC2A1. The aim of the CancerSEA database is to help researchers better understand various functional states of cancer cells at the single-cell level. This database contained 41,900 cancer single cells from 25 cancers, a total of 280 cell groups, and summarized 14 functional statuses of cancer cells.

2.8. Pan-Cancer Analysis of Correlation of SLC2A1 Expression with Tumor Cell Infiltration

TME plays an important role in the occurrence and development of cancers. First, we used three algorithms, ESTIMATEScore, MCP-counter score, and EPIC [18–20], to evaluate the tumor immune infiltration in pan-cancer from the TCGA dataset via the SangerBox website (http://vip.sangerbox.com/home.html, accessed on 14 July 2022), which is a useful online platform for TCGA data analysis. Second, we compared the differences in ImmuneScore, StromalScore, and ESTIMATEScore between patients from the low-SLC2A1 and high- SLC2A1 groups with Wilcoxon signed-rank test. In addition, Spearman's correlation analysis was used to evaluate the relationship between SLC2A1 and the tumor immune infiltration evaluated by the MCP counter score and EPIC algorithms.

2.9. Correlation between SLC2A1 and Immune Checkpoint Genes, Tumor Mutation Burden (TMB), and Microsatellite Instability (MSI) in Pan-Cancer

According to a previous study [21], we collected 60 immune checkpoint (ICP) genes, which included 36 immune stimulators and 24 immune inhibitors among. Using the SangerBox tools, we analyzed the correlation between SLC2A1 expression and ICP genes. TMB [22] and MSI [23] are effective biomarkers for cancer immunotherapy. The correlations between SLC2A1 expression and TMB and MSI were also explored via the SangerBox website.

2.10. Statistical Analysis

We used R version 4.1.0 to perform the statistical analysis. Survival analysis was carried out according to Kaplan–Meier analysis, the log-rank test, and Cox regression analysis. We compared the continuous variables using Student's t-test or the Wilcoxon rank-sum test, as appropriate. Categorical clinicopathological variables were compared using the chi-square test or Fisher's exact test. Correlation analysis was performed by Pearson correlation analysis. A p-value of less than 0.05 was considered statistically significant (ns, $p ≥ 0.05$; *, $p < 0.05$; **, $p < 0.01$; ***, $p < 0.001$; ****, $p < 0.0001$).

3. Results

3.1. Pan-Cancer Expression Landscape of SLC2A1

To preliminarily understand the expression of SLC2A1 in cancers, we first evaluated SLC2A1 mRNA expression in the TCGA-GTEx pan-cancer dataset. The results revealed that SLC2A1 expression was significantly upregulated in 22 cancer types: ACC, BLCA, BRCA, CESC, CHOL, COAD, ESCA, GBM, HNSC, KIRC, LGG, LIHC, LUAD, LUSC, OV, PAAD, READ, STAD, TGCT, THCA, UCEC, and UCS. In comparison, low SLC2A1 expression was observed in five kinds of tumors: DLBC, KICH, LAML, SKCM, and THYM (Figure 1). For paired tumor and normal tissues in TCGA pan-cancer, SLC2A1 levels was were significantly higher in BRCA, CHOL, COAD, ESCA, KIRC, LIHC, LUAD, LUSC, READ, STAD, THCA, and UCEC, but lower in KICH and PRAD (Figure S1).

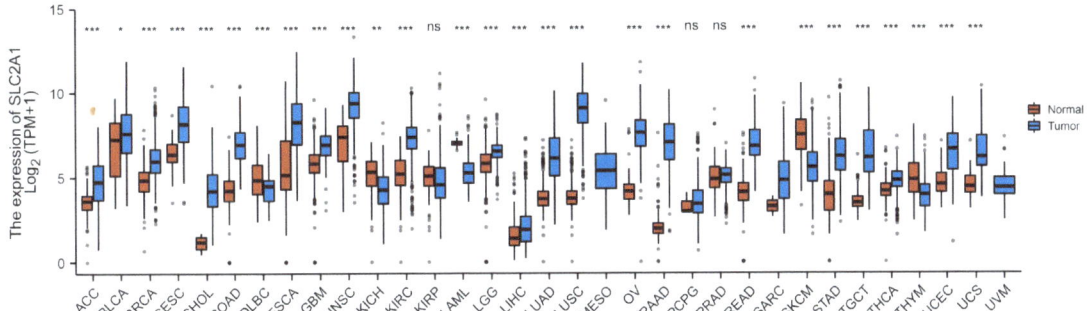

Figure 1. SLC2A1 expression in pan-cancer. ACC, adrenocortical carcinoma; BLCA, bladder urothelial carcinoma; BRCA, breast invasive carcinoma; CESC, cervical squamous cell carcinoma and endocervical adenocarcinoma; CHOL, cholangiocarcinoma; COAD, colon adenocarcinoma; DLBC, lymphoid neoplasm diffuse large B-cell lymphoma; ESCA, esophageal carcinoma; GBM, glioblastoma multiforme; HNSC, head and neck squamous cell carcinoma; KICH, kidney chromophobe; KIRC, kidney renal clear cell carcinoma; KIRP, kidney renal papillary cell carcinoma; LAML, acute myeloid leukemia; LGG, brain lower grade glioma; LIHC, liver hepatocellular carcinoma; LUAD, lung adenocarcinoma; LUSC, lung squamous cell carcinoma; MESO, mesothelioma; OV, ovarian serous cystadenocarcinoma; PAAD, pancreatic adenocarcinoma; PCPG, pheochromocytoma and paraganglioma; PRAD, prostate adenocarcinoma; READ rectum adenocarcinoma; SARC, sarcoma; SKCM, skin cutaneous melanoma; STAD, stomach adenocarcinoma; TGCT, testicular germ cell tumor; THCA, thyroid carcinoma; THYM, Thymoma; UCEC, uterine corpus endometrial carcinoma; UCS, uterine carcinosarcoma; UVM uveal melanoma(ns, $p \geq 0.05$; *, $p < 0.05$; **, $p < 0.01$; ***, $p < 0.001$).

To further validate the differential mRNA expression of SLC2A1, we comprehensively searched the GEO database and found a total of 20 relative datasets for the validation of the SLC2A1 pan-cancer analysis. As shown in Figure 2A–T, we confirmed that SLC2A1 was significantly highly expressed in 19 cancer types: ACC, BLCA, BRCA, CESC, CHOL, COAD, ESCA, HNSC, KIRC, LIHC, LUAD, LUSC, OV, PAAD, READ, STAD, TGCT, THCA, and UCEC; SLC2A1 expression was significantly lower in SKCM. Furthermore, we collected 30 pairs of samples with LUAD, 30 pairs of samples with COAD, and 30 pairs of samples with ESCA in the Sixth Affiliated Hospital of Sun Yat-Sen University. We detected the expression of SLC2A1 in the paired samples by qPCR. The results showed that the expression of SLC2A1 in LUAD ($p < 0.0001$), COAD ($p < 0.0001$), and ESCA ($p < 0.0001$) tissues was much higher than that in paired normal tissues (Figure 2U–W). The above results strongly suggested that SLC2A1 is overexpressed in most cancer tissues.

3.2. Association between SLC2A1 Expression and Clinicopathologic Parameters in Pan-Cancer

To explore the association between SLC2A1 expression and the clinicopathologic parameter of cancers, we performed differential analysis of SLC2A1 expression among different pathological stages of patients in pan-cancer. The results revealed that the expression of SLC2A1 was significantly higher in higher stages in most tumors, including ACC, CESC, COAD, COADREAD, PAAD, KIRP, LIHC, LUAD, TGCT, UCEC, and UVM (Figure 3A–K). The above results indicated that the expression of SLC2A1 is higher as pathological stage advances in most cancers

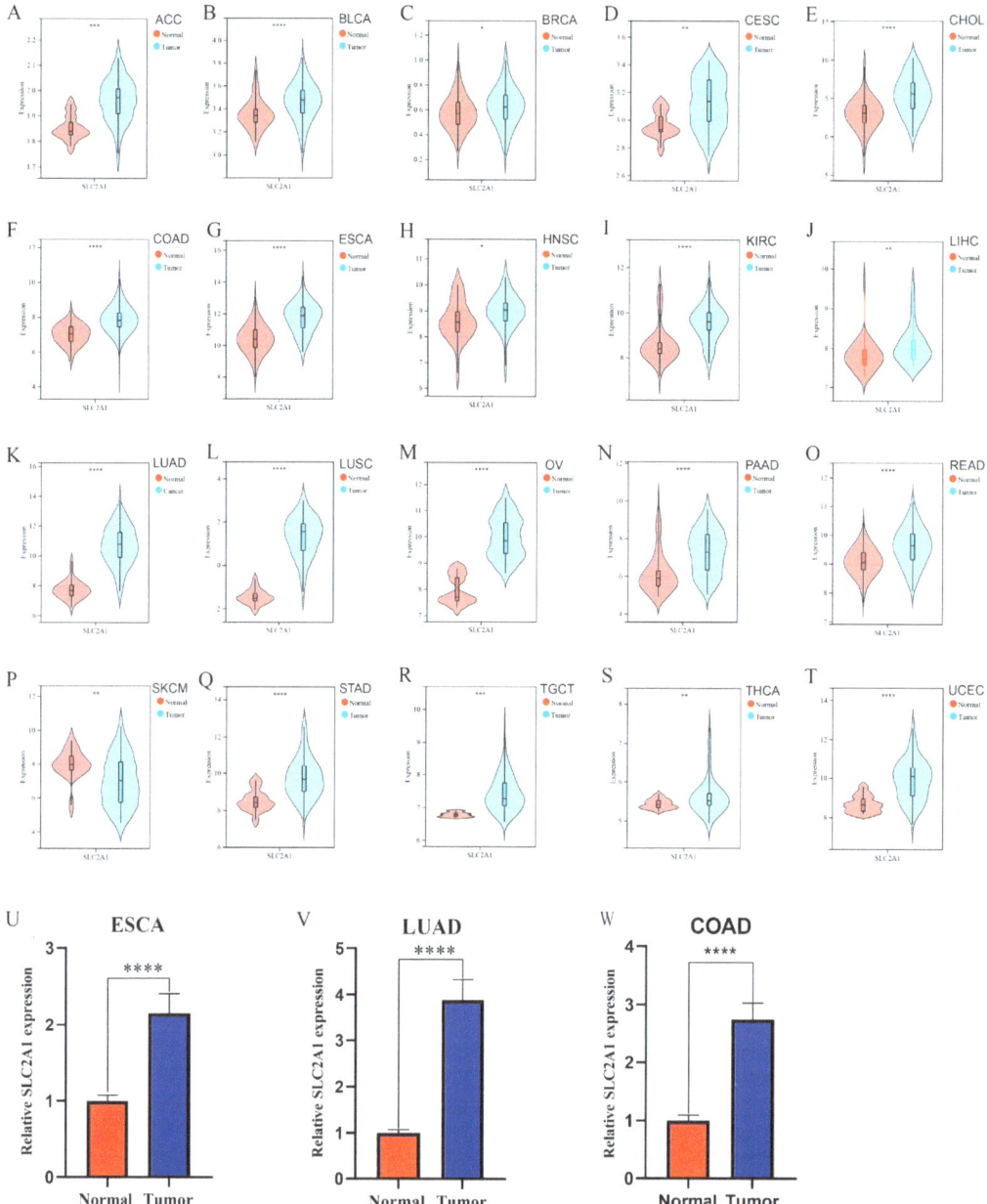

Figure 2. Validation of expression of SLC2A1 in pan-cancer. We used 20 GEO datasets for validation (**A–T**); SLC2A1 expression in 30 pairs of ESCA tissues and their normal counterparts was measured by qPCR (**U**); SLC2A1 expression in 30 pairs of LUAD tissues and their normal counterparts was measured by qPCR (**V**); SLC2A1 expression in 30 pairs of COAD tissues and their normal counterparts was measured by qPCR (**W**) (*, $p < 0.05$; **, $p < 0.01$; ***, $p < 0.001$; ****, $p < 0.0001$).

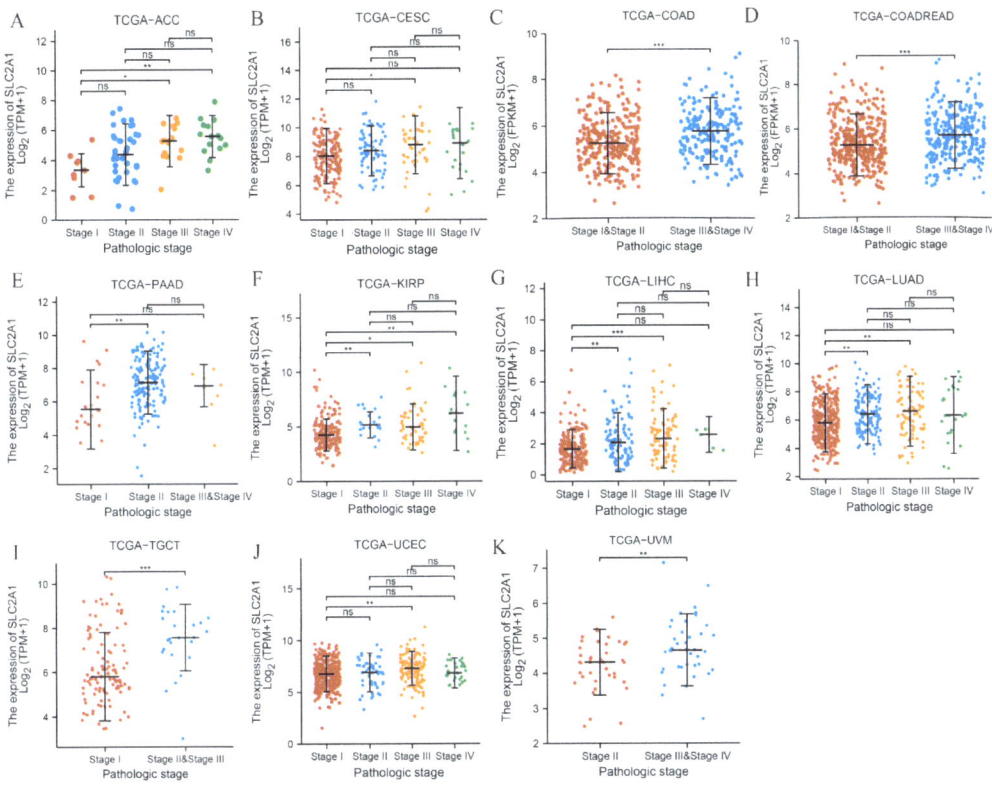

Figure 3. Pan-cancer differential expression of SLC2A1 in different pathologic stages in indicated tumor types from TCGA database (**A–K**) (ns, $p \geq 0.05$; *, $p < 0.05$; **, $p < 0.01$; ***, $p < 0.001$).

3.3. Protein Level Analysis of SLC2A1

The previous results confirmed that *SLC2A1* is highly expressed in most cancers at the mRNA level, but whether *SLC2A1* is also highly expressed at the protein level needed further exploration. We used the HPA database to verify the protein expression level of SLC2A1. The subcellular localization of SLC2A1 in cancer cells indicated that it is predominantly expressed in the plasma membrane (Figure 4A). The HPA database included 20 types of immunohistochemistry data on cancers. We found that SLC2A1 was strongly or medium stained in most cancers, but was negative or weakly stained in most normal tissues. The detailed information was as follows: lung (weak) vs. LUAD (strong), liver (negative) vs. LIHC (strong), testis (weak) vs. TGCT (strong), cervix (negative) vs. CESC (strong), thyroid (weak) vs. THCA (medium), colon (negative) vs. COAD (strong), ovary (weak) vs. OV (strong), brain (negative) vs. GBMLGG (strong), bladder (negative) vs. BLCA (strong), skin (weak) vs. SKCM (strong), pancreas (weak) vs. PAAD (strong), breast (negative) vs. BRCA (strong), kidney (weak) vs. KIRC (strong), tongue (negative) vs. HNSC (strong), and stomach (weak) vs. STAD (strong) (Figure 4B–P). The above results indicated that SLC2A1 is highly expressed in most cancers at the protein level. In addition, we analyzed the protein expression of SLC2A1 of 2002 patients across 14 cancer subtypes in the CPTAC samples based on UALCAN data. In the CPTAC samples, we found 11 proteome-based subtypes (s1–s11), and the statistical results between 2 of the 11 subtypes are shown in Table S4. High SLC2A1 expression strongly correlated with proteome-based subtype s8 (Figure 5). These findings suggested that SLC2A1 may have an important regulatory role in the progression of various cancers and may be related to the immune system process, extracellular region, and glycolysis.

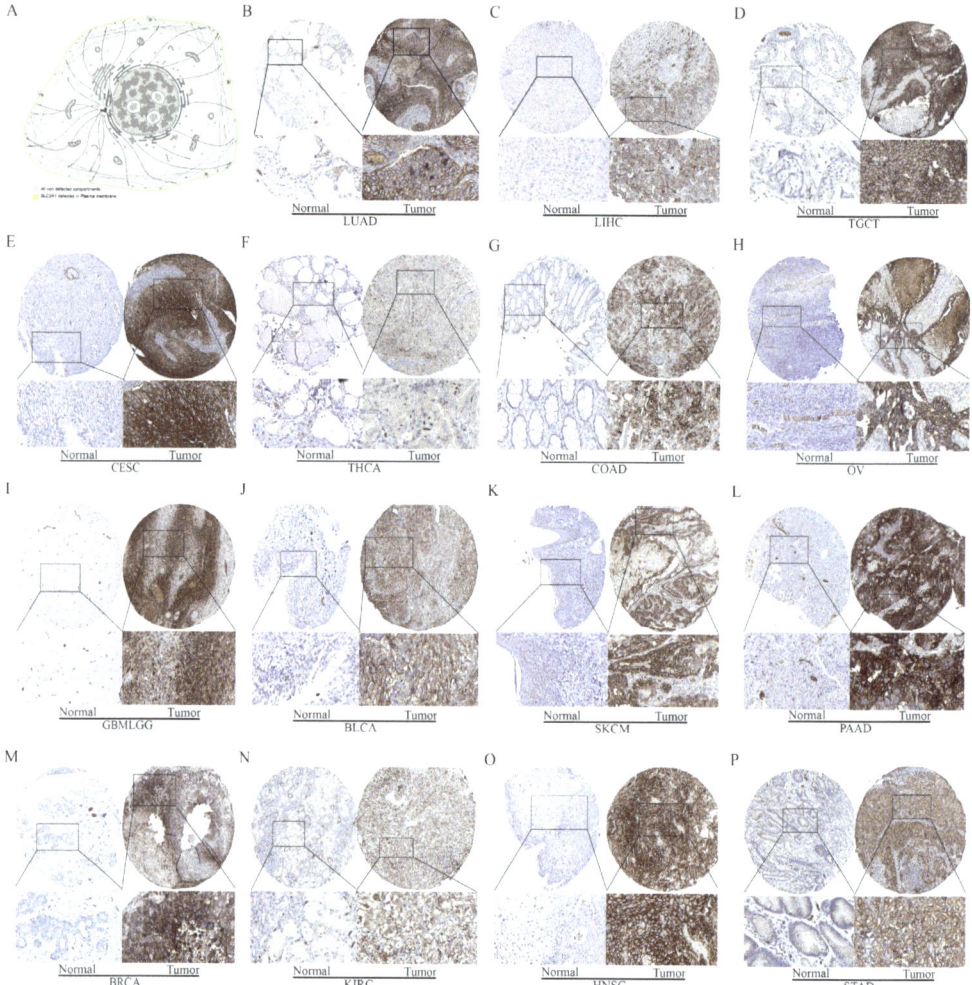

Figure 4. Protein level analysis of SLC2A1 in pan-cancer. Subcellular localization of SLC2A1 in cancer cells per the HPA database (**A**); immunohistochemical data of SLC2A1 in pan-cancer from HPA dataset (**B–P**).

3.4. Diagnostic Value of SLC2A1 in Pan-Cancer

Although we found that SLC2A1 is highly expressed in cancers compared with in normal tissues, whether SLC2A1 has diagnostic value for cancers still need further analysis. We evaluated the diagnostic value of SLC2A1 in pan-cancer by using ROC curves. AUC > 0.7 is considered high accuracy [24]. The results identified 24 cancer types (AUC > 0.7): ACC (AUC = 0.751), BRCA (AUC = 0.820), CESC (AUC = 0.814), COAD (AUC = 0.968), COADREAD (AUC = 0.962), ESCA (AUC = 0.841), GBM (AUC = 0.821), GBMLGG (AUC = 0.775), KIRC (AUC = 0.893), LAML (AUC = 0.929), LGG (AUC = 0.762), LUAD (AUC = 0.917), LUSC (AUC = 0.996), HNSC (AUC = 0.903), OV(AUC = 0.973), PAAD (AUC = 0.986), READ (AUC = 0.975), SKCM (AUC = 0.850), STAD (AUC = 0.903), TGCT (AUC = 0.960), THCA (AUC = 0.745, THYM (AUC = 0.732), UCEC (AUC = 0.865), and UCS (AUC = 0.889) (Figure 6A–X). Notably, SLC2A1 had very high accuracy in predicting COAD, COADREAD, LAML, LUAD, LUSC, HNSC, OV, PAAD, READ, STAD, and TGCT (AUC > 0.9). These results suggested that SLC2A1 may have valid pan-cancer diagnostic value.

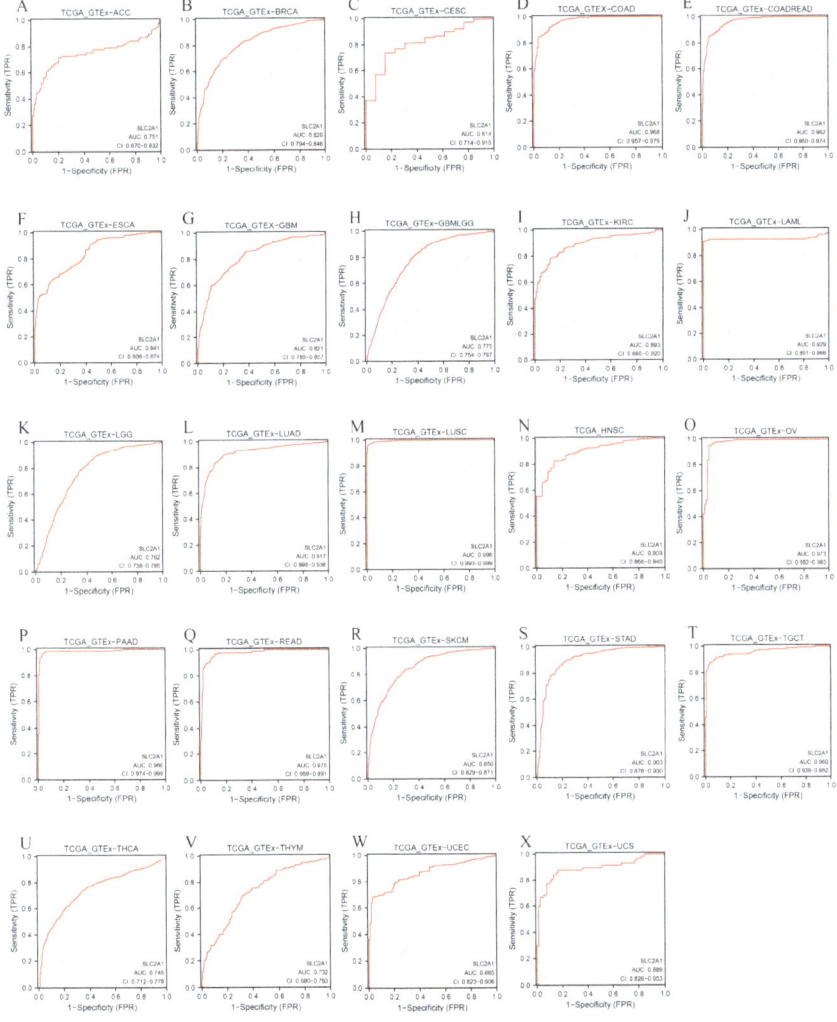

Figure 5. Protein expression of SLC2A1 across pan-cancer subtype in CPTAC samples based on UALCAN data.

Figure 6. Receiver operating characteristic (ROC) curve for SLC2A1 expression in pan-cancer (**A–X**).

3.5. Prognostic Value of SLC2A1 in Pan-Cancer

Whether the high expression of SLC2A1 in cancers affects the prognosis of patients is an issue of concern to researchers. We used two methods, Kaplan–Meier and univariate Cox regression analyses, to evaluate the prognostic value of SLC2A1 in pan-cancer. First, the results of Kaplan–Meier analysis showed that SLC2A1 was a hazard factor for the OS of patients with ACC, BLCA, CESC, GBMLGG, HNSC, KICH, KIPAN, KIRP, LGG, LIHC, LUAD, MESO, OV, PAAD, SARC, SKCM, SKCM-M, and THYM (Figure 7A–R). Second, we used univariate Cox regression analysis to evaluate the OS, PFI, DSS, and DFI of the patients. The results of OS analysis revealed that SLC2A1 acted as a hazard factor for patients with LIHC, LUAD, KIRP, MESO, ACC, PAAD, KICH, SARC, CESC, BLCA, and SKCM (Figure 8A). The results of PFI analysis showed that SLC2A1 acted as a hazard factor for patients with ACC, KICH, KIRP, PAAD, LUAD, MESO, SARC, and BLCA (Figure 8B). The results of DSS analysis indicated that SLC2A1 acted as a hazard factor for patients with KIRP, LUAD, PAAD, MESO, ACC, KICH, LIHC, SARC, and BLCA (Figure S2A). The results of DFI analysis showed that SLC2A1 acted as a hazard factor for patients with PAAD, LUAD, COAD, ACC, MESO, KIRC, and TGCT (Figure S2B). The above results suggested that patients with high expression of SLC2A1 have a poor prognosis in most cancers.

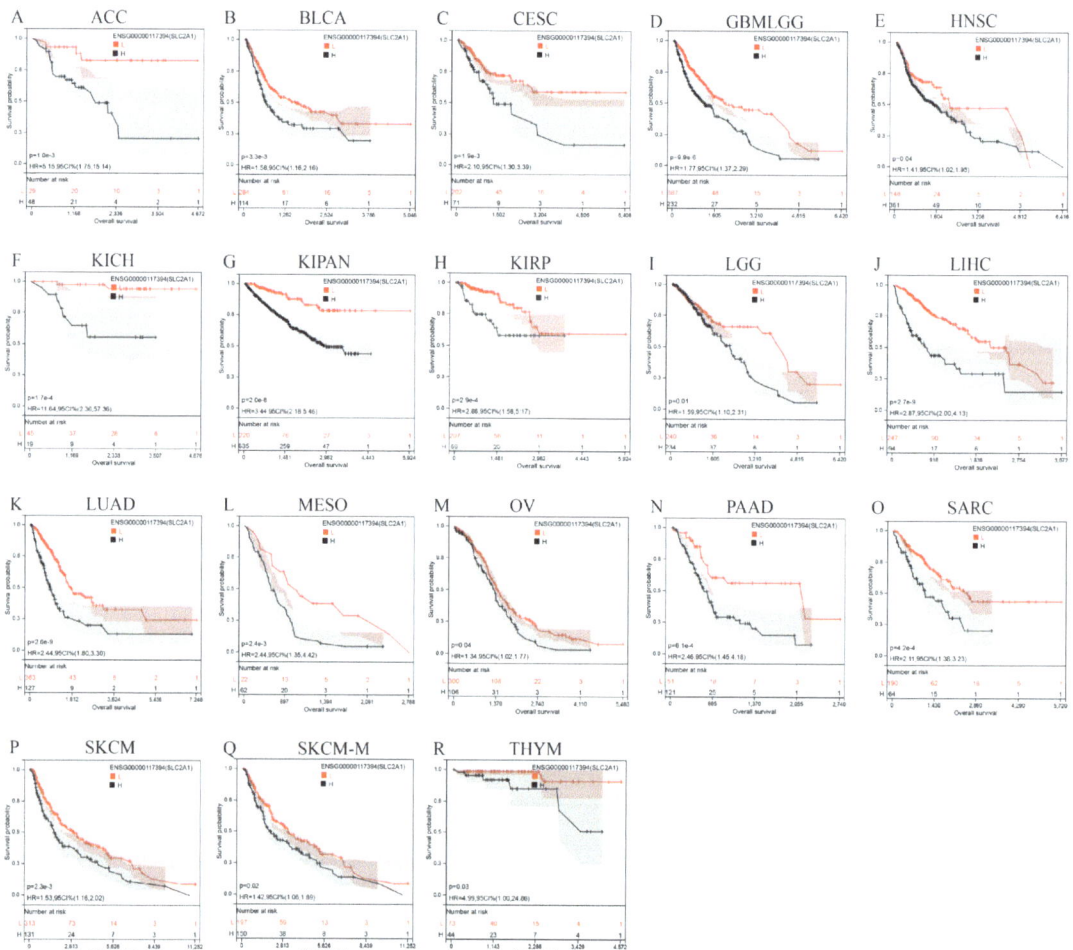

Figure 7. Pan-cancer Kaplan–Meier overall survival of SLC2A1 in indicated tumor types from TCGA database (**A–R**).

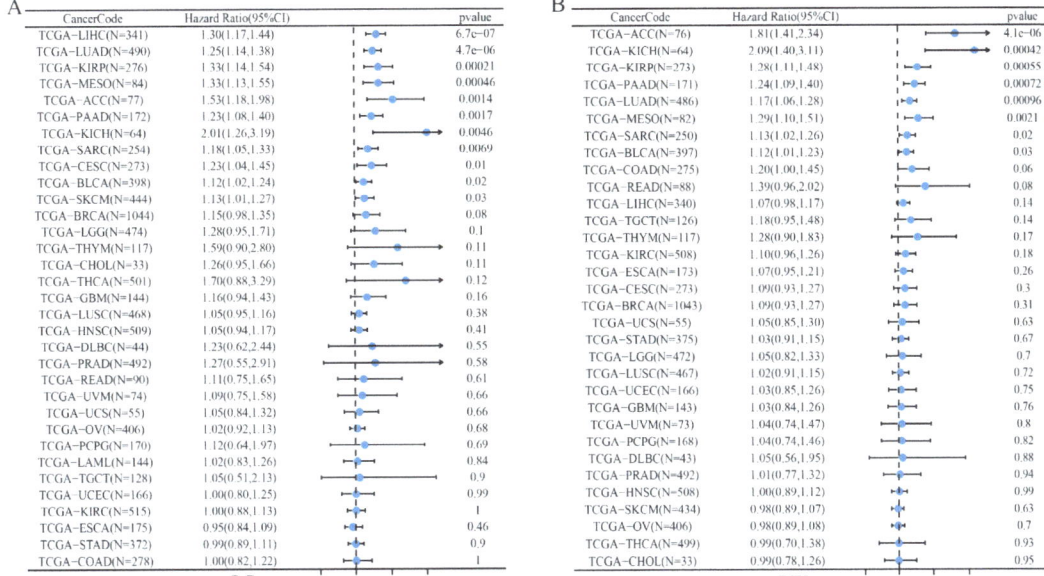

Figure 8. Univariate Cox regression analysis of SLC2A1. Forest map shows univariate Cox regression results of SLC2A1 for OS (**A**) and PFI (**B**) in pan-cancer.

3.6. Genetic Alteration Analysis of SLC2A1

The above results indicated that SLC2A1 is highly expressed in most cancers, and carries a poor prognosis. Genetic alteration is one of the key factors that affects gene expression [25]. Thus, we analyzed he genetic alteration status of SLC2A1 in the TCGA pan-cancer cohorts. We included a total of 10,967 pan-cancer patients in the cBioPortal in the study. OncoPrint showed that the overall genetic alteration rate of SLC2A1 in cancers was relatively low (only 1.8%) (Figure S3A). As shown in Figure S3B, 24 of 32 types of cancer had *SLC2A1* gene alteration data. The highest alteration frequency of SLC2A1 appeared in the ovarian carcinoma patients with "amplification" as the primary type. Additionally, amplification was the main genetic alteration type in some other cancers, such as BLCA, ESCA, SARC, LUSC, BRCA, LUAD, MESO, ACC, and LIHC, whose frequency ranged from 1% to 4%. The types and sites of the SLC2A1 mutations are further presented in Figure S3C. The results showed 80 mutation sites in the SLC2A1 gene, and the missense mutation of SLC2A1 was the main type of genetic mutation. These findings suggested that the genetic alteration status of SLC2A1 may not be the cause of the high expression of SLC2A1 in cancer tissues.

3.7. Epigenetic Analysis of SLC2A1

Epigenetic modifications, such as DNA promoter methylation and RNA m6A methylation, regulate the gene expression, thus affecting the growth and development of cancers [26]. Therefore, to explore the cause of the high expression level of SLC2A1 in cancers, we analyzed DNA promoter methylation and RNA methylation. First, we investigated DNA promoter methylation of SLC2A1 in pan-cancer by using the UALCAN database. We used 24 types of cancers in the UALCAN database to analyze the methylation of SLC2A1. The results showed that DNA methylation significantly differed in nine types of cancers compared with normal tissues. We observed a significant decrease in the methylation level of SLC2A1 in BLCA, KIRC, LIHC, LUAD, LUSC, UCEC, TGCT, and THCA (Figure 9A,C–I), and a significant increase in the level in COAD (Figure 9B). The above results suggested that SLC2A1 gene promoter methylation may be one of the reasons for the high expression level of SLC2A1 in some cancers. Moreover, we explored the correlation between SLC2A1 and m6A-methylation-related genes in pan-cancer, and the results demonstrated that most of the m6A-methylation-related genes positively correlated with the expression of SLC2A1 in 33 TCGA cancers, which suggested that m6A methylation plays an important role in the epigenetic modification of SLC2A1 (Figure 10).

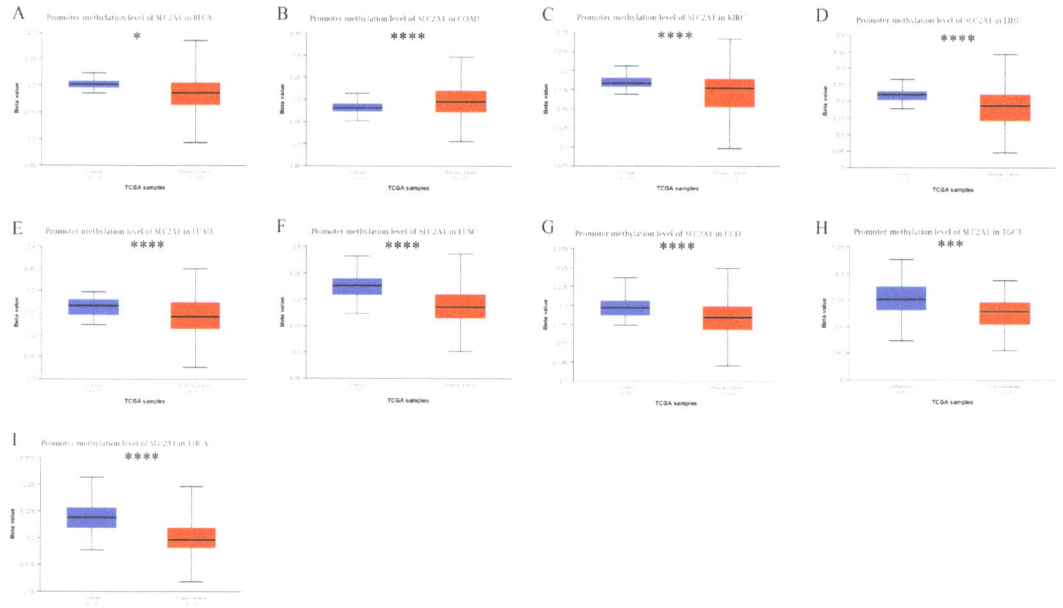

Figure 9. Promoter methylation level of SLC2A1 in pan-cancer: BLCA (**A**), COAD (**B**), KIRC (**C**), LIHC (**D**), LUAD (**E**), LUSC (**F**), UCEC (**G**), TGCT (**H**), and THCA (**I**) (*, $p < 0.05$; ***, $p < 0.001$; ****, $p < 0.0001$).

3.8. Functional Enrichment Analysis of SLC2A1

To comprehensively explore the mechanism underlying SLC2A1 leading to the poor prognosis of cancer patients, we used LUAD as an example to perform GO, KEGG, and GSEA analyses. We regarded the median value of SLC2A1 as the cut-off point. First, during GO and KEGG analyses, we detected 346 DEGs (FDR < 0.05 and $|\log 2FC| \geq 1$), of which 154 genes were downregulated and 192 genes were upregulated (Figure S4A). The heat map showed the top 50 upregulated and downregulated DEGs related to SLC2A1 (Figure S4B). Under the condition of p.adj < 0.05, q-value < 0.05, and count $\geq$ 2, we found that SLC2A1-related DEGs are involved in 269 biological process (GO-BP), 56 in cell component (GO-CC), 10 in molecular function (GO-MF), and 14 in KEGG (Table S5). The bubble graph demonstrated the top 10 messages for GO-BP, GO-CC, GO-MF, and KEGG (Figure 11A–D). The GO functional annotations showed that SLC2A1-related DEGs are mainly involved in the cell-cycle regulation, neutrophil mediated immunity, neutrophil activation, etc. The results of KEGG pathway analysis demonstrated that SLC2A1-related DEGs are primarily associated with cell cycle, glycolysis/gluconeogenesis, carbon metabolism, etc. Second, using the REACTOME and HALLMARK gene sets, we performed GSEA to identify the functional enrichment of high and low SLC2A1 expression. The results of GSEA with $|NES| > 1$, p.adj < 0.05 and q-value (FDR) < 0.25 are shown in Tables S6 and S7. The HALLMARK enrichment term showed that SLC2A1 is mainly associated with epithelial–mesenchymal transition (NES = 2.235, P = 0.003, FDR < 0.001), glycolysis (NES = 2.167, P = 0.003, FDR < 0.001), and hypoxia (NES = 2.059, P = 0.003, FDR < 0.001), (Figure 12A–C). The REACTOME enrichment term showed that SLC2A1 is mainly associated with cell-cycle checkpoints (NES = 2.455, P = 0.010, FDR = 0.006), mitotic metaphase and anaphase (NES = 2.410, P = 0.011, FDR = 0.006), and DNA repair (NES = 2.244, P = 0.011, FDR = 0.006) (Figure 12D–F). In addition, single-cell analysis can provide a profound understanding of the biological characteristics of cancer. We analyzed the correlation between SLC2A1 and 14 functional states in pan-caner by using the single-cell CancerSEA database. The results showed that SLC2A1 is mainly positively related to hypoxia, angiogenesis, epithelial–mesenchymal transition (EMT), and metastasis, and negatively related to DNA repair (Figure 12G). Collectively, the above results suggested that SLC2A1 affects the growth and development of cancers through multiple mechanisms, including immune regulation.

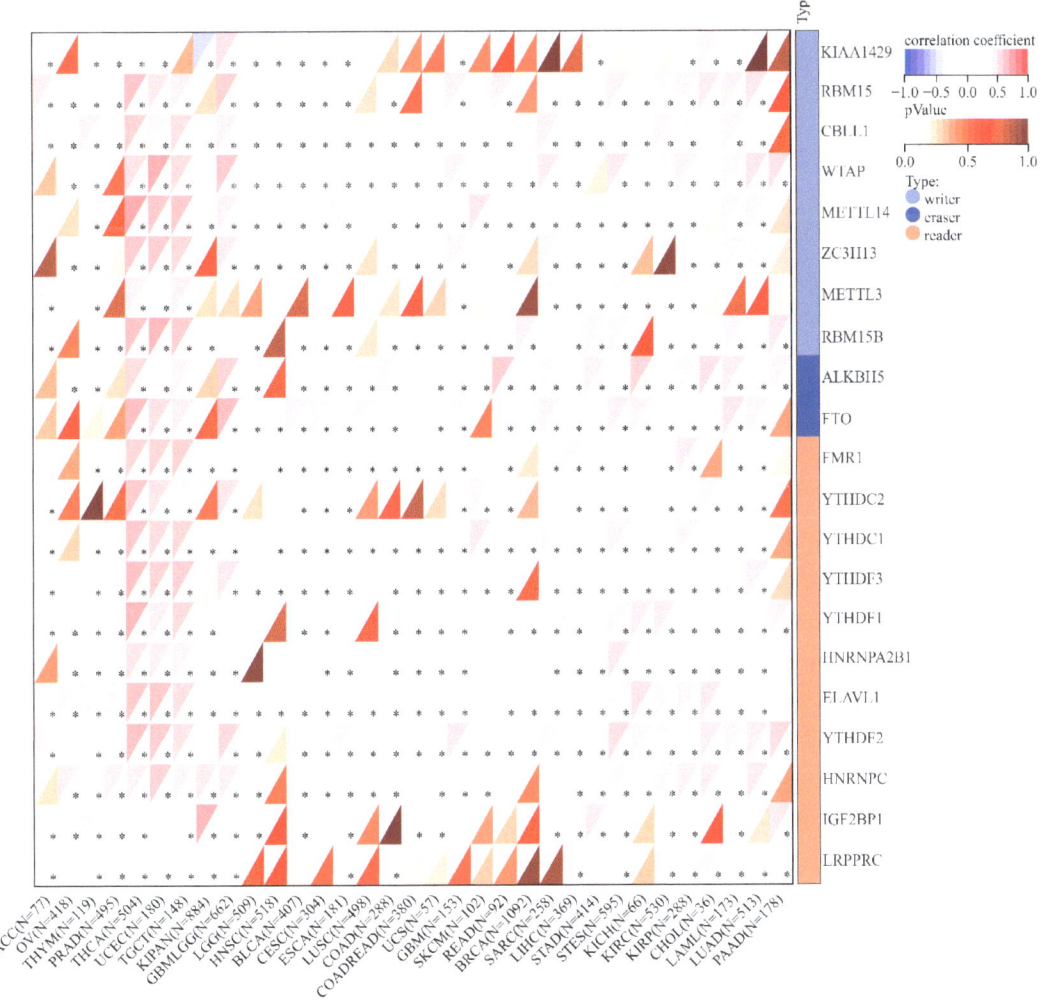

Figure 10. Relationship between SLC2A1 expression and RNA m6A-methylation-related genes in pan-cancer (*, $p < 0.05$).

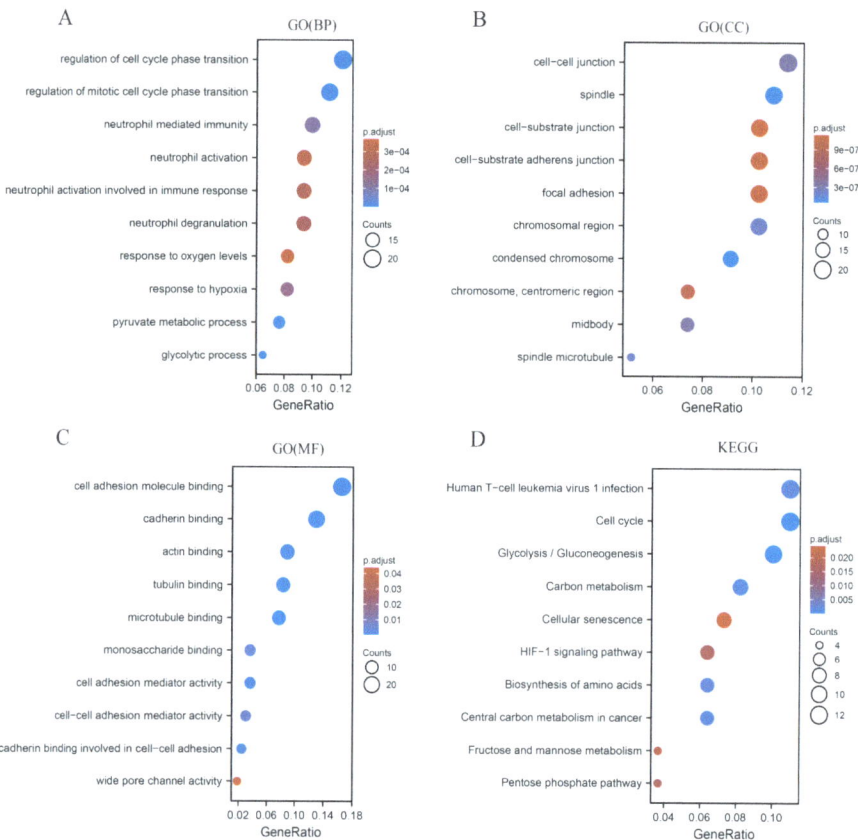

Figure 11. GO (**A–C**) and KEGG (**D**) functional enrichment analyses of SLC2A1-related DEGs in TCGA LUAD.

3.9. Immune Cell Infiltration Analysis of SLC2A1

The above results of function enrichment analysis and the protein expression of SLC2A1 across pan-cancer subtypes in the CPTAC samples suggested that SLC2A1 may be related to immune regulation, so we conducted an immune cell infiltration analysis, We used three algorithms (ESTIMATEscore, EPIC, and MCPcounter) to explore the relationship between SLC2A1 expression and immune cell infiltration of TME. First, using the ESTI-MATEscore, we found high expression levels of SLC2A1 are related to low ImmuneScore, low StromalScore, and low ESTIMATEScore in most cancers, such as ACC, BLCA, BRCA, ESCA, HNSC, LUAD, OSCC, PAAD, PRAD, SARC, SKCM, STAD, TGCT, UCEC, and UCS (Figure S5A–O). Second, using the EPIC algorithm, we found that SLC2A1 expression is positively correlated with cancer-associated fibroblasts (CAFs) in most cancers. SLC2A1 expression is negatively correlated with CD8+ T cells in 9 types of cancers (LUSC, TGCT, HNSC, CESC, LUAD, LAML, SKCM, THYM, and GBM), but positively with CD8+ T cells in 4 types of cancers (PRAD, KIPAN, UVM, and CHOL) (Figure 13A). Third, using the MCPcounter algorithm, we found that SLC2A1 expression is positively correlated with neutrophils and CAFs in most cancers. SLC2A1 expression is negatively correlated with CD8+ T cells in 11 types of cancers (LUSC, TGCT, THYM, HNSC, BRCA, SKCM, STES, GBMLGG, GBM, PAAD, and ESCA), but positively with CD8+ T cells in 5 types of cancers (KIPAN, LIHC, LAML, PCPG, and CHOL) (Figure 13B). The above results indicated that SLC2A1 has an impact on the infiltration of immune cells in the TME of most cancers and is especially positively correlated with neutrophils and CAFs in the TME.

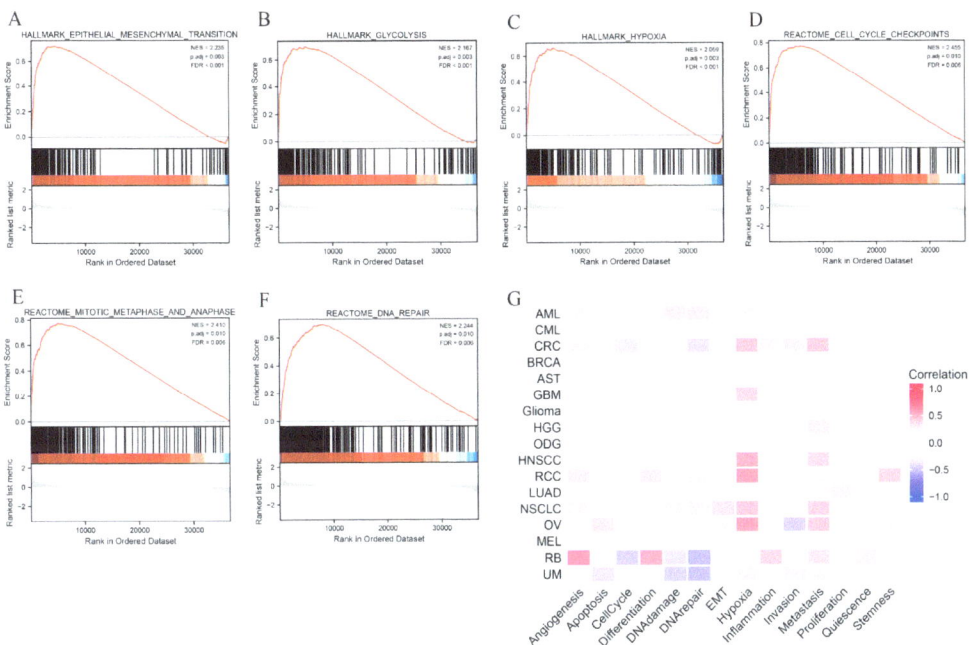

Figure 12. GSEA of SLC2A1-related DEGs based on HALLMARK gene sets (**A–C**) and based on REACTOME gene sets (**D–F**); single-cell analysis based on the CancerSEA database (**G**).

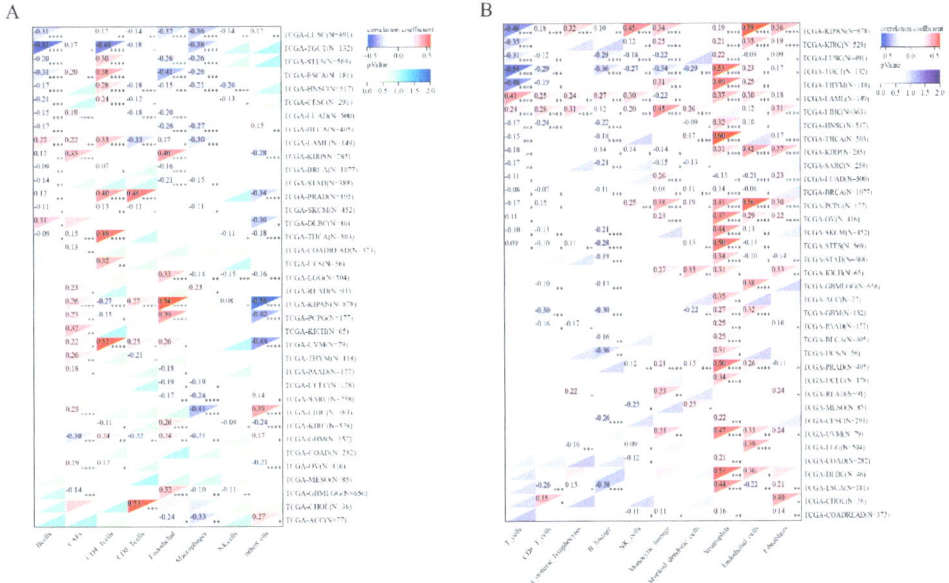

Figure 13. Correlation between SLC2A1 and immune cell infiltration. Heatmap represents correlation between SLC2A1 expression and immune cell infiltration using the EPIC (**A**) and MCPcounter (**B**) algorithms (*, $p < 0.05$; **, $p < 0.01$; ***, $p < 0.001$; ****, $p < 0.0001$).

3.10. SLC2A1 Related to Immune Checkpoint (ICP) Genes, TMB, and MSI in Human Cancers

Immune surveillance affects the growth and development of cancer cells, and cancer cells evade immune responses by taking advantage of ICP [27]. ICP genes are divided into two major categories: immunoinhibitors and immunostimulators. As such, we investigated the associations between SLC2A1 expression and the two main types of immune modulators in human cancers to explore the potential function of SLC2A1 in immunotherapy. The results showed a certain correlation between SLC2A1 and immune modulators in all 33 tumor types. We found that the expression of SLC2A1 is positively correlated with most immunoinhibitors and immunostimulators in LAML, LIHC, UVM, THCA, PCPG, PRAD, OV, READ, KIRC, KIPAN, DLBC, and THYM. In contrast, the expression of SLC2A1 is negatively correlated with most immunoinhibitors and immunostimulators in TGCT, ESCA, STES, HNSC, and LUSC. Notably, SLC2A1 is remarkably positively correlated with CD274 (PD-L1) and CTLA4 in most cancers (Figure 14). These findings suggested that SLC2A1 may affect the immune checkpoint blockade treatment response in human cancers.

TMB and MSI are two new biomarkers that reflect the response of immunotherapy. So, we explored the correlation between SLC2A1 expression and TMB, and MSI. The expression of SLC2A11 is significantly positively correlated with TMB in most cancers, including PAAD, ACC, LUAD, THYM, GBM, SARC, STAD, CESC, BRCA, GBMLGG, STES, and HNSC, but negatively correlated with TMB in SKCM (Figure 15A). We also investigated the correlation of the SLC2A1 expression with MSI in pan-cancer: ACC, UVM, TGCT, SARC, STAD, and STES exhibited positive correlations; DLBC, KIPAN, GBMLGG, and PRAD exhibited negative correlations (Figure 15B). The above results indicated that SLC2A1 may be used to predict the response to immunotherapy.

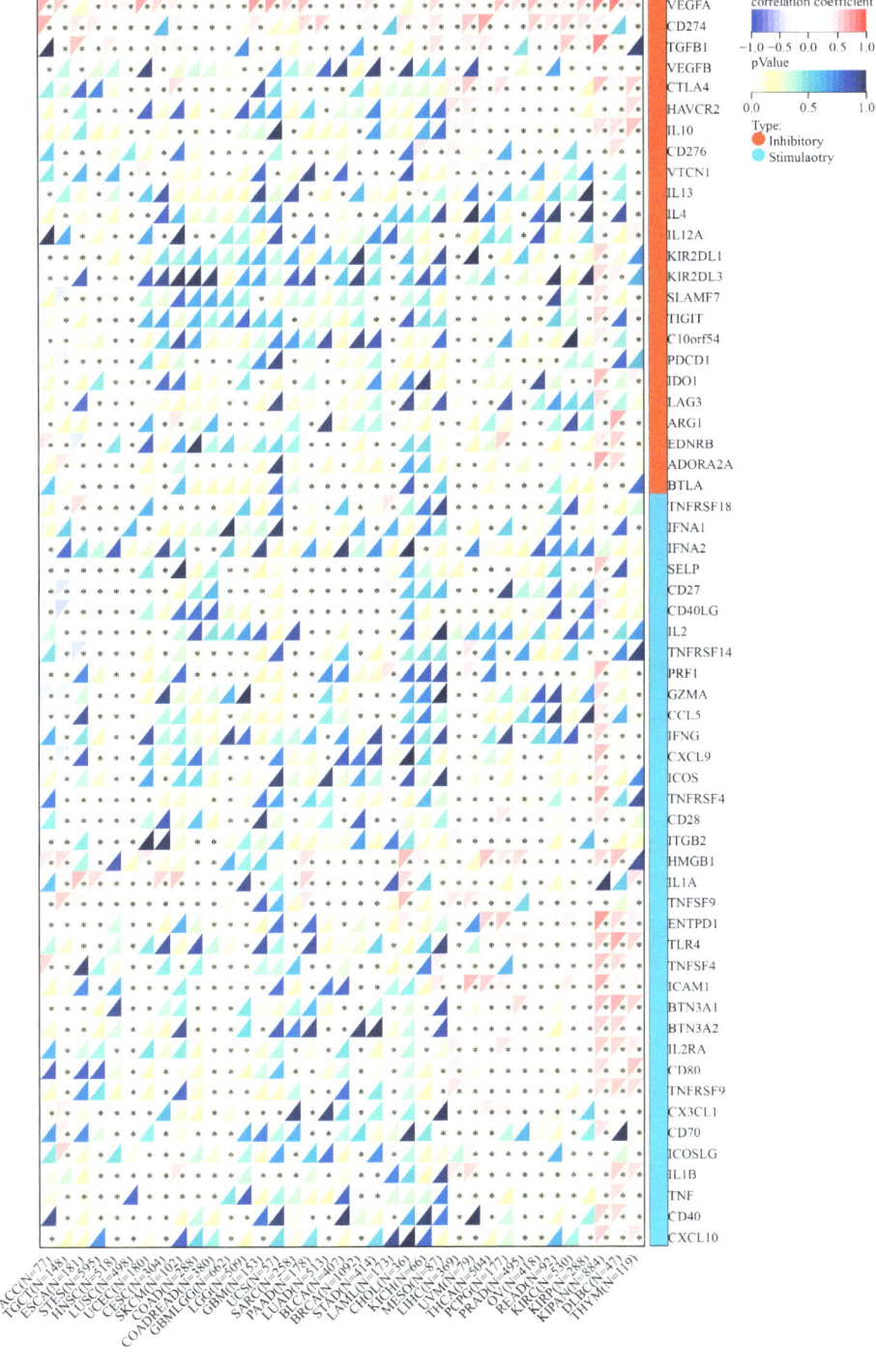

Figure 14. Correlation between SLC2A1 and ICP genes (*, $p < 0.05$).

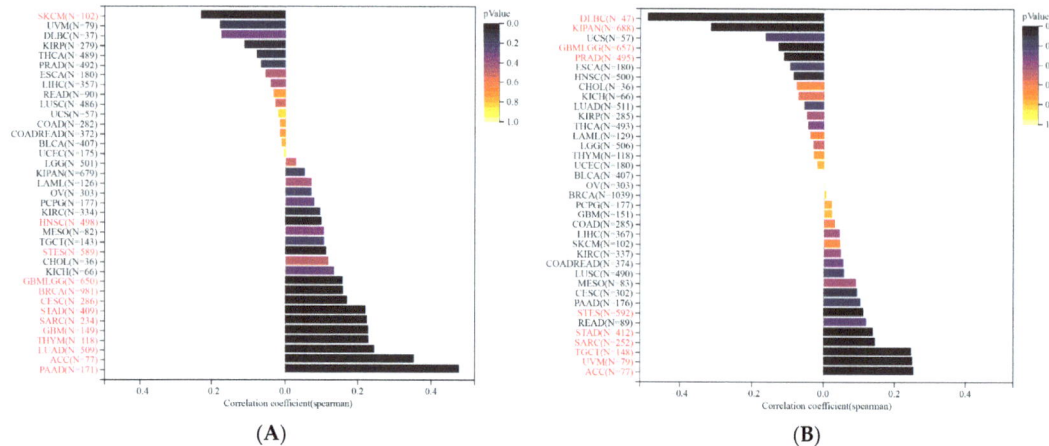

Figure 15. Correlation of SLC2A1 expression with TMB (**A**) and MSI (**B**) in pan-cancer.

4. Discussion

The increase in glycolysis is one of the main characteristics of glycometabolism in cancer cells [28]. The *SLC2A1* gene is one of the key genes in cancer glycometabolism, which promotes the glycolysis of cancer cells, thus affecting their growth and metastasis [29,30]. Studies on SLC2A1 in pan-cancer analysis were previously lacking. This is the first study in which the role of SLC2A1 at the pan-cancer level was explored.

In our study, based on the TCGA-GTEx pan-cancer dataset, we found that SLC2A1 is highly expressed in most cancers compared with normal tissues, which we further confirmed via the GEO datasets, protein expression data from the HPA database, and our own data. Additionally, the expression of SLC2A1 is significantly upregulated in higher pathologic stages in various cancers. Previous studies have reported that SLC2A1 is highly expressed in a variety of cancers, such as BLCA, LUAD, LIHC, CESC, COAD, OV, UCEC, BRCA, STAD, ESCA, and PAAD [11–15,31–37]. These results are consistent with our research results. In addition, the results of the ROC analysis of pan-cancers revealed that the AUC values of most cancers were greater than 0.7. Therefore, our results suggested that SLC2A1 may play an important role in the growth and metabolism of cancers, and they support the possibility of SLC2A1 being used as a biomarker for the diagnosis of pan-cancer.

The evaluation of the prognostic value of SLC2A1 is an indispensable part of our study. We assessed the prognostic value of SLC2A1 in pan-cancer by using Kaplan–Meier and Cox regression analyses. The results showed that SLC2A1 is a hazard factor for the OS of patients in most cancers. Mortality from noncancerous causes may not reflect tumor biology, aggressiveness, or response to therapy. Additionally, a longer follow-up time is required for using OS. Therefore, to more accurately reflect the impact of SLC2A1 on the prognosis of patients, we further conducted a univariate COX analysis for PFI, DFI, and DSS of patients. The results also showed that SLC2A1 is a hazard factor for the PFI, DFI and DSS of patients in various cancers. These results indicated that high SLC2A1 expression mainly plays a hazardous role in patient prognosis for most cancer types. The high expression of SLC2A1 in cancers is often associated with poor prognosis [38,39].

To study why SLC2A1 is highly expressed in pan-cancer, we performed genetic alteration, DNA promoter methylation, and RNA m6A methylation analyses. We found that the overall mutation rate of SLC2A1 in pan-cancer is only 1.8%, which could not explain the high transcriptome expression of SLC2A1 in most cancers. Klepper et al. reported that Glut1 deficiency syndromes are due to SLC2A1 genetic variation [40]. Therefore, we think that genetic alteration is not the main cause of the high expression of SLC2A1. In addition, DNA promoter methylation can regulate gene expression without changing the DNA sequence, which is one of the main forms of DNA epigenetic modification [41]. A higher level of DNA promoter methylation means lower expression of the corresponding gene [42]. We found hypomethylation in the SLC2A1 promoter region in various cancer tissues, which might, to some extent, explain the SLC2A1 mRNA overexpression in the corresponding cancers. Furthermore, RNA m6A methylation is an important mechanism affecting the regulation of RNA expression. We collected 21 RNA m6A-methylation-related genes and performed pan-cancer correlation analysis between SLC2A1 and m6A-methylation-related genes, finding that they are significantly correlated in pan-cancer. This indicated that the mechanism of m6A methylation may play a vital role in the regulation of SLC2A1 expression in cancer tissues. Shen et al. demonstrated that the m6A-IGF2BP2/3-dependent mechanism inhibits the mRNA degradation of SLC2A1 in colorectal cancer [43]. Some other mechanisms may lead to the overexpression of SLC2A1, for example, histone modification on chromosomes [44] or RNA m1A/m5C modification [45]. We did not consider these potential mechanisms in this study.

The mechanism of SLC2A1 in pan-cancer has rarely been explored. LUAD is one of the most common cancer types. In our study, we found that SLC2A1 is highly expressed in LUAD, and was related to a poor prognosis in terms of OS, PFI, DSS, and DFI, so we took LUAD as the representative tumor in the GO, KEGG, and GSEA analyses of SLC2A1. The results showed that SLC2A1 is mainly associated with hypoxia, EMT, glycolysis, cell-cycle regulation, DNA repair, and neutrophil-mediated immunity. Single-cell sequencing can help us better understand the biological features of cancers, to achieve the goal of more precise cancer treatment [46,47]. In our study, we used the single-cell database CancerSEA to explore the function of SLC2A1 in pan-cancer. We discovered that SLC2A1 is remarkably positively related to hypoxia, EMT, and metastasis, and negatively related to DNA repair, which was roughly consistent with the bulk analysis. Most of these functions of SLC2A1 have been studied in various types of cancers. For example, hypoxia induces GLUT1 overexpression in various cancers [48]; Azadeh Nilchian et al. revealed that overexpression of GLUT1 can make breast cancer cells produce stable EMT and promote proliferation during chronic TGF-β1 exposure [49]; Zhang et al. revealed that GLUT1 S-palmitoylation mediated by DHHC9 promotes glycolysis and tumorigenesis in glioblastoma [50]. Takahashi et al. reported that Glut-1 knockdown also induces cell-cycle arrest in pancreas cancer cells [51]; Kim et al. found that increased GLUT1 expression can repair damaged DDR in SALL4-deficient human cancer cells [52]. In summary, SLC2A1 may be overexpressed in cancers tissues by hypoxia and promote cancer-cell proliferation and metastasis by regulating cancer glycometabolism, the cell-cycle checkpoint, DNA repair process, and EMT.

The TME plays a key role in the support of tumor progression, invasiveness, and metastasis [53]. In our study, we found that high SLC2A1 expression strongly correlates with proteome-based subtypes s8. A previous study [16] demonstrated that s8 is related to the immune system process, extracellular region, and glycolysis. Therefore, we explored the relationship of SLC2A1 expression with immune cell infiltration by using three algorithms (ESTIMATEScore, EPIC, and MCPcounter). We found that high expression of SLC2A1 corresponds to low immune, stromal and ESTIMATE scores in the TME in most cancer types, which indicated that SLC2A1 might be mainly expressed by cancer cells. In addition, SLC2A1 is positively correlated with the neutrophils and CAFs in the TME in most cancers. Neutrophils and CAFs in the TME promote tumor proliferation and metastasis [54–56]. Thus, SLC2A1 may promote tumor proliferation and metastasis by affecting neutrophils and CAFs in the TME. Ancey et al. revealed that the radiotherapy resistance of lung cancer depends on GLUT1-mediated glucose uptake in tumor-associated neutrophils [54]. Sun et al. discovered that phosphorylating GLUT1 enhances glycolytic activity of the CAFs in breast cancer to promote cancer-cell invasion by activating the TGFβ1/p38 MAPK/MMP2/9 signaling axis [57]. CD8+ T cells are an important component of cancer immunity. Our findings showed that SLC2A1 is positively correlated with CD8+ T cells in some cancer types, but negatively correlated in other cancer types, suggesting that the effect of SLC2A1 on CD8+ T cells in the TME is complex.

ICP genes affect the immune cell infiltration of the TME and cancer immunotherapy [58]. As such, we analyzed the relationship between the SLC2A1 expression and ICP genes. The results showed a certain correlation between SLC2A1 and ICP genes in all 33 tumors. This indicated that SLC2A1 has an impact on immune function in the TME. Notably, SLC2A1 is remarkably positively correlated with CD274 (PD-L1) and CTLA4 in most cancers. Young Wha Koh et al. demonstrated that PD-L1 protein and mRNA expressions are correlated with GLUT1 expression in lung adenocarcinoma [59]. PD-L1 and CTLA4 are the essential biomarkers of T cell exhaustion [60]. The definition of T-cell exhaustion is that the T-cell functions of patients with common chronic infection or cancer is impaired or even lost. Therefore, the expression of SLC2A1 results in the T-cell exhaustion of the TME. MSI and TMB are the biomarkers for predicting cancer immunotherapy response [22,23]. We performed a correlation analysis between SLC2A1 and TMB and MSI, and we found that SLC2A1 expression is significantly correlated with TMB in 13 cancer types and with MSI in 10 cancer types. Additionally, PD-L1 and CTLA4 are the main targets of clinical immunotherapy. This indicated that SLC2A1 may be considered as a biomarker to predict the response to immunotherapy.

The limitations in our study should be considered when generalizing the findings. First, our results were mainly generated from bioinformatics analysis. In vivo and in vitro experiments are needed to prove our results regarding the potential function of SLC2A1. Second, the microarray and sequencing data from different databases might have caused systematic bias. Third, the data used in this study were retrospective. Our results should thus be further confirmed by prospective studies in the future. Finally, no anti-SLC2A1 therapeutic monoclonal antibodies have yet been evaluated in clinical trials. Therefore, we have no specific and complete cases with data to identify the benefit of anti-SLC2A1-targeting drugs in the survival of cancer.

5. Conclusions

SLC2A1 may play a crucial role in cancer cell proliferation and metastasis through multiple mechanisms, such as regulating the cell-cycle checkpoint, DNA repair process, EMT, CAFs and neutrophils in the TME, and T-cell exhaustion. SLC2A1 might serve as a novel pan-cancer diagnostic and prognostic biomarker and provide an opportunity to develop new immunotherapy strategies.

Supplementary Materials: The following supporting information can be downloaded at: https://www.mdpi.com/article/10.3390/cancers14215344/s1, Figure S1: SLC2A1 expression in TCGA cancers and adjacent normal tissues(ns, $p \geq 0.05$; *, $p < 0.05$; **, $p < 0.01$; ***, $p < 0.001$); Figure S2: Univariate Cox regression analysis of SLC2A1. Forest map shows the univariate Cox regression results of SLC2A1 for DSS (A) and DFI (B) in pan-cancer; Figure S3. SLC2A1 genetic alterations in pan-cancer analyzed using cBioPortal database. OncoPrint of SLC2A1 genetic alterations in pan-cancer (different colors mean different types of genetic alterations) (A); SLC2A1 alteration types and frequency of pan-cancer (B); mutation types and sites of SLC2A1 gene (C); Figure S4: Identification of DEGs related to SLC2A1. Volcano plot depicts the 346 DEGs ($|\log2FC| > 1$; FDR < 0.05) in TCGA LUAD group of high vs. low expression of SLC2A1 (A); heatmap shows top 50 upregulated and downregulated DEGs (B); Figure S5: Differences in TME between high-SLC2A1 and low-SLC2A1 were evaluated by ESTIMATEScore algorithm(ns, $p \geq 0.05$; *, $p < 0.05$; **, $p < 0.01$; ***, $p < 0.001$); Table S1: Abbreviations of all cancer types; Table S2: Basic information of GEO datasets in the study; Table S3: Pan-cancer proteome-based subtypes (s1 to s11) in UALCAN database; Table S4: Pan-cancer proteinomic analysis of SLC2A1; Table S5: GO/KEGG analysis of SLC2A1-related DEGs; Table S6: GSEA of SLC2A1 based on HALLMARK gene sets; Table S7: GSEA of SLC2A1 based on REACTOME gene sets.

Author Contributions: H.Z. and X.Q. conceived and designed the study. H.Z., G.L., Y.Z., X.Y. and W.C. performed the data analysis. H.Z., X.Q., G.L. and S.H. analyzed and interpreted the results. H.Z. wrote the original manuscript. H.Z. and H.L. reviewed and revised the manuscript. All authors have read and agreed to the published version of the manuscript.

Funding: This study was funded by Supporting funds for scientific research of the Sixth Affiliated Hospital, Sun Yat-sen University, grant number P20200217202404781.

Institutional Review Board Statement: The study was conducted in accordance with the Declaration of Helsinki, and approved by the clinical research ethics committee of the Sixth Affiliated Hospital of Sun Yat-sen University (2022ZSLYEC-351, 12 August 2022).

Informed Consent Statement: Informed consent was obtained from all subjects involved in the study. Written informed consent was obtained from the patients to publish this paper.

Data Availability Statement: Publicly available datasets were analyzed in this study. TCGA and GTEx data can be found here: (UCSC) Xena browser (https://xena.ucsc.edu/, accessed on 14 July 2022) and the Genotype-Tissue Expression (GTEx) database (https://www.gtexportal.org/home/-index.html, accessed on 14 July 2022); GSE2088, GSE13507, GSE10927, GSE39001, GSE26566, GSE18520, GSE53757, GSE62452, GSE87211, GSE15605, GSE33630, GSE3218, GSE17025, GSE47861, GSE68468, GSE53625, GSE13601, GSE57927, GSE75037, and GSE26899 datasets from GEO database(https://www.ncbi.nlm.nih.gov/geo, accessed on 14 July 2022). The original contributions presented in the study are included in the article. Further inquiries can be directed to the corresponding authors.

Acknowledgments: We thank Sangerbox tools and Xiantao Academic Tools for providing technical advice on our bioinformatics analysis.

Conflicts of Interest: The authors declare no conflict of interest.

References

1. Luo, Q.; Zhang, L.; Luo, C.; Jiang, M. Emerging Strategies in Cancer Therapy Combining Chemotherapy with Immunotherapy. *Cancer Lett.* **2019**, *454*, 191–203. [CrossRef] [PubMed]
2. Yang, Y. Cancer Immunotherapy: Harnessing the Immune System to Battle Cancer. *J. Clin. Investig.* **2015**, *125*, 3335–3337. [CrossRef] [PubMed]
3. Marcus, L.; Lemery, S.J.; Keegan, P.; Pazdur, R. FDA Approval Summary: Pembrolizumab for the Treatment of Microsatellite Instability-High Solid Tumors. *Clin. Cancer Res.* **2019**, *25*, 3753–3758. [CrossRef] [PubMed]
4. Li, F.; Wu, T.; Xu, Y.; Dong, Q.; Xiao, J.; Xu, Y.; Li, Q.; Zhang, C.; Gao, J.; Liu, L.; et al. A Comprehensive Overview of Oncogenic Pathways in Human Cancer. *Brief. Bioinform.* **2020**, *21*, 957–969. [CrossRef]
5. Boroughs, L.K.; DeBerardinis, R.J. Metabolic Pathways Promoting Cancer Cell Survival and Growth. *Nat. Cell Biol.* **2015**, *17*, 351–359. [CrossRef]
6. Pavlova, N.N.; Thompson, C.B. The Emerging Hallmarks of Cancer Metabolism. *Cell Metab.* **2016**, *23*, 27–47. [CrossRef]
7. Biswas, S.K. Metabolic Reprogramming of Immune Cells in Cancer Progression. *Immunity* **2015**, *43*, 435–449. [CrossRef]
8. Cao, S.; Chen, Y.; Ren, Y.; Feng, Y.; Long, S. GLUT1 Biological Function and Inhibition: Research Advances. *Future Med. Chem.* **2021**, *13*, 1227–1243. [CrossRef]
9. Masoud, G.N.; Li, W. HIF-1α Pathway: Role, Regulation and Intervention for Cancer Therapy. *Acta Pharm. Sin. B* **2015**, *5*, 378–389. [CrossRef]
10. Pereira, K.M.A.; Chaves, F.N.; Viana, T.S.A.; Carvalho, F.S.R.; Costa, F.W.G.; Alves, A.P.N.N.; Sousa, F.B. Oxygen Metabolism in Oral Cancer: HIF and GLUTs (Review). *Oncol. Lett.* **2013**, *6*, 311–316. [CrossRef]
11. Avanzato, D.; Pupo, E.; Ducano, N.; Isella, C.; Bertalot, G.; Luise, C.; Pece, S.; Bruna, A.; Rueda, O.M.; Caldas, C.; et al. High USP6NL Levels in Breast Cancer Sustain Chronic AKT Phosphorylation and GLUT1 Stability Fueling Aerobic Glycolysis. *Cancer Res.* **2018**, *78*, 3432–3444. [CrossRef] [PubMed]
12. Sun, H.-W.; Yu, X.-J.; Wu, W.-C.; Chen, J.; Shi, M.; Zheng, L.; Xu, J. GLUT1 and ASCT2 as Predictors for Prognosis of Hepatocellular Carcinoma. *PLoS ONE* **2016**, *11*, e0168907. [CrossRef] [PubMed]
13. Berlth, F.; Mönig, S.; Pinther, B.; Grimminger, P.; Maus, M.; Schlösser, H.; Plum, P.; Warnecke-Eberz, U.; Harismendy, O.; Drebber, U.; et al. Both GLUT-1 and GLUT-14 Are Independent Prognostic Factors in Gastric Adenocarcinoma. *Ann. Surg. Oncol.* **2015**, *22* (Suppl. S3), 822–831. [CrossRef] [PubMed]
14. Goldman, N.A.; Katz, E.B.; Glenn, A.S.; Weldon, R.H.; Jones, J.G.; Lynch, U.; Fezzari, M.J.; Runowicz, C.D.; Goldberg, G.L.; Charron, M.J. GLUT1 and GLUT8 in Endometrium and Endometrial Adenocarcinoma. *Mod. Pathol.* **2006**, *19*, 1429–1436. [CrossRef]
15. Smolle, E.; Leko, P.; Stacher-Priehse, E.; Brcic, L.; El-Heliebi, A.; Hofmann, L.; Quehenberger, F.; Hrzenjak, A.; Popper, H.H.; Olschewski, H.; et al. Distribution and Prognostic Significance of Gluconeogenesis and Glycolysis in Lung Cancer. *Mol. Oncol.* **2020**, *14*, 2853–2867. [CrossRef]
16. Zhang, Y.; Chen, F.; Chandrashekar, D.S.; Varambally, S.; Creighton, C.J. Proteogenomic Characterization of 2002 Human Cancers Reveals Pan-Cancer Molecular Subtypes and Associated Pathways. *Nat. Commun.* **2022**, *13*, 2669. [CrossRef]
17. Jiang, X.; Liu, B.; Nie, Z.; Duan, L.; Xiong, Q.; Jin, Z.; Yang, C.; Chen, Y. The Role of M6A Modification in the Biological Functions and Diseases. *Signal Transduct. Target. Ther.* **2021**, *6*, 74. [CrossRef]

18. Yoshihara, K.; Shahmoradgoli, M.; Martínez, E.; Vegesna, R.; Kim, H.; Torres-Garcia, W.; Treviño, V.; Shen, H.; Laird, P.W.; Levine, D.A.; et al. Inferring Tumour Purity and Stromal and Immune Cell Admixture from Expression Data. *Nat. Commun.* **2013**, *4*, 2612. [CrossRef]
19. Becht, E.; Giraldo, N.A.; Lacroix, L.; Buttard, B.; Elarouci, N.; Petitprez, F.; Selves, J.; Laurent-Puig, P.; Sautès-Fridman, C.; Fridman, W.H.; et al. Estimating the Population Abundance of Tissue-Infiltrating Immune and Stromal Cell Populations Using Gene Expression. *Genome Biol.* **2016**, *17*, 218. [CrossRef]
20. Racle, J.; de Jonge, K.; Baumgaertner, P.; Speiser, D.E.; Gfeller, D. Simultaneous Enumeration of Cancer and Immune Cell Types from Bulk Tumor Gene Expression Data. *Elife* **2017**, *6*, e26476. [CrossRef]
21. Thorsson, V.; Gibbs, D.L.; Brown, S.D.; Wolf, D.; Bortone, D.S.; Ou Yang, T.-H.; Porta-Pardo, E.; Gao, G.F.; Plaisier, C.L.; Eddy, J.A.; et al. The Immune Landscape of Cancer. *Immunity* **2018**, *48*, 812–830.e14. [CrossRef] [PubMed]
22. Sha, D.; Jin, Z.; Budczies, J.; Kluck, K.; Stenzinger, A.; Sinicrope, F.A. Tumor Mutational Burden as a Predictive Biomarker in Solid Tumors. *Cancer Discov.* **2020**, *10*, 1808–1825. [CrossRef] [PubMed]
23. Bonneville, R.; Krook, M.A.; Kautto, E.A.; Miya, J.; Wing, M.R.; Chen, H.Z.; Reeser, J.W.; Yu, L.; Roychowdhury, S. Landscape of Microsatellite Instability Across 39 Cancer Types. *JCO Precis. Oncol.* **2017**, *1*, 1–15. [CrossRef]
24. Nahm, F.S. Receiver Operating Characteristic Curve: Overview and Practical Use for Clinicians. *Korean J. Anesthesiol.* **2022**, *75*, 25–36. [CrossRef] [PubMed]
25. Matharu, N.; Ahituv, N. Modulating Gene Regulation to Treat Genetic Disorders. *Nat. Rev. Drug Discov.* **2020**, *19*, 757–775. [CrossRef]
26. Chen, Y.; Hong, T.; Wang, S.; Mo, J.; Tian, T.; Zhou, X. Epigenetic Modification of Nucleic Acids: From Basic Studies to Medical Applications. *Chem Soc. Rev.* **2017**, *46*, 2844–2872. [CrossRef]
27. Muenst, S.; Läubli, H.; Soysal, S.D.; Zippelius, A.; Tzankov, A.; Hoeller, S. The Immune System and Cancer Evasion Strategies: Therapeutic Concepts. *J. Intern. Med.* **2016**, *279*, 541–562. [CrossRef]
28. Li, Z.; Zhang, H. Reprogramming of Glucose, Fatty Acid and Amino Acid Metabolism for Cancer Progression. *Cell. Mol. Life Sci.* **2016**, *73*, 377–392. [CrossRef]
29. Ooi, A.T.; Gomperts, B.N. Molecular Pathways: Targeting Cellular Energy Metabolism in Cancer via Inhibition of SLC2A1 and LDHA. *Clin. Cancer Res.* **2015**, *21*, 2440–2444. [CrossRef]
30. Ancey, P.-B.; Contat, C.; Meylan, E. Glucose Transporters in Cancer—from Tumor Cells to the Tumor Microenvironment. *FEBS J.* **2018**, *285*, 2926–2943. [CrossRef]
31. Massari, F.; Ciccarese, C.; Santoni, M.; Iacovelli, R.; Mazzucchelli, R.; Piva, F.; Scarpelli, M.; Berardi, R.; Tortora, G.; Lopez-Beltran, A.; et al. Metabolic Phenotype of Bladder Cancer. *Cancer Treat. Rev.* **2016**, *45*, 46–57. [CrossRef] [PubMed]
32. Wang, X.; He, H.; Rui, W.; Zhang, N.; Zhu, Y.; Xie, X. TRIM38 Triggers the Uniquitination and Degradation of Glucose Transporter Type 1 (GLUT1) to Restrict Tumor Progression in Bladder Cancer. *J. Transl. Med.* **2021**, *19*, 508. [CrossRef] [PubMed]
33. Kim, B.W.; Cho, H.; Chung, J.-Y.; Conway, C.; Ylaya, K.; Kim, J.-H.; Hewitt, S.M. Prognostic Assessment of Hypoxia and Metabolic Markers in Cervical Cancer Using Automated Digital Image Analysis of Immunohistochemistry. *J. Transl. Med.* **2013**, *11*, 185. [CrossRef] [PubMed]
34. Zhao, J.; Chen, Y.; Liu, F.; Yin, M. Overexpression of MiRNA-143 Inhibits Colon Cancer Cell Proliferation by Inhibiting Glucose Uptake. *Arch. Med. Res.* **2018**, *49*, 497–503. [CrossRef]
35. Cho, H.; Lee, Y.S.; Kim, J.; Chung, J.-Y.; Kim, J.-H. Overexpression of Glucose Transporter-1 (GLUT-1) Predicts Poor Prognosis in Epithelial Ovarian Cancer. *Cancer Investig.* **2013**, *31*, 607–615. [CrossRef]
36. Zhao, X.; Huang, Q.; Koller, M.; Linssen, M.D.; Hooghiemstra, W.T.R.; de Jongh, S.J.; van Vugt, M.A.T.M.; Fehrmann, R.S.N.; Li, E.; Nagengast, W.B. Identification and Validation of Esophageal Squamous Cell Carcinoma Targets for Fluorescence Molecular Endoscopy. *Int. J. Mol. Sci.* **2021**, *22*, 9270. [CrossRef]
37. Sung, J.-Y.; Kim, G.Y.; Lim, S.-J.; Park, Y.-K.; Kim, Y.W. Expression of the GLUT1 Glucose Transporter and P53 in Carcinomas of the Pancreatobiliary Tract. *Pathol. Res. Pract.* **2010**, *206*, 24–29. [CrossRef]
38. Osugi, J.; Yamaura, T.; Muto, S.; Okabe, N.; Matsumura, Y.; Hoshino, M.; Higuchi, M.; Suzuki, H.; Gotoh, M. Prognostic Impact of the Combination of Glucose Transporter 1 and ATP Citrate Lyase in Node-Negative Patients with Non-Small Lung Cancer. *Lung Cancer* **2015**, *88*, 310–318. [CrossRef]
39. Yu, M.; Zhou, Q.; Zhou, Y.; Fu, Z.; Tan, L.; Ye, X.; Zeng, B.; Gao, W.; Zhou, J.; Liu, Y.; et al. Metabolic Phenotypes in Pancreatic Cancer. *PLoS ONE* **2015**, *10*, e0115153. [CrossRef]
40. Klepper, J.; Akman, C.; Armeno, M.; Auvin, S.; Cervenka, M.; Cross, H.J.; de Giorgis, V.; Della Marina, A.; Engelstad, K.; Heussinger, N.; et al. Glut1 Deficiency Syndrome (Glut1DS): State of the Art in 2020 and Recommendations of the International Glut1DS Study Group. *Epilepsia Open* **2020**, *5*, 354–365. [CrossRef]
41. Mehdi, A.; Rabbani, S.A. Role of Methylation in Pro- and Anti-Cancer Immunity. *Cancers* **2021**, *13*, 545. [CrossRef] [PubMed]
42. Wang, M.; Ngo, V.; Wang, W. Deciphering the Genetic Code of DNA Methylation. *Brief. Bioinform.* **2021**, *22*, bbaa424. [CrossRef] [PubMed]
43. Shen, C.; Xuan, B.; Yan, T.; Ma, Y.; Xu, P.; Tian, X.; Zhang, X.; Cao, Y.; Ma, D.; Zhu, X.; et al. M6A-Dependent Glycolysis Enhances Colorectal Cancer Progression. *Mol. Cancer* **2020**, *19*, 72. [CrossRef]
44. Lawrence, M.; Daujat, S.; Schneider, R. Lateral Thinking: How Histone Modifications Regulate Gene Expression. *Trends Genet.* **2016**, *32*, 42–56. [CrossRef]

45. Zhao, B.S.; Roundtree, I.A.; He, C. Post-Transcriptional Gene Regulation by MRNA Modifications. *Nat. Rev. Mol. Cell Biol.* **2017**, *18*, 31–42. [CrossRef] [PubMed]
46. Lei, Y.; Tang, R.; Xu, J.; Wang, W.; Zhang, B.; Liu, J.; Yu, X.; Shi, S. Applications of Single-Cell Sequencing in Cancer Research: Progress and Perspectives. *J. Hematol. Oncol.* **2021**, *14*, 91. [CrossRef]
47. Dusny, C.; Grünberger, A. Microfluidic Single-Cell Analysis in Biotechnology: From Monitoring towards Understanding. *Curr. Opin. Biotechnol.* **2020**, *63*, 26–33. [CrossRef]
48. Tirpe, A.A.; Gulei, D.; Ciortea, S.M.; Crivii, C.; Berindan-Neagoe, I. Hypoxia: Overview on Hypoxia-Mediated Mechanisms with a Focus on the Role of HIF Genes. *Int. J. Mol. Sci.* **2019**, *20*, E6140. [CrossRef]
49. Nilchian, A.; Giotopoulou, N.; Sun, W.; Fuxe, J. Different Regulation of Glut1 Expression and Glucose Uptake during the Induction and Chronic Stages of TGFβ1-Induced EMT in Breast Cancer Cells. *Biomolecules* **2020**, *10*, E1621. [CrossRef]
50. Zhang, Z.; Li, X.; Yang, F.; Chen, C.; Liu, P.; Ren, Y.; Sun, P.; Wang, Z.; You, Y.; Zeng, Y.-X.; et al. DHHC9-Mediated GLUT1 S-Palmitoylation Promotes Glioblastoma Glycolysis and Tumorigenesis. *Nat. Commun.* **2021**, *12*, 5872. [CrossRef]
51. Takahashi, M.; Nojima, H.; Kuboki, S.; Horikoshi, T.; Yokota, T.; Yoshitomi, H.; Furukawa, K.; Takayashiki, T.; Takano, S.; Ohtsuka, M. Comparing Prognostic Factors of Glut-1 Expression and Maximum Standardized Uptake Value by FDG-PET in Patients with Resectable Pancreatic Cancer. *Pancreatology* **2020**, *20*, 1205–1212. [CrossRef] [PubMed]
52. Kim, J.; Xu, S.; Xiong, L.; Yu, L.; Fu, X.; Xu, Y. SALL4 Promotes Glycolysis and Chromatin Remodeling via Modulating HP1α-Glut1 Pathway. *Oncogene* **2017**, *36*, 6472–6479. [CrossRef] [PubMed]
53. Hinshaw, D.C.; Shevde, L.A. The Tumor Microenvironment Innately Modulates Cancer Progression. *Cancer Res.* **2019**, *79*, 4557–4566. [CrossRef] [PubMed]
54. Ancey, P.-B.; Contat, C.; Boivin, G.; Sabatino, S.; Pascual, J.; Zangger, N.; Perentes, J.Y.; Peters, S.; Abel, E.D.; Kirsch, D.G.; et al. GLUT1 Expression in Tumor-Associated Neutrophils Promotes Lung Cancer Growth and Resistance to Radiotherapy. *Cancer Res.* **2021**, *81*, 2345–2357. [CrossRef]
55. Biffi, G.; Tuveson, D.A. Diversity and Biology of Cancer-Associated Fibroblasts. *Physiol. Rev.* **2021**, *101*, 147–176. [CrossRef]
56. Kaltenmeier, C.; Yazdani, H.O.; Morder, K.; Geller, D.A.; Simmons, R.L.; Tohme, S. Neutrophil Extracellular Traps Promote T Cell Exhaustion in the Tumor Microenvironment. *Front. Immunol.* **2021**, *12*, 785222. [CrossRef]
57. Sun, K.; Tang, S.; Hou, Y.; Xi, L.; Chen, Y.; Yin, J.; Peng, M.; Zhao, M.; Cui, X.; Liu, M. Oxidized ATM-Mediated Glycolysis Enhancement in Breast Cancer-Associated Fibroblasts Contributes to Tumor Invasion through Lactate as Metabolic Coupling. *EBioMedicine* **2019**, *41*, 370–383. [CrossRef]
58. Topalian, S.L.; Drake, C.G.; Pardoll, D.M. Immune Checkpoint Blockade: A Common Denominator Approach to Cancer Therapy. *Cancer Cell* **2015**, *27*, 450–461. [CrossRef]
59. Koh, Y.W.; Lee, S.J.; Han, J.-H.; Haam, S.; Jung, J.; Lee, H.W. PD-L1 Protein Expression in Non-Small-Cell Lung Cancer and Its Relationship with the Hypoxia-Related Signaling Pathways: A Study Based on Immunohistochemistry and RNA Sequencing Data. *Lung Cancer* **2019**, *129*, 41–47. [CrossRef]
60. Wherry, E.J. T Cell Exhaustion. *Nat. Immunol.* **2011**, *12*, 492–499. [CrossRef]

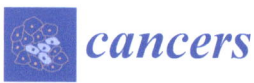

Article

A Novel Role of SMG1 in Cholesterol Homeostasis That Depends Partially on p53 Alternative Splicing

Muyang Li [1,*], Fredrick Philantrope [1], Alexandra Diot [2], Jean-Christophe Bourdon [2] and Patricia Thompson [1,*]

[1] Department of Pathology, Renaissance School of Medicine, Stony Brook University, New York, NY 11794, USA; fphilantrope@gmail.com
[2] Division of Cancer Research, University of Dundee, Ninewells Hospital and Medical School, Dundee DD1 9SY, Scotland, UK; a.z.diot@dundee.ac.uk (A.D.); j.bourdon@dundee.ac.uk (J.-C.B.)
* Correspondence: muyanglee@gmail.com (M.L.); Patricia.Thompson@cshs.org (P.T.)

Simple Summary: p53 isoforms have been reported in various tumor types. Both p53β and p53γ were recently reported to retain functionalities of full-length p53α. A role for p53 and p53 loss in cholesterol metabolism has also emerged. We show that SMG1, a phosphatidylinositol 3-kinase-related kinase, when inhibited in p53 wild-type MCF7 and HepG2 cells, significantly alters the expression of cholesterol pathway genes, with a net increase in intracellular cholesterol and an increased sensitivity to Fatostatin in MCF7. We confirm a prior report that SMG1 inhibition in MCF7 cells promotes expression of p53β and show the first evidence for increases in p53γ. Further, induced p53β expression, confirmed with antibody, explained the loss of SMG1 upregulation of the ABCA1 cholesterol exporter where p53γ had no effect on ABCA1. Additionally, upregulation of ABCA1 upon SMG1 knockdown was independent of upregulation of nonsense-mediated decay target RASSF1C, previously suggested to regulate ABCA1 via a "RASSF1C-miR33a-ABCA1" axis.

Citation: Li, M.; Philantrope, F.; Diot, A.; Bourdon, J.-C.; Thompson, P. A Novel Role of SMG1 in Cholesterol Homeostasis That Depends Partially on p53 Alternative Splicing. *Cancers* 2022, *14*, 3255. https://doi.org/10.3390/cancers14133255

Academic Editor: Paola Tucci

Received: 31 May 2022
Accepted: 29 June 2022
Published: 2 July 2022

Publisher's Note: MDPI stays neutral with regard to jurisdictional claims in published maps and institutional affiliations.

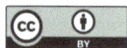

Copyright: © 2022 by the authors. Licensee MDPI, Basel, Switzerland. This article is an open access article distributed under the terms and conditions of the Creative Commons Attribution (CC BY) license (https://creativecommons.org/licenses/by/4.0/).

Abstract: SMG1, a phosphatidylinositol 3-kinase-related kinase (PIKK), essential in nonsense-mediated RNA decay (NMD), also regulates p53, including the alternative splicing of p53 isoforms reported to retain p53 functions. We confirm that SMG1 inhibition in MCF7 tumor cells induces p53β and show p53γ increase. Inhibiting SMG1, but not UPF1 (a core factor in NMD), upregulated several cholesterol pathway genes. SMG1 knockdown significantly increased ABCA1, a cholesterol efflux pump shown to be positively regulated by full-length p53 (p53α). An investigation of RASSF1C, an NMD target, increased following SMG1 inhibition and reported to inhibit miR-33a-5p, a canonical ABCA1-inhibiting miRNA, did not explain the ABCA1 results. ABCA1 upregulation following SMG1 knockdown was inhibited by p53β siRNA with greatest inhibition when p53α and p53β were jointly suppressed, while p53γ siRNA had no effect. In contrast, increased expression of MVD, a cholesterol synthesis gene upregulated in p53 deficient backgrounds, was sensitive to combined targeting of p53α and p53γ. Phenotypically, we observed increased intracellular cholesterol and enhanced sensitivity of MCF7 to growth inhibitory effects of cholesterol-lowering Fatostatin following SMG1 inhibition. Our results suggest deregulation of cholesterol pathway genes following SMG1 knockdown may involve alternative p53 programming, possibly resulting from differential effects of p53 isoforms on cholesterol gene expression.

Keywords: SMG1; p53β; ABCA1; cholesterol; mevalonate; RASSF1C; miR-33a-5p; statin

1. Introduction

SMG1 (suppressor with morphogenetic effect on genitalia), the most recently characterized phosphatidylinositol 3-kinase-related kinase (PIKK) family member, is highly conserved across organisms [1]. Similar to structurally homologous PIKK proteins ATM and ATR, SMG1 plays a role in genome stress response (GSR) including activity to phosphorylate p53 on serine 15 [2–5]. Phosphorylation of p53 is a key step in stabilizing p53, making it more resistant to ubiquitination-mediated degradation by MDM2 [6]. SMG1 is best characterized for its role as an essential kinase in the phosphorylation of the DNA/RNA helicase UPF1, via a SMG1-SMG8-SMG9 complex, which is the first and rate-limiting step of nonsense-mediated RNA decay (NMD) [7–9]. NMD is a RNA quality control and gene regulatory mechanism that mediates the recognition and rapid clearance of mRNAs harboring premature termination codon (PTC) [10]. Thus, SMG1 functions uniquely in NMD and overlaps that of ATM and ATR to phosphorylate p53. With this duality of function, SMG1 has emerged in recent years as a putative tumor suppressor [4,11,12] and cancer drug target [13], though the relative importance of SMG1 in tumor biology remains unclear.

Since the late 1980s [14,15], the presence of p53 isoforms derived from alternative splicing have been observed in a variety of human cancers [16]. Experimental works support both distinct and overlapping functions of p53 isoforms with full-length p53 (p53α) [17–20]. To date, nine p53 mRNAs and at least thirteen p53 peptide variants have been reported (reviewed in [21]). On the 5′ of p53 gene, there are two promotors, P1 and P2, and two internal ribosome entry sites (IRES), ATG40 and ATG160. P1 initiates two distinct forms of p53 mRNAs, fully spliced mRNAs and intron-2 retaining mRNAs. These two types of mRNA translate into two types of N-terminal variants: the most prevalent full-length p53, which is translated from fully spliced mRNA; Δ40p53, which can be translated from ATG40 of either fully spliced mRNA or the intron-2 retaining mRNA. Both Δ133 and Δ160 are launched by P2 (which serves as introns and exons in P1-initiated mRNAs), while Δ160 begins with the alternative start codon ATG160. On the C-terminus, p53 has three distinct C-termini (Figure 2A). Despite the full-length α, β and γ, result from two 'cryptic' exons, 9β and 9γ, and the stop codons following them. Both 9β and 9γ have putative PTCs hypothesized as targets of NMD [22]. This is supported by Tang et al. who showed that inhibiting two NMD pathway components, SMG7 or UPF1, increased the expression of p53β [22]. More recent, Gudikote et. al. showed that pharmacologic inhibition of NMD or inhibition of UPF1 increased the expression of p53β and p53γ in MDM2 overexpressing and p53 mutant cell lines [23]. These investigators postulate that p53β and p53γ isoforms 'restore' p53 functionality in p53 deficient cells. However, Chen et. al. [24] provided evidence suggesting that SMG1 directly suppresses alternative splicing of p53 intron 9 by binding p53 pre-mRNA near exon 8–10. Loss of SMG1 was found to promote binding of ribosomal protein L26 (RPL26) to p53 pre-mRNA and to the recruitment of the Serine/Arginine-rich splicing factors (SRSFs), SRSF7, and expression of p53β protein. Earlier work from Tang et. al. [25] also supports a role for splicing factors. In their studies, downregulation of SRSF3 in early passage fibroblasts was mechanistically linked to alternative splicing of p53β and replicative senescence.

We are similarly interested in the effects of SMG1 on p53, p53 isoforms and their function. This includes their role in the context of work from the Prives laboratory [26,27] that identified a link between p53 and cholesterol synthesis and transport including effects on the expression of the ATP binding cassette transporter A1 (ABCA1), a transmembrane protein transporter of cholesterol [28]. The Prives group was the first to show that loss (knockout) of wild type p53 or missense mutations in p53 resulted in ABCA1 mRNA downregulation, whereas stabilization of wildtype p53 with Nutlin-3 (inhibitor of Mdm2) increased ABCA1 at the RNA and protein level. Intriguingly, loss of p53 or ABCA1 promoted sterol regulatory element-binding protein 2 (SREBP2) maturation from its uncleaved precursor and upregulation of mevalonate pathway genes involved in cholesterol synthesis. In contrast, the accumulation of wild-type p53 following Nutlin-3 treatment suppressed mevalonate (MVA) pathway signals. A follow-up study concluded that p53 inhibits cholesterol synthesis in a SREBP2 independent manner by transcriptionally suppressing squalene epoxidase (SQLE), a rate-limiting enzyme in sterol synthesis [29]. Findings from these studies have been replicated in vivo in mouse models.

On interest in SMG1, as well as NMD, as a therapeutic target for cancer [30,31] and findings that overexpression of p53β in advanced stage breast cancers is associated with better patient outcomes [32], we confirm that SMG1 knockdown increases p53β isoform protein with specific antibody. Further, we show the first evidence that SMG1 inhibition also increases transcription of the p53γ isoform. Similarly to Chen et al., we did not find an increase in p53β after targeting UPF1 for NMD-only effects. Interestingly, inhibition of SMG1, but not UPF1 in MCF7 and HepG2 cells, led to a significant alteration in cholesterol homeostasis, including increased expression of both the MVA pathway genes and ABCA1. On hypothesized effects of p53 to modulate cholesterol synthesis in tumor cells, we investigated SMG1 induced p53β and p53γ isoforms for effects on ABCA1 and cholesterol pathway genes and on the sensitivity of MCF7 to cholesterol lowering drugs following SMG1 knockdown.

2. Materials and Methods

2.1. Cell Culture and Transfection

MCF7(HTB-22), HepG2 (HB-806), and NCI-H1299 (CRL-5803) were purchased from ATCC. MCF7 was cultured in DMEM (high glucose, Gibco) with 10%FBS and 1% pen-strep. HepG2 (HB-806) and H1299 was cultured in RPMI-1640 (Gibco) with 10%FBS and 1% pen-strep. For experiments shorter than 72 h and/or with cytotoxic treatments (plasmid transfection, drug treatment, etc), cells were plated in 6-well or 24-well plates at a starting confluency of 70%. For experiments longer than 96 h (siRNA transfection), cells were plated at a lower starting confluency of 30% to prevent overconfluent.

Pre-designed siRNAs were purchased from GE Dharmacon™ (non-targeting, SMG1, GAPDH, UPF1) and Thermo Fisher Silencer Select™ (ABCA1, SREBP2, SMG1, RASSF1). Customized siRNAs of p53 isoforms were synthesized following previous publication [33]. See Supplemental List S2 for details. All siRNAs were transfected with Lipofectamine™ RNAiMAX (Thermo Fisher, Waltham, MA, USA) following official protocol.

Plasmids and plasmids/siRNA combination are transfected via Lipofectamine™ 3000 (Thermo Fisher). Due to the cytotoxicity, we used reduced amount of transfection reagent and higher seeding density. For example, to transfect MCF7 plated in 6-well plate, 6 μL reagent and 2.5 μg of DNA are used per well, and 80% confluency is required at time of transfection.

2.2. Cell Viability Analysis

Viability was assayed by Cell Counting Kit-8 as described by the manufacturer (CCK-8, Dojindo, Rockville, MD, USA). Briefly, CCK-8 reagent was added to cell culture medium directly and incubated for 2 h at 37 °C. Absorbance at 450 nM was measured by microplate reader. Living cell counts was determined using the linear proportional from control standard curve.

2.3. Western Blots

For proteins with molecular weight (MW) > 200 kDa, NuPAGE™ 3–8% tris-acetate 3–8% gels (Invitrogen, Waltham, MA, USA) and HiMark™ Pre-stained Protein Standard (Invitrogen) were used. Gels were transferred to nitrocellulose membranes via ultra-low voltage overnight transfer (12 V, ~100 mA, 20 h). For proteins with MW < 200 kDa, 10% tris-glycine gels (Invitrogen) and DualColor protein standard (Bio-rad, Hercules, CA, USA) were used instead. Primary antibodies (see Supplemental List S2 for a list of antibodies used) were diluted in 5% BSA 0.1%TBST and incubated overnight at 4 °C with gentle rocking. After primary antibody incubation, membranes were washed in 0.05% TBST three times, 10min each, followed by 1h incubation in Secondary antibody diluent. After a second series of wash, membranes were incubated in Clarity ECL substrates (Bio-rad) for 5min. Images were acquired by ChemDoc MP image system (Bio-rad).

2.4. Real-Time PCR and miRNA Assay

All pre-designed Taqman probes were purchased from Applied Biosciences (see Supplemental List S2 for Assay IDs). cDNA was synthesized with High-Capacity cDNA

Reverse Transcription kit and RT-PCR were performed on the StepOnePlus system (Applied Biosciences, Waltham, MA, USA). All RT-PCRs were run in triplicate.

Mature microRNAs, miR-33a-5p and 3p, were first isolated by mirVana™ miRNA Isolation Kit (Invitrogen), then reverse transcribed by Taqman advanced miRNA cDNA synthesis kit (Applied Biosciences) following official protocol. Briefly, a poly-A tail and a universal 5′ adapter is ligated to 20 nt mature miRNAs sequentially, followed by reversed transcription and a miRNA-specific amplification. The RT-PCR step can be performed as standard Taqman RT-PCR using miRNA specific probes.

2.5. Transcriptome and Analysis

Total RNA was extracted, and RNA Integrity Number (RIN) was measured by Bioanalyzer. Library preparation (poly-A enriched, non-directional) and sequencing (20 M raw reads, paired-end 150 bp, total 6 G raw data per sample) was done by Novogene America (Sacramento, CA, USA). HISAT2 [34] was used for alignment, followed by Differential Expression Analysis (DEseq2) [35] and Gene Set Enrichment Analysis (GSEA) [36].

2.6. Cholesterol Staining and Analysis

To initially visualize uptake of cholesterol, a fluorescent tagged cholesterol—BODIPY-cholesterol was used. Cells were incubated in medium supplemented with 5% lipoprotein depleted serum (KalenBio, Montgomery Village, MD, USA) and 2 µM BODIPY-cholesterol (Cayman) for 48 h. Living cell fluorescent images were captured using EVOS FL Auto system (Thermo Fisher). Next, individual cells were manually outlined, and fluorescence intensity measured using the EVOS build-in software. Calculate corrected total cell fluorescence (CTCF) = Integrated Density − (Area of Selected Cell × Mean Fluorescence of Background readings).

For a more quantitative assessment, intracellular cholesterol levels were also assessed using Amplex Red by total cholesterol/total protein ratio as previously described [37]. Cells plated in 6-well plates were washed three times with PBS and then harvested in 200 µL Amplex reaction buffer (contains mild detergent) by scraping. The lysate was sonicated (5 s on and 5 s off, three cycles) to fully disrupt membranes and centrifuged at 14,000 g for 15 min. Protein concentrations were determined by Pierce BCA assay and cholesterol concentration was measured by Amplex Red cholesterol assay following official protocols.

3. Results

3.1. SMG1 Is an Unrecognized Cholesterol Metabolism Regulator

With interest in the global effects of SMG1 knockdown, we conducted a small-scale exploratory transcriptome investigation and discovered a previously unknown link between SMG1 and cholesterol metabolism. In gene set enrichment analysis (GSEA) (Figure 1A), SMG1 siRNA treatment of the wtp53 breast cancer cell line MCF7 results in altered expression of several genes involved in cholesterol homeostasis compared to non-target siRNA treated controls. Specifically, a number of genes involved in the MVA pathway (i.e., *MVD*, *MVK*, *LSS*, *HMGCS1*, and *FDFT1*), are increased in the SMG1 siRNA treated group, as seen in the DESeq2 (Supplemental List S1) and GSEA results (Figure 1A, right panel). On the contrary, cholesterol homeostasis was not among enriched gene sets in UPF1 siRNA treated cells. Follow-up confirmatory time-course gene expression profiling of two important cholesterol regulatory genes, *ABCA1* and *SREBP2*, as well as mevalonate diphosphate decarboxylase (*MVD*), a key MVA pathway enzyme gene, was also studied. *SREBP2* and *MVD* expression increased over time after siRNA transfection consistent with our GSEA exploratory results. Somewhat unexpectedly, we also observed a significant and consistent increase in the expression of the *ABCA1*, a reverse cholesterol transporter (Figure 1B). *ABCA1* expression was consistently 10-fold higher 5 days after siRNA transfection across multiple experiments. ABCA1 operates as a cholesterol pump in a cholesterol-rich environment because it transfers cholesterol from the endoplasmic reticulum as well as phospholipid from the Golgi apparatus across cell membranes. This contrasts with the increased MVA pathway (Figure 1C), which implies a low-cholesterol environment and the production of additional cholesterols. Considering that observed effects on cholesterol pathway genes may result from NMD pathway inhibition following SMG1 knockdown, UPF1 siRNA treated cells were included as NMD pathway controls. Significant inhibition of UPF1 with siRNA was confirmed by RT-PCR (Figure 1C) and Western blot (Figure 2D). UPF1 knockdown resulted in an increase in *ABCA1* (~4-fold) and *MVD* (~1.7-fold) transcripts (Appendix A Figure A1). These data support a possible role for NMD pathway inhibition in the upregulation of cholesterol homeostasis genes though the magnitude of increase was consistently less than that observed with SMG1 inhibition across multiple experiments. Notably, UPF1 knockdown reliably leads to a 3-fold increase in SMG1 expression and vice versa, at both the mRNA and protein levels (Figures 1C and 2D). Knockdown of SMG1 in HepG2, a hepatocellular carcinoma cell line, resulted in similar increases in MVA pathway genes and in *ABCA1*, though to a lesser extent (Figure 1D). To our knowledge, SMG1 inhibition has not previously been link to effects on cholesterol metabolism, and the simultaneous regulation of *ABCA1* and the MVA pathway genes is inconsistent with previous work demonstrating their counter regulation in cholesterol homeostasis [26].

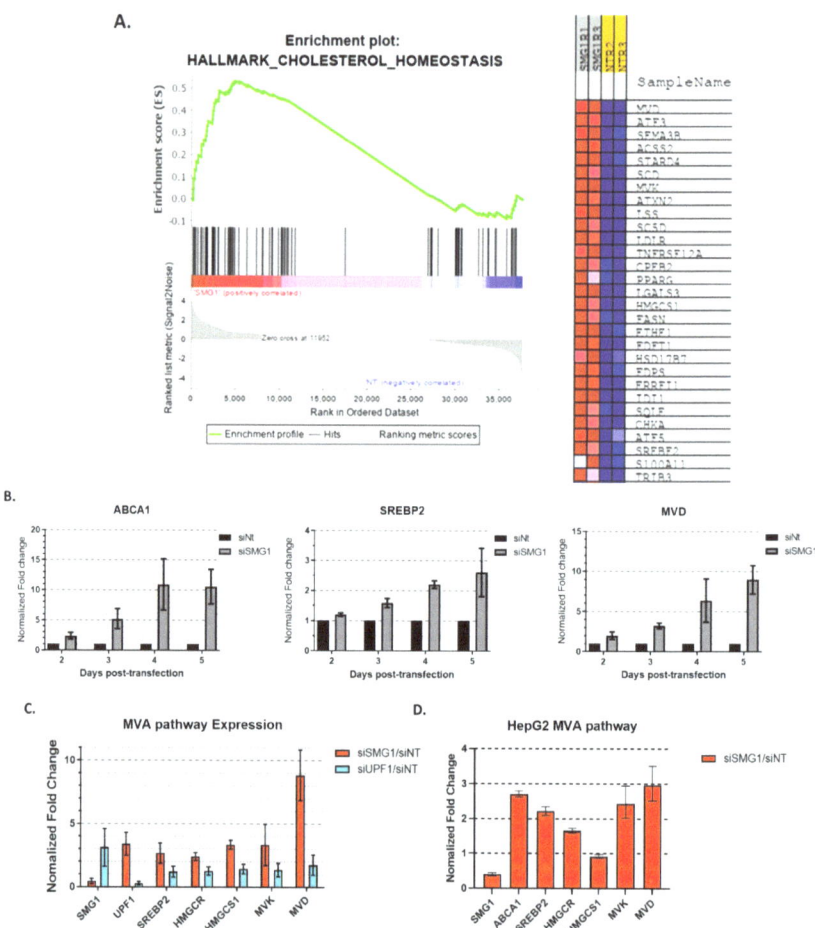

Figure 1. SMG1, but not NMD pathway, represses cholesterol metabolism. (**A**) Summary results of an exploratory gene set enrichment analysis from RNA-Seq data from RNA collected from MCF7 cells

cells 5 days after transfection with SMG1 siRNA (1:1 mix of Silencer® Select, s223560 and S223562, Thermo Fisher) or non-targeting siRNA (ON-TARGETplus SMARTPool of four siRNAs, GE DHARMACON). Cholesterol Homeostasis was the most enriched gene set following SMG1 knockdown (p-value = 0.022, FDR = 0.226); All the 29 Core Enrichment genes are listed. (**B**) Confirmational summary RT-PCR results of cholesterol pathway genes *ABCA1, SREBP2, MVD* from three independent time-course experiments (duplicated or triplicated each) of RNA collected from siSMG1 and siNT transfected MCF7 at 48-, 72-, 96-, and 120-h. (**C**) RT-PCR results for *SMG1, UPF1, SREBP2, HMGCR, HMGCS1, MVK* and *MVD* from RNA collected from MCF7 cells 5 days post-transfection with siSMG1, siNT or siRNA targeting UFP1 (ON-TARGETplus SMARTPool of four siRNAs, GE DHARMACON). Results are summary of three independent experiments (duplicated each). (**D**) RT-PCR results from a single triplicated experiment for *SMG1, ABCA1, SREBP2, HMGCR, HMGCS1, MVK* and *MVD* from RNA collected from HepG2 cells 4 days post-transfection with siSMG1 or siNT. Results in (**C**) and (**D**) are normalized to siNT for both siSMG1 and siUPF1 treated cells. Error bars represent Mean ± SD. For all RT-PCR studies, individual samples are run in triplicate.

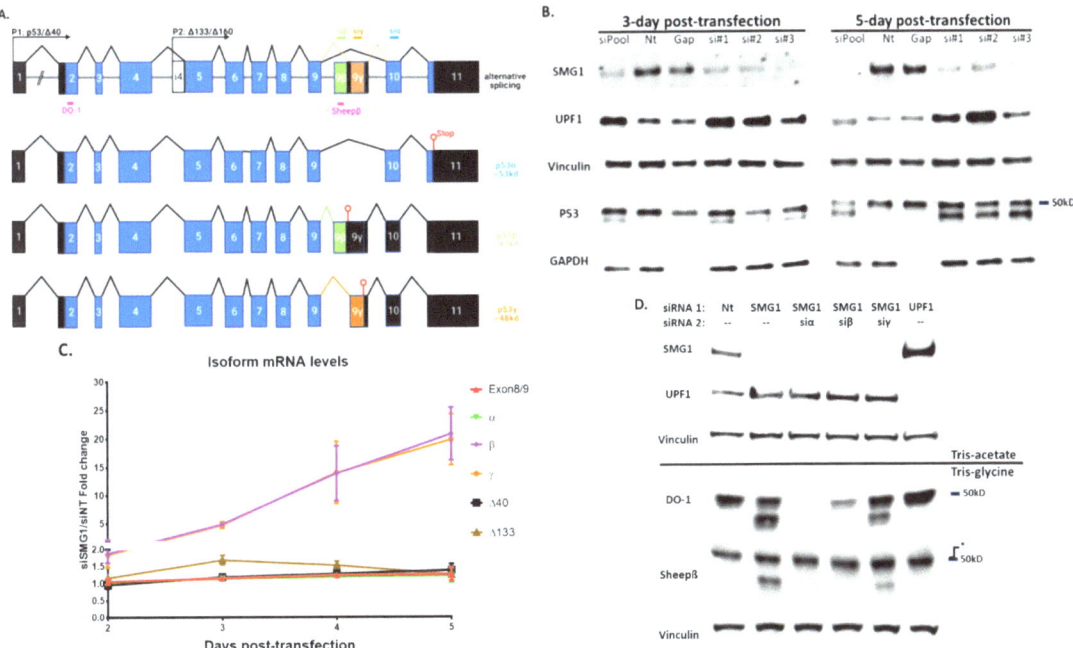

Figure 2. SMG1 knockdown induces p53β isoform. (**A**) Top: Schema depicting p53 alternative splicing isoforms, siRNA target exons and epitopes of p53 antibodies. Bottom: three mRNAs represent three types of C-terminus variants. Created with Biorender.com. (**B**) Proteins of p53 and p53 isoforms detected with DO-1 antibody in MCF7 p53[+/+] cells 3 and 5 days after transfection with siRNAs. siPool and Gap, Dharmacon™ ON-TARGETPlus validated 4-siRNA pool targeting SMG1 and GAPDH, respectively. NT is a 4-siRNA pool of no-target control siRNAs from the same vendor. si#1 and si#2 are Silencer™ select validated SMG1 siRNAs and si#3 is a 1:1 mix of si#1 and si#2. All other experiments utilized the si#3 mixture with the highest knockdown efficiency. Vinculin is the loading control. (**C**) RT-PCR analysis of p53 isoform mRNA expression in MCF7 cells following transfection with siSMG1 or siNT at 48-, 72-, 96-, and 120 h. Cells were harvested, and RNA collected at indicated times post-transfection. Taqman primers were specific to N-term variants (Δ40 or Δ133) or C-term variants (α, β or γ) or total spliced p53 (Exon8/9). The results of three separate experiments

(duplicated or triplicated each) are summarized. Results for siSMG1 are normalized to siNT. (**D**) p53 isoform protein expression by Western blot 5 days post transfection of MCF7 cells with siRNA combinations. Results for p53 antibody DO-1 (recognizes amino acids 20-25 in exon 2) and a Sheep-host β specific antibody (recognizes amino acids peptide TLQDQTSFQKENC in exon 9β; see Appendix A Figure A2) are shown. * Asterisk indicates a known cross reactivity band that is unaffected by any p53 siRNA. Siα targets p53 mRNA exon 10, which is common in all isoforms, and mainly silences p53α; siβ and siγ targets β/γ specific c-termini, respectively (see Supplemental List S2 for sequences). * Asterisk indicates a known cross reactivity band that is unaffected by any p53 siRNA. Two types of electrophoresis gels, tris-acetate and tris-glycine were used to achieve best separation based on protein MW (see Methods 2.3 for details). Error bars represent Mean ± SD. For all RT-PCR studies, individual samples are run in triplicate. Original Western blots, view Supplemental Figures.

3.2. Loss of SMG1 Alternates p53 Isoform Splicing

Previous investigations [2–5] demonstrated that SMG1 is a classical PIKK family protein that phosphorylates p53 in response to genome stress. Additionally, a report by Chen and Kasten described a 'SMG1-RPL26-SRSF7' model that resulted in alternative p53 splicing and the production of the p53 C-terminal isoform, p53β [24]. Similar to their finding, using a series of siRNA combinations to knock down SMG1 and the most prevalent N-terminal antibody DO-1, we detected a putative isoform of p53 in the absence of a genome stressor (Figure 2B). To identify the specific alternative splice variants of p53 induced by SMG1 knockdown, we utilized isoform specific Taqman probes [33], isoform specific siRNAs [21] and p53 isoform antibodies (generous gifts from Dr. Jean-Christophe Bourdon, see Appendix A Figure A2 for validation) (Figure 2A). The RT-PCR results demonstrated a significant increase in the expression of *p53β* and *p53γ* mRNA following SMG1 knockdown, with > 10-fold increase in both transcripts 120 h post-transfection (Figure 2C). Furthermore, with the combination of isoform specific siRNA and isoform specific antibodies, we were able to confirm that the 'extra' band we observed on Western blot following SMG1 knockdown (Figure 2B) represents p53β but not p53γ (Figure 2D). We were unable to detect p53γ protein by Western blot despite significantly upregulated transcript. This may reflect the low stability of p53γ protein previously reported by Camus et al. and related to E3 ligase activity [38]. However, the use of the proteosome inhibitor MG-132 did not increase either p53β or p53γ in our studies. UPF1 knockdown (NMD control) increased *p53β* and *p53γ* mRNA level by 2- and 1.7-fold, respectively (Appendix A Figure A3) with no detectable p53β or p53γ protein (Figure 2D). Taken together, these observations support Chen and Kasten's findings but contradict, at least partially, reports that UPF1 knockdown induces p53β at both the mRNA and protein levels [22,23], as discussed further in the discussion section.

3.3. P53 Isoforms Modulate the Expression of ABCA1 Differently with No Effects on SREBP2 or MVD

Lacking a clear mechanism for SMG1 inhibition to increase both *ABCA1* expression and MVA synthesis genes, and with published studies supporting p53's non-canonical effects on lipid and cholesterol metabolisms [39,40], including the findings from the Prives' laboratory for a 'p53-ABCA1-SREBP2' metabolic axis [26], we asked if SMG1 knockdown effects on p53 isoform expression could explain any of our results. After demonstrating that SMG1 inhibition leads to an increase in p53 alternative splicing, we co-transfected MCF7 cells with SMG1 siRNA and the individual isoform-specific siRNAs and quantified *ABCA1*, *SREBP2*, and *MVD* mRNA levels. Under these conditions, interestingly, p53β siRNA alone or in any combination with p53α or p53γ significantly abrogated the effect of SMG1 inhibition on the upregulation of *ABCA1*, whereas p53α siRNA alone slightly reduced *ABCA1* expression ($p = 0.1$), and p53γ siRNA alone had no activity to blunt *ABCA1* transcript upregulation following SMG1 inhibition (Figure 3A). In contrast, none of the isoform specific siRNAs altered *SREBP2* or *MVD* expression, indicating that the effect of SMG1 knockdown on MVA pathway may be distinct from SMG1 effects on the expression of alternative p53 isoforms. Representative Western blot studies also show that siRNA targeting of the p53β transcript blunted the increase in ABCA1 protein expression upon SMG1 inhibition (Figure 3B), supporting the findings from the mRNA studies.

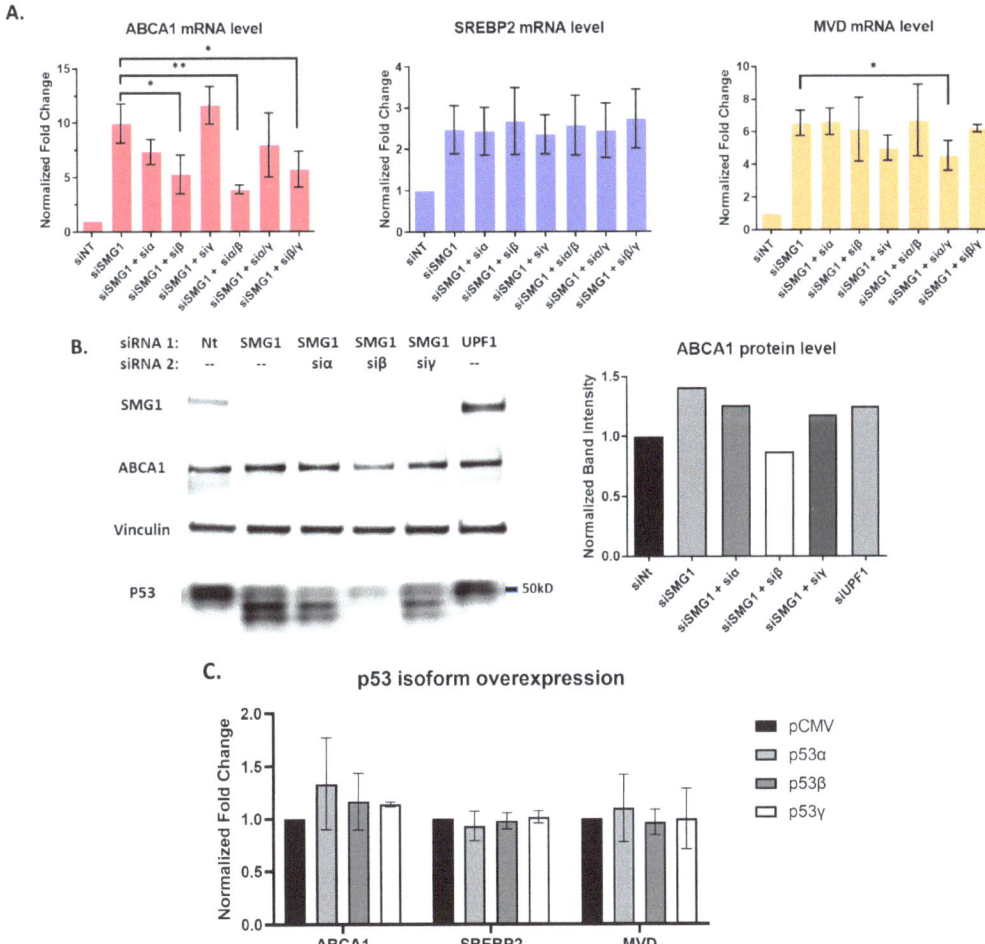

Figure 3. p53 isoforms differentially influence *ABCA1* expression following SMG1 knockdown but are unrelated to SMG1 effects on MVA pathway. (**A**) Summary RT-PCR results from three experiments for *ABCA1*, *SREBP2* and *MVD* mRNA expression from RNA collected from MCF7 cells 5 days after transfection with different siRNAs targeting SMG1 and SMG1 in combination with siRNAs targeting p53α, p53β, p53γ or the combination of p53α + p53β, p53α + p53γ, and p53β + p53γ. non-target siRNA (siNT) is included as a control. (**B**) Representative Western blot results for ABCA1 protein showing MCF7 cells treated with the different combinations of siRNAs as in panel A harvested 5 days post-transfection. The DO-1 (aa 20–25) p53 specific antibody was used examine alternative splicing. The bar plot on the right shows band intensity of ABCA1 normalized by the vinculin band intensity as a loading control. (**C**) Summary RT-PCR results from three independent experiments for *ABCA1*, *SREBP2*, and *MVD* mRNA expression from RNA collected from MCF7 that were harvested 2 days post-transfection with p53 isoform plasmids and compared to pCMV vector control. *p*-values shown for siSMG1 versus the different combinations of siSMG1 and p53 isoform siRNA(s) are from unpaired t-test. * = $p < 0.05$; ** $p < 0.01$. Error bars represent Mean ± SD. For all RT-PCR studies, individual samples are run in triplicate. Original Western blots, view Supplemental Figures.

Based on these results, we investigated whether the overexpression of individual p53 isoform showed distinct regulation of *ABCA1*, *SREBP2*, or *MVD* expression. Using the wtp53 MCF7 cell line, we were unable to replicate earlier studies that reported direct activation of *ABCA1* following upregulated wtp53 in HCT116 and SK-HEP-1 cell lines [26]. While one or two experiments support a modest increase in ABCA1 levels following forced overexpression of p53α and p53β (no change with p53γ), the increase was not significant, and *SREBP2* as well as *MVD* mRNA levels remained unchanged (Figure 3C). To summarize, alterations in alternative splicing of p53 following siRNA knockdown of SMG1 could partially explain increased expression of *ABCA1*. The upregulation of *SREBP2* and the MVA pathway following SMG1 inhibition could not be linked to alternative splicing and p53 isoforms in MCF7.

3.4. miR-33a, the Canonical ABCA1 Inhibitor Is Not Perturbated by Loss of SMG1

In canonical models of *ABCA1* gene regulation [41–44], microRNA-33a-5p, embedded in the *SREBP2* gene intron-2 and complementary to *ABCA1* 3′ untranslated region (3′ UTR), inhibits *ABCA1* expression (Figure 4A). While no link between SMG1 and miR-33a-5p has previously been reported, a recent study implicated the putative NMD target, Ras association domain-containing protein 1C (*RASSF1C*) as an inhibitor of miR-33a-5p [45]. Thus, we hypothesized that NMD inhibition following SMG1 silencing may result in an increase in RASSF1C and act on ABCA1 via miR-33a-5p inhibition. RASSF1C mRNA and protein levels were found to increase significantly as expected in response to SMG1 knockdown in MCF7 cell (Figure 4B,C). *RASSF1C* mRNA increased > 10-fold 5 days following transfection with siRNA targeting SMG1, while only slightly increased (1.4-fold) with UPF1 siRNA (Figure 4B). In line with the mRNA expression, SMG1 knockdown, but not UPF1 knockdown, induced a band on Western blot at the expected molecular weight detected by RASSF1 antibody (Figure 4C; see Appendix A Figure A4 for antibody validation). These data show that *RASSF1C* upregulation in MCF7 cells was specific to SMG1 knockdown and not observed with UPF1 inhibition despite clear inhibition of UPF1 at the protein level.

Mature microRNAs are short (22 nt) single-stranded non-coding RNAs that act as an active component of the RNA interfering mechanism. These mature microRNAs are difficult to stabilize and cannot be probed using conventional RT-PCR. We utilized a workflow specifically designed for mature microRNAs (see Methods) to probe the *ABCA1* inhibitor miR-33a-5p. Initially, we measured miR-33a-5p levels 5 days after siSMG1 or siUPF1 transfection and found no significant changes (Figure 4D). Given the possibility that miRNA disruption may occur earlier post-transfection, we next validated that the levels of miR-33a-5p were unaffected 2 or 3 days after transfection of MCF7 cells with SMG1 siRNA versus control siRNA (Appendix A Figure A5), indicating that the increase in *RASSF1C* was not associated with a decrease in miR-33a-5p as previously reported [45]. To explore this further in our model on concerns over the detectability of miR-33a-5p, we more directly examined the activity of RASSF1C on *ABCA1* expression in MCF7. As reported by others [46,47], *RASSF1A*, the major isoform of *RASSF1C*, is silent in most cancer cell lines and our RT-PCR trials cannot detect its expression in MCF7, H1299, or HepG2 (failed to amplify under any circumstances). Thus, we used a RASSF1 siRNA that targets a single exon shared by all RASSF1 isoforms. The RASSF1 siRNA successfully reduced total *RASSF1* and *RASSF1C* levels but showed no effect on *ABCA1* expression or on miR-33a-5p levels either alone or in combination with SMG1 inhibition with siRNA (Figure 4E). These data show that NMD inhibition via SMG1 knockdown results in increased RASSF1C in MCF7 but that the increase in *ABCA1* transcription could not be explained by any effect of RASSF1C via inhibitory activity on miR-33a-5p.

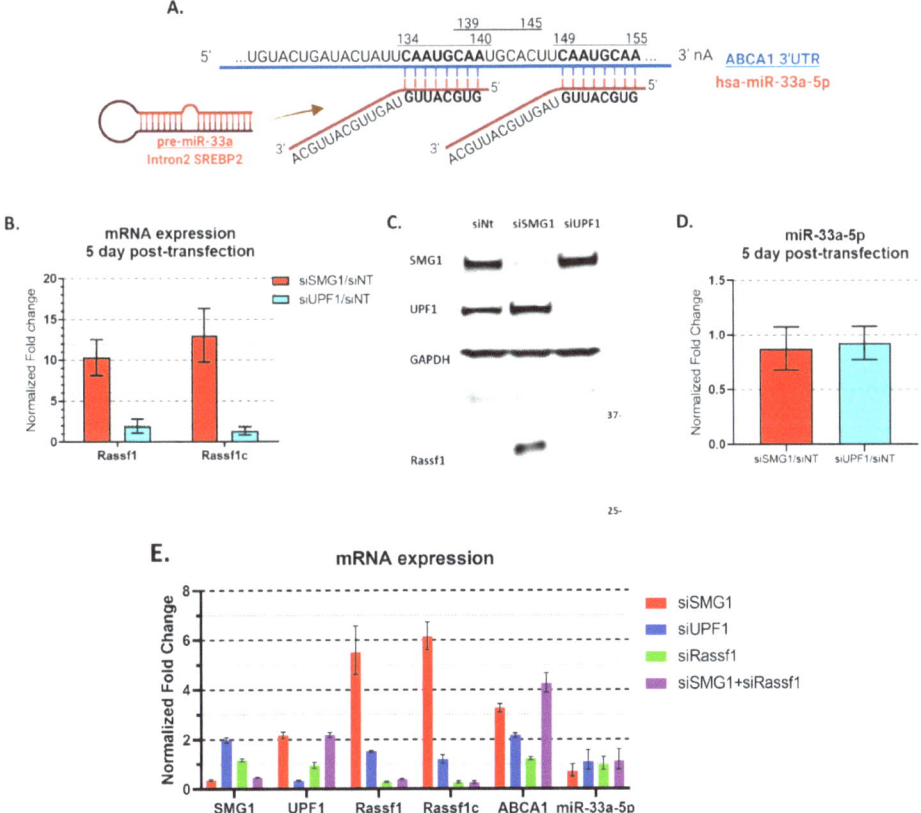

Figure 4. No effect of SMG1 inhibition on the expression of mir−33a−5p. (**A**) Schematic of miR−33a−5p and ABCA1 complementary sequences. miRNA−33a−5p, located in intron−2 of the SREBP2 gene, is complementary to 3′ UTR of ABCA1 and inhibits ABCA1 expression [41–44]. Created with Biorender.com. (**B**) Summary RT-PCR results from three experiments (duplicated each) for RASSF1 and RASSF1C mRNA levels in MCF7 cells 5 days post transfection with siSMG1, siUPF1 or siNT. (**C**) Western blot results for RASSF1C (probed with Rassf1 [EPR7127], Abcam; see Appendix A Figure A4 for validation) on Western blots of a representative experiment showing MCF7 cells treated with different siRNAs. Cells are harvested 5 days post-transfection. (**D**) Summary RT-PCR for two experiments (duplicated each) for miR−33a−5p from RNA collected from MCF7 cells 5 days post transfection with siRNA targeting SMG1, UPF1 and non-target controls. miR−33a−5p cDNA were synthesized via TaqMan™ Advanced miRNA cDNA Synthesis Kit (Applied Biosystems), probed by TaqMan Advanced miRNA Assays and normalized by miR−16−5p. (**E**) Representative RT-PCR mir−33a−5p results for a single triplicated experiment for MCF7 cells 3 days post-transfection with siSMG1, siUPF1, siRASSF1 or the combination of siSMG1 and siRASSF1. Error bars represent Mean ± SD. For all RT-PCR studies, individual samples are run in triplicate. Original Western blots, view Supplemental Figures.

3.5. Loss of SMG1 Increased Intracellular Cholesterol Level

Having consistently observed upregulation of *ABCA1*, a reverse cholesterol transporter, and MVA synthesis genes following SMG1 knockdown, we examined the more direct effect of SMG1 inhibition on intracellular cholesterol levels. Following siRNA transfection, MCF7 cells were cultured in serum depleted of lipoproteins and supplemented with fluorescent BODIPY-cholesterol. After 2 days, the fluorescent cells were observed via fluorescence microscopy. In comparison to non-targeting siRNA treated control cells, which exhibited a typical MCF7 flat-sheet morphology, SMG1 siRNA targeted cells had a rounded shape with less extracellular matrix (Figure 5A). Additionally, SMG1-siRNA targeted cells exhibited significantly increased fluorescent signal confirmed by corrected total cell fluorescence (CTCF) analysis (Figure 5B). To confirm and quantify the apparent increase in intracellular cholesterol level observed with image analysis following SMG1 knockdown, we utilized an Amplex Red cholesterol fluorometric method to quantify both free and esterified cholesterol (or total cholesterol). The cholesterol values were normalized against the protein concentration, yielding a cholesterol-to-protein ratio, as previously described [37]. In line with the CTCF analysis, SMG1 siRNA treated cells had higher level of intracellular cholesterol than non-targeted siRNA treated cells (Figure 5C). However, a combination of SMG1 and p53β siRNAs did not significantly differ from SMG1 siRNA alone, implying that changes in *ABCA* levels may not have a direct effect on cholesterol levels. Combining results from these two methods, we concluded that inhibition of SMG1 results in an increase in intracellular cholesterol levels, despite the 10-fold increase in *ABCA1* gene expression.

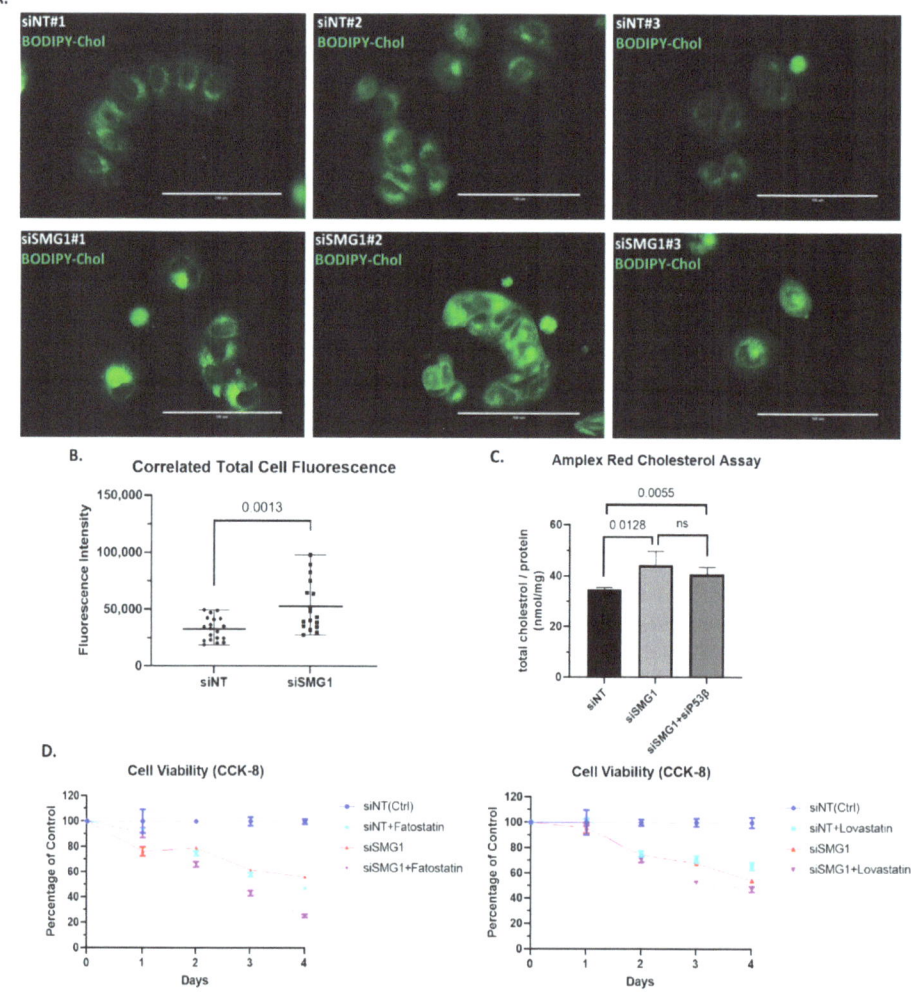

Figure 5. SMG1 knockdown increases intracellular cholesterol levels and sensitizes MCF7 cells to Fatostatin, and less degree to Lovastatin. (**A**) Representative images of the immunofluorescence staining

of BODIPY-cholesterol in MCF7 grown in 35mm glass bottom dishes. Images were acquired 4 days post-transfection with siSMG1 or siNT, using an EVOS FL Auto Fluorescence Inverted Microscope Imaging System. For each siRNA treatment group, three randomly selected areas of interest are shown (Bottom right scale bar, 100μM). (**B**) Captured images are summarized as a corrected total cell fluorescence (CTCF) statistic. Intensities of cells, as well as background intensity were measured by EVOS software. CTCF = cell intensity − (background intensity × area of outlined cell). 19 cells in siNT group, and 17 cells in siSMG1 group were counted. Presents Error bar shows Mean with Range. (**C**) Total intracellular cholesterol level was quantified in MCF7 cells 4 days post-transfection with siRNA targeting NT, SMG1 and SMG1 + p53β by Amplex Red cholesterol assay; four replications per treatment group. Total protein, measured by Pierce BCA assay, was used as an input reference (see Method 2.6 for details). ns, not significant. (**D**) To assess SMG1 inhibition effects on MCF7 sensitivity to cholesterol lowering agents, MCF7 cells were plated in 24-well plates and transfected 24 h later with siRNA targeting NT or SMG1 and then treated with Fatostatin (25 μM), Lovastatin(25 μM) or DMSO (control) as indicated. Each treatment group was performed in triplicate. Post-treatment viability was assessed every 24 h using the colorimetric CCK-8 cell viability assay until posttreatment day 4.

Given that loss of SMG1 expression results in an increase in intracellular cholesterol levels, we wish to establish whether this increases cancer cell sensitivity to inhibitors of cholesterol synthesis. To our surprise, MCF7 cells treated with siRNA to SMG1 were more sensitive to the growth inhibitory effects of Fatostatin, an inhibitor of SREBP activation, than to Lovastatin, a clinically approved HMG-CoA reductase inhibitor (Figure 5D). Fatostatin is known as a specific inhibitor of SREBP cleavage-activating protein (SCAP), a required protein for SREBP activation, but also has SREBP-independent effects [48,49]. This raises the possibility that the observed co-efficiency of Fatostatin and SMG1 knockdown is due to factor other than an SREBP2–MVA pathway.

4. Discussion

Here, we confirm that inhibiting PIKK SMG1, but not the core NMD factor UPF1, in p53 wildtype MCF7 mammary cells induces the expression of p53β with the first evidence for concomitant upregulation of p53γ. Coincident with SMG1 knockdown and alternative splicing of p53, we demonstrate a significant upregulation in cholesterol synthesis gene expression not observed with UFP1 targeting. We show that the effects of SMG1 knockdown on cholesterol pathway genes is explained by the upregulation of the p53 exon 9 isoforms including an increase in *ABCA1* following the expression of p53β. Noting that Amaar and Reeves recently reported [45] that *RASS1C*, a known NMD target upregulated by SMG1 knockdown, has activity to inhibit miR-33a-5p, a validated microRNA and canonical inhibitor of *ABCA1* housed in intron 2 of the *SREBP2* gene [41–44], we examined this alternative mechanism but found no evidence to support a role for the NMD target RASSF1C in *ABCA1* expression.

Like Chen et. al., [24] our results indicate that SMG1 loss significantly alters the expression of p53 isoforms from exon 9 and alters the expression of p53 target genes. Our work extends the effect of SMG1 loss to alterations in the expression of several cholesterol pathway genes mediated in part through upregulation of p53β and p53γ isoforms. One unexpected observation was the concurrent upregulation of both *ABCA1* and *SREBP2-MVA* mRNA upon SMG1 knockdown. In earlier work, ABCA1 has been identified as positively regulated by p53 [26] while MVA pathway genes have been shown to be upregulated in p53 null or mutant backgrounds [27] with some, but not all, studies showing dependence on SREBP2 [29]. We suspect that the concurrent increase in cholesterol transport genes and MVA synthesis following SMG1 loss reflects deregulation of p53 target gene control mediated through alternative splicing and altered function of p53αThe observation that p53β is mediating the increase in *ABCA1* following inhibition of SMG1; a function ascribed to full-length p53 [26]. The activity of p53β on *ABCA1* supports Heymach [23] premise that the exon 9 derived isoforms share overlapping functionalities with full-length p53α to compensate for p53 loss. This idea is supported by Chen et al. [24] who demonstrated that p53β when overexpressed had activity to regulate subsets of p53 target genes some independent of and some dependent on the presence of p53α. Our story with p53γ, which could not be detected on Western blot presumably a result of lower stability [38], is less clear. Induction of p53γ appears to explain the effects of SMG1 inhibition to increase MVD (MVA pathway gene) but showed no activity to increase *SREBP2* expression. This result suggests that p53γ activity is distinct from p53β. Notably, our data also do not support a role for any of the p53 isoforms in the increase in expression of the *SREBP2* gene following SMG1 inhibition.

Importantly, and a limitation of our study, the mRNA for p53α does not contain a p53α 'specific' sequence for exclusive siRNA targeting. In previous studies [21] and in these new results, targeting of exon 10 with siRNA shows preferential activity to inhibit p53α and thus, siRNA targeting exon 10 is commonly referred to as a siRNA to p53α. In contrast, selective siRNAs can be, and have been designed and validated, against exon 9-9β for p53β silencing and exon 9-9γ for p53γ silencing [21]. Exon 10 however is also part of the 3' untranslated region of p53β and p53γ. Theoretically, siRNA targeting of exon 10 could inhibit the expression of p53β and p53γ. Indeed, when we ectopically express p53β and p53γ both are slightly decreased with siRNA targeting exon 10. We interpret these results cautiously as evidence that the siRNA targeting of exon 10 predominantly suppresses p53α with slight inhibition of p53β and p53γ. Thus, in Figure 3A,B, the effect of siα (siRNA to exon 10) to reverse the effect of SMG1 knockdown on ABCA1 could result from inhibiting p53α alone, p53β, or both. Because we observed that the combined treatment of siRNA to exon 10 (siα) and siRNA to p53β (siβ) blunted the effect of SMG1 inhibition to a greater extent on ABCA1 expression (and siα and siγ to blunt the activity of SMG1 inhibition to increase MVD), our main conclusions are that p53β has activity to target gene ABCA1 and p53γ to impact MVD and that their activity on these gene targets likely depends on p53α. This is consistent with findings that p53β impacts the expression of a subset of p53 target genes in 'collaboration' and not through physical contact with p53α [24].

Observing an increase in intracellular cholesterol and altered p53 expression, we wanted to know if loss of SMG1 increased the sensitivity of MCF7 to cholesterol lowering drugs similar to reports for p53 null/mutant cells [26,27]. SMG1 knockdown appeared to sensitize MCF7 cells more to Fatostatin, an inhibitor of SREBP activation, than to Lovastatin, a competitive inhibitor of 3-hydroxy-3-methylglutaryl-coenzyme A (HMG-CoA) reductase and the rate-limiting enzyme in cholesterol synthesis. Because Fatostatin has been reported to have non-selective activity to inhibit endoplasmic reticulum to Golgi transport [49], it is possible that increased sensitivity to Fatostatin is related to the unfolded protein response induced by inhibiting NMD [50]. Additional work is needed to separate p53 deregulation from NMD in response to lipid-lowering drugs following SMG1 inhibition.

Despite the observation that p53 isoforms are differentially expressed in development and in different organs, tissue types and in human tumors, their study has received limited attention. This reflects several technical challenges. The widely used DO-1 antibody can detect only one of the four N-terminal variants, and any C-terminal variants detected are widely ignored as "background" "shades" or "doubling bands" due to molecular weights close to p53α (full-length p53). While Fahraeus (Δ40p53), Harris (Δ133p53), Lane and Bourdon (all p53 isoforms), as well as several reports by others evaluating expression in different tumor types (reviewed in [16]) have provided some initial insights about p53 alternative splicing and biological effects, the role and control of p53 isoforms in normal and in tumor biology remain poorly understood. Several commercially available p53 antibodies targeting various epitopes have been discontinued. Antibodies specific for p53 isoforms are difficult to develop due to near identical amino acid sequences. Both the C-terminal variants, β and γ, have very short unique peptide sequences, 10 and 15 amino acids, respectively. These C-termini are also actively post-translationally modified, making it more difficult to develop high-quality specific antibodies. With evidence that p53β and p53γ impact the expression of p53 target genes including cell metabolism, a significant need exists for isoform specific tools and model systems to better define the role of p53 isoforms in cellular functions remains.

5. Conclusions

Our studies support findings that SMG1 is acting as a major regulator of p53 exon 9 isoform expression [24,32], and the studies of Bourdon and others [19,51] that the gene targets and cellular outcomes of 'p53' are determined by a more complex complement of p53 isoforms than what is currently understood. Our results demonstrate a role for p53β in the upregulation of ABCA1 following SMG1 inhibition with evidence that p53γ may explain increases in MVA pathway genes following loss of SMG1. Similarly to Chen et al., [24] we find strikingly different effects of SMG1 inhibition on the p53 exon 9 isoforms in MCF7 cells, compared to reported UPF1 inhibition in other cell lines [22,23]. One possibility is that, despite high efficiency inhibition of UPF1, the NMD pathway in MCF7 is not completely inhibited by targeting UPF1 alone. This is interesting as it agrees with the findings from Heymach [23] whose has suggested that 'p53 deficiency' increases the sensitivity of cell lines to NMD inhibitors as a druggable vulnerability. Our work partly supports the premise that p53β and p53γ isoforms may partly restore p53 functionality in a p53 deficient state though in balance, following SMG1 inhibition MCF7 cells have increased intracellular cholesterol and are more vulnerable to lipid lowering drugs more like p53 null or mutant cells. Importantly, with the broadening interests in NMD [23] and SMG1 [13] as drug candidates, a better understanding of the regulation and function of p53 and p53 isoform will be important for predicting the consequences of targeted interventions on these pathways.

Supplementary Materials: The following supporting information can be downloaded at: https://www.mdpi.com/article/10.3390/cancers14133255/s1, Supplemental List S1: DEseq2 results; Supplemental List S2: Material List. Supplemental Figures: original Western blots.

Author Contributions: Conceptualization, M.L. and P.T.; methodology, M.L., F.P., and J.-C.B.; Validation, M.L. and F.P.; resource (p53 isoform antibodies), A.D. and J.-C.B.; formal analysis, M.L. and F.P.; investigation, M.L.; resources, P.T.; data curation, M.L.; writing—original draft preparation, M.L.; writing—review and editing, P.T.; visualization, M.L.; supervision, P.T.; project administration, M.L. and P.T.; funding acquisition, P.T. All authors have read and agreed to the published version of the manuscript.

Funding: This research received no external funding.

Data Availability Statement: The data presented in this study are available in the article and Supplementary Materials.

Acknowledgments: Special thanks to Jason Newton from Biology, Virginia Commonwealth University for his generous help with the optimization of Amplex Red Cholesterol Assay.

Conflicts of Interest: The authors declare no conflict of interest.

Appendix A

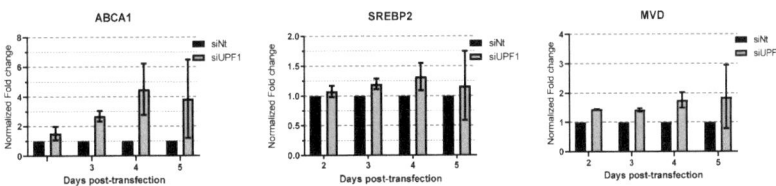

Figure A1. RT-PCR results of cholesterol pathway genes *ABCA1, SREBP2, MVD* from two independent time-course experiments (duplicated each) of RNA collected at 48-, 72-, 96- and 120-h post-transfection with siUPF1 and siNT. Error bars represent Mean ± SD. For all RT-PCR studies, individual samples are run in triplicate.

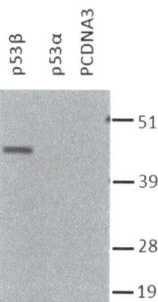

Figure A2. Western blot analyses demonstrating specificity of p53 specific antibody. Data are shown for H1299 p53$^{-/-}$ cells transfected with 1 µg of pcDNA3 plasmid expressing p53β, p53α, or pCDNA3 (empty vector). Cells were harvested 24 h after transfection. The protein extract (5µg) was analyzed by Western blot using a p53β antibody raised in sheep against peptide TLQDQTSFQKENC conjugated to KLH protein. After three injections of the p53β specific peptide/KLH conjugate, serum was harvested and the p53β antibody purified by chromatography on peptide a TLQDQTSFQKENC-Sepharose bead column as previously described [19].

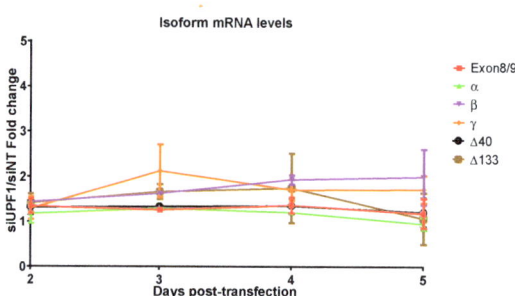

Figure A3. Summary RT-PCR analysis from two experiments (duplicated each) of p53 isoform mRNA expression following MCF7 transfection with siUPF1 or siNT at 48-, 72-, 96-, and 120 h. Cells were harvested at indicated time post-transfection. Results for siUPF1 are shown normalized to siNT. Taqman primers are the same as those in Figure 2B. Error bars represent Mean ± SD. For all RT-PCR studies, individual samples are run in triplicate.

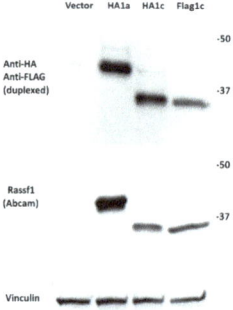

Figure A4. Western blotting verification of RASSF1 antibody and overexpressed isoforms. H1299 cells were transfected with HA-tagged RASSF1A (Addgene#1980), HA-tagged RASSF1C (Addgene#1981), FLAG-tagged RASSF1C (Addgene#1977) or empty vector and harvested 2 days post-transfection. HA or FLAG tags were probed by Anti-HA: Anti Flag mixed antibodies. RASSF1A and C were probed by RASSF1 antibody (EPR7127, Abcam). Vinculin was probed as loading control.

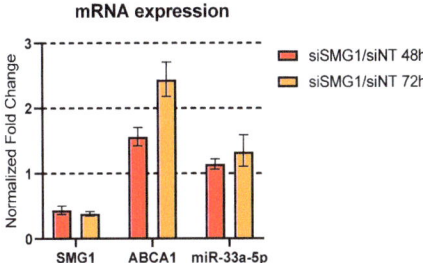

Figure A5. Representative RT-PCR results for *SMG1*, *ABCA1* and miR-33a-5p expression levels in RNA collected from MCF7 cells from a single triplicated experiment 48- and 72-h post-transfection. Error bars represent Mean ± SD. For all RT-PCR studies, individual samples are run in triplicate.

References

1. Lloyd, J.P.; Davies, B. SMG1 is an ancient nonsense-mediated mRNA decay effector. *Plant J.* **2013**, *76*, 800–810. [CrossRef] [PubMed]
2. Brumbaugh, K.M.; Otterness, D.M.; Geisen, C.; Oliveira, V.; Brognard, J.; Li, X.; Lejeune, F.; Tibbetts, R.S.; Maquat, L.E.; Abraham, R.T. The mRNA surveillance protein hSMG-1 functions in genotoxic stress response pathways in mammalian cells. *Mol. Cell* **2004**, *14*, 585–598. [CrossRef] [PubMed]
3. Gewandter, J.S.; Bambara, R.A.; O'Reilly, M.A. The RNA surveillance protein SMG1 activates p53 in response to DNA double-strand breaks but not exogenously oxidized mRNA. *Cell Cycle* **2011**, *10*, 2561–2567. [CrossRef]
4. Gubanova, E.; Issaeva, N.; Gokturk, C.; Djureinovic, T.; Helleday, T. SMG-1 suppresses CDK2 and tumor growth by regulating both the p53 and Cdc25A signaling pathways. *Cell Cycle* **2013**, *12*, 3770–3780. [CrossRef] [PubMed]
5. Gehen, S.C.; Staversky, R.J.; Bambara, R.A.; Keng, P.C.; O'Reilly, M.A. hSMG-1 and ATM sequentially and independently regulate the G1 checkpoint during oxidative stress. *Oncogene* **2008**, *27*, 4065–4074. [CrossRef] [PubMed]
6. Shieh, S.-Y.; Ikeda, M.; Taya, Y.; Prives, C. DNA Damage-Induced Phosphorylation of p53 Alleviates Inhibition by MDM2. *Cell* **1997**, *91*, 325–334. [CrossRef]
7. Yamashita, A. Role of SMG-1-mediated Upf1 phosphorylation in mammalian nonsense-mediated mRNA decay. *Genes Cells* **2013**, *18*, 161–175. [CrossRef]
8. Yamashita, A.; Izumi, N.; Kashima, I.; Ohnishi, T.; Saari, B.; Katsuhata, Y.; Muramatsu, R.; Morita, T.; Iwamatsu, A.; Hachiya, T.; et al. SMG-8 and SMG-9, two novel subunits of the SMG-1 complex, regulate remodeling of the mRNA surveillance complex during nonsense-mediated mRNA decay. *Genes Dev.* **2009**, *23*, 1091–1105. [CrossRef]
9. He, F.; Jacobson, A. Nonsense-Mediated mRNA Decay: Degradation of Defective Transcripts Is Only Part of the Story. *Annu. Rev. Genet.* **2015**, *49*, 339–366. [CrossRef]
10. Lykke-Andersen, S.; Jensen, T.H. Nonsense-mediated mRNA decay: An intricate machinery that shapes transcriptomes. *Nat. Rev. Mol. Cell Biol.* **2015**, *16*, 665–677. [CrossRef]
11. Gubanova, E.; Brown, B.; Ivanov, S.V.; Helleday, T.; Mills, G.B.; Yarbrough, W.G.; Issaeva, N. Downregulation of SMG-1 in HPV-positive head and neck squamous cell carcinoma due to promoter hypermethylation correlates with improved survival. *Clin. Cancer Res.* **2012**, *18*, 1257–1267. [CrossRef] [PubMed]
12. Roberts, T.L.; Ho, U.; Luff, J.; Lee, C.S.; Apte, S.H.; MacDonald, K.P.; Raggat, L.J.; Pettit, A.R.; Morrow, C.A.; Waters, M.J.; et al. Smg1 haploinsufficiency predisposes to tumor formation and inflammation. *Proc. Natl. Acad. Sci. USA* **2013**, *110*, E285–E294. [CrossRef] [PubMed]
13. Gopalsamy, A.; Bennett, E.M.; Shi, M.; Zhang, W.G.; Bard, J.; Yu, K. Identification of pyrimidine derivatives as hSMG-1 inhibitors. *Bioorg. Med. Chem. Lett.* **2012**, *22*, 6636–6641. [CrossRef] [PubMed]
14. Matlashewski, G.; Lamb, P.; Pim, D.; Peacock, J.; Crawford, L.; Benchimol, S. Isolation and characterization of a human p53 cDNA clone: Expression of the human p53 gene. *EMBO J.* **1984**, *3*, 3257–3262. [CrossRef] [PubMed]
15. Wolf, D.; Rotter, V. Major deletions in the gene encoding the p53 tumor antigen cause lack of p53 expression in HL-60 cells. *Proc. Natl. Acad. Sci. USA* **1985**, *82*, 790–794. [CrossRef]
16. Bourdon, J.C. p53 and its isoforms in cancer. *Br. J. Cancer* **2007**, *97*, 277–282. [CrossRef]
17. Ghosh, A.; Stewart, D.; Matlashewski, G. Regulation of human p53 activity and cell localization by alternative splicing. *Mol. Cell. Biol.* **2004**, *24*, 7987–7997. [CrossRef]
18. Courtois, S.; Caron de Fromentel, C.; Hainaut, P. p53 protein variants: Structural and functional similarities with p63 and p73 isoforms. *Oncogene* **2004**, *23*, 631–638. [CrossRef]
19. Bourdon, J.C.; Fernandes, K.; Murray-Zmijewski, F.; Liu, G.; Diot, A.; Xirodimas, D.P.; Saville, M.K.; Lane, D.P. p53 isoforms can regulate p53 transcriptional activity. *Genes Dev.* **2005**, *19*, 2122–2137. [CrossRef]

20. Fujita, K.; Mondal, A.M.; Horikawa, I.; Nguyen, G.H.; Kumamoto, K.; Sohn, J.J.; Bowman, E.D.; Mathe, E.A.; Schetter, A.J.; Pine, S.R.; et al. p53 isoforms Delta133p53 and p53beta are endogenous regulators of replicative cellular senescence. *Nat. Cell Biol.* **2009**, *11*, 1135–1142. [CrossRef]
21. Joruiz, S.M.; Bourdon, J.C. p53 Isoforms: Key Regulators of the Cell Fate Decision. *Cold Spring Harb. Perspect. Med.* **2016**, *6*, a026039. [CrossRef] [PubMed]
22. Cowen, L.E.; Tang, Y. Identification of nonsense-mediated mRNA decay pathway as a critical regulator of p53 isoform beta. *Sci. Rep.* **2017**, *7*, 17535. [CrossRef] [PubMed]
23. Gudikote, J.P.; Cascone, T.; Poteete, A.; Sitthideatphaiboon, P.; Wu, Q.; Morikawa, N.; Zhang, F.; Peng, S.; Tong, P.; Li, L.; et al. Inhibition of nonsense-mediated decay rescues p53beta/gamma isoform expression and activates the p53 pathway in MDM2-overexpressing and select p53-mutant cancers. *J. Biol. Chem.* **2021**, *297*, 101163. [CrossRef] [PubMed]
24. Chen, J.; Crutchley, J.; Zhang, D.D.; Owzar, K.; Kastan, M.B. Identification of a DNA Damage-Induced Alternative Splicing Pathway That Regulates p53 and Cellular Senescence Markers. *Cancer Discov.* **2017**, *7*, 766–781. [CrossRef]
25. Tang, Y.; Horikawa, I.; Ajiro, M.; Robles, A.I.; Fujita, K.; Mondal, A.M.; Stauffer, J.K.; Zheng, Z.M.; Harris, C.C. Downregulation of splicing factor SRSF3 induces p53beta, an alternatively spliced isoform of p53 that promotes cellular senescence. *Oncogene* **2013**, *32*, 2792–2798. [CrossRef]
26. Moon, S.H.; Huang, C.H.; Houlihan, S.L.; Regunath, K.; Freed-Pastor, W.A.; Morris, J.P.T.; Tschaharganeh, D.F.; Kastenhuber, E.R.; Barsotti, A.M.; Culp-Hill, R.; et al. p53 Represses the Mevalonate Pathway to Mediate Tumor Suppression. *Cell* **2019**, *176*, 564–580.e519. [CrossRef]
27. Freed-Pastor, W.A.; Mizuno, H.; Zhao, X.; Langerod, A.; Moon, S.H.; Rodriguez-Barrueco, R.; Barsotti, A.; Chicas, A.; Li, W.; Polotskaia, A.; et al. Mutant p53 disrupts mammary tissue architecture via the mevalonate pathway. *Cell* **2012**, *148*, 244–258. [CrossRef]
28. Vedhachalam, C.; Duong, P.T.; Nickel, M.; Nguyen, D.; Dhanasekaran, P.; Saito, H.; Rothblat, G.H.; Lund-Katz, S.; Phillips, M.C. Mechanism of ATP-binding cassette transporter A1-mediated cellular lipid efflux to apolipoprotein A-I and formation of high density lipoprotein particles. *J. Biol. Chem.* **2007**, *282*, 25123–25130. [CrossRef]
29. Sun, H.; Li, L.; Li, W.; Yang, F.; Zhang, Z.; Liu, Z.; Du, W. p53 transcriptionally regulates SQLE to repress cholesterol synthesis and tumor growth. *EMBO Rep.* **2021**, *22*, e52537. [CrossRef]
30. Bongiorno, R.; Colombo, M.P.; Lecis, D. Deciphering the nonsense-mediated mRNA decay pathway to identify cancer cell vulnerabilities for effective cancer therapy. *J. Exp. Clin. Cancer Res.* **2021**, *40*, 376. [CrossRef]
31. Nogueira, G.; Fernandes, R.; Garcia-Moreno, J.F.; Romao, L. Nonsense-mediated RNA decay and its bipolar function in cancer. *Mol. Cancer* **2021**, *20*, 72. [CrossRef] [PubMed]
32. Chen, J.; Zhang, D.; Qin, X.; Owzar, K.; McCann, J.J.; Kastan, M.B. DNA-Damage-Induced Alternative Splicing of p53. *Cancers* **2021**, *13*, 251. [CrossRef] [PubMed]
33. Sumitra Deb, S.P.D. *p53 Protocols: Methods in Molecular Biology*; Humana: Louisville, KY, USA, 2013; Volume 962.
34. Kim, D.; Paggi, J.M.; Park, C.; Bennett, C.; Salzberg, S.L. Graph-based genome alignment and genotyping with HISAT2 and HISAT-genotype. *Nat. Biotechnol.* **2019**, *37*, 907–915. [CrossRef]
35. Anders, S.; Huber, W. Differential expression analysis for sequence count data. *Genome Biol.* **2010**, *11*, R106. [CrossRef]
36. Subramanian, A.; Tamayo, P.; Mootha, V.K.; Mukherjee, S.; Ebert, B.L.; Gillette, M.A.; Paulovich, A.; Pomeroy, S.L.; Golub, T.R.; Lander, E.S.; et al. Gene set enrichment analysis: A knowledge-based approach for interpreting genome-wide expression profiles. *Proc. Natl. Acad. Sci. USA* **2005**, *102*, 15545–15550. [CrossRef]
37. Newton, J.; Palladino, E.N.D.; Weigel, C.; Maceyka, M.; Graler, M.H.; Senkal, C.E.; Enriz, R.D.; Marvanova, P.; Jampilek, J.; Lima, S.; et al. Targeting defective sphingosine kinase 1 in Niemann-Pick type C disease with an activator mitigates cholesterol accumulation. *J. Biol. Chem.* **2020**, *295*, 9121–9133. [CrossRef]
38. Camus, S.; Menendez, S.; Fernandes, K.; Kua, N.; Liu, G.; Xirodimas, D.P.; Lane, D.P.; Bourdon, J.C. The p53 isoforms are differentially modified by Mdm2. *Cell Cycle* **2012**, *11*, 1646–1655. [CrossRef] [PubMed]
39. Laubach, K.; Zhang, J.; Chen, X. The p53 Family: A Role in Lipid and Iron Metabolism. *Front. Cell Dev. Biol.* **2021**, *9*, 715974. [CrossRef]
40. Parrales, A.; Iwakuma, T. p53 as a Regulator of Lipid Metabolism in Cancer. *Int. J. Mol. Sci.* **2016**, *17*, 2074. [CrossRef]
41. Marquart, T.J.; Allen, R.M.; Ory, D.S.; Baldan, A. miR-33 links SREBP-2 induction to repression of sterol transporters. *Proc. Natl. Acad. Sci. USA* **2010**, *107*, 12228–12232. [CrossRef]
42. Herrera-Merchan, A.; Cerrato, C.; Luengo, G.; Dominguez, O.; Piris, M.A.; Serrano, M.; Gonzalez, S. miR-33-mediated downregulation of p53 controls hematopoietic stem cell self-renewal. *Cell Cycle* **2010**, *9*, 3277–3285. [CrossRef] [PubMed]
43. Najafi-Shoushtari, S.H.; Kristo, F.; Li, Y.; Shioda, T.; Cohen, D.E.; Gerszten, R.E.; Naar, A.M. MicroRNA-33 and the SREBP host genes cooperate to control cholesterol homeostasis. *Science* **2010**, *328*, 1566–1569. [CrossRef] [PubMed]
44. Rayner, K.J.; Suarez, Y.; Davalos, A.; Parathath, S.; Fitzgerald, M.L.; Tamehiro, N.; Fisher, E.A.; Moore, K.J.; Fernandez-Hernando, C. MiR-33 contributes to the regulation of cholesterol homeostasis. *Science* **2010**, *328*, 1570–1573. [CrossRef] [PubMed]
45. Amaar, Y.G.; Reeves, M.E. RASSF1C regulates miR-33a and EMT marker gene expression in lung cancer cells. *Oncotarget* **2019**, *10*, 123–132. [CrossRef]

46. Burbee, D.G.; Forgacs, E.; Zochbauer-Muller, S.; Shivakumar, L.; Fong, K.; Gao, B.; Randle, D.; Kondo, M.; Virmani, A.; Bader, S.; et al. Epigenetic inactivation of RASSF1A in lung and breast cancers and malignant phenotype suppression. *J. Natl. Cancer Inst.* **2001**, *93*, 691–699. [CrossRef]
47. Dammann, R.; Schagdarsurengin, U.; Strunnikova, M.; Rastetter, M.; Seidel, C.; Liu, L.; Tommasi, S.; Pfeifer, G.P. Epigenetic inactivation of the Ras-association domain family 1 (RASSF1A) gene and its function in human carcinogenesis. *Histol. Histopathol.* **2003**, *18*, 665–677. [CrossRef]
48. Gholkar, A.A.; Cheung, K.; Williams, K.J.; Lo, Y.C.; Hamideh, S.A.; Nnebe, C.; Khuu, C.; Bensinger, S.J.; Torres, J.Z. Fatostatin Inhibits Cancer Cell Proliferation by Affecting Mitotic Microtubule Spindle Assembly and Cell Division. *J. Biol. Chem.* **2016**, *291*, 17001–17008. [CrossRef]
49. Shao, W.; Machamer, C.E.; Espenshade, P.J. Fatostatin blocks ER exit of SCAP but inhibits cell growth in a SCAP-independent manner. *J. Lipid Res.* **2016**, *57*, 1564–1573. [CrossRef]
50. Karam, R.; Lou, C.H.; Kroeger, H.; Huang, L.; Lin, J.H.; Wilkinson, M.F. The unfolded protein response is shaped by the NMD pathway. *EMBO Rep.* **2015**, *16*, 599–609. [CrossRef]
51. Marcel, V.; Fernandes, K.; Terrier, O.; Lane, D.P.; Bourdon, J.C. Modulation of p53beta and p53gamma expression by regulating the alternative splicing of TP53 gene modifies cellular response. *Cell Death Differ.* **2014**, *21*, 1377–1387. [CrossRef]

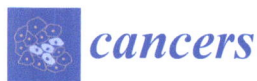

Article

Ascorbate Plus Buformin in AML: A Metabolic Targeted Treatment

Cristina Banella [1,2,†], Gianfranco Catalano [1,3,†], Serena Travaglini [1,3], Elvira Pelosi [4], Tiziana Ottone [1,3], Alessandra Zaza [1,3], Gisella Guerrera [5], Daniela Francesca Angelini [5], Pasquale Niscola [6], Mariadomenica Divona [7], Luca Battistini [5], Maria Screnci [8], Emanuele Ammatuna [9], Ugo Testa [4], Clara Nervi [10], Maria Teresa Voso [1,3,*] and Nelida Ines Noguera [1,3,*]

1. Neurooncoemtology Units, Santa Lucia Foundation, I.R.C.C.S., 00143 Rome, Italy; cristina.banella@meyer.it (C.B.); gianfranco.catalano@uniroma2.it (G.C.); serenatravaglini@live.it (S.T.); tiziana.ottone@uniroma2.it (T.O.); zazaalessandra96@gmail.com (A.Z.)
2. Department of Health Sciences, Meyer Children's University Hospital, 50139 Florence, Italy
3. Department of Biomedicine and Prevention, University of Rome Tor Vergata, 00133 Rome, Italy
4. Department of Hematology, Oncology and Molecular Medicine, Istituto Superiore di Sanità, 00161 Rome, Italy; elvira.pelosi@iss.it (E.P.); ugo.testa@iss.it (U.T.)
5. Neuroimmunology and Flow Cytometry Units, Santa Lucia Foundation, I.R.C.C.S., 00143 Rome, Italy; g.guerrera@hsantalucia.it (G.G.); df.angelini@hsantalucia.it (D.F.A.); l.battistini@hsantalucia.it (L.B.)
6. Hematology Unit, Saint' Eugenio Hospital, University of Rome Tor Vergata, 00144 Rome, Italy; pniscola@aslrmc.it
7. Policlinico Tor Vergata, University of Rome Tor Vergata, 00133 Rome, Italy; mariadomenica.divona@ptvonline.it
8. Banca Regionale Sangue Cordone Ombelicale UOC Immunoematologia e Medicina Trasfusionale, Policlinico Umberto I, 00161 Roma, Italy; m.screnci@policlinicoumberto1.it
9. Department of Hematology, University Medical Center Groningen, 9713 GZ Groningen, The Netherlands; e.ammatuna@umcg.nl
10. Department of Medical and Surgical Sciences and Biotechnologies, University of Roma La Sapienza, 04100 Latina, Italy; clara.nervi@uniroma1.it
* Correspondence: voso@med.uniroma2.it (M.T.V.); nelida.ines.noguera@uniroma2.it (N.I.N.); Tel.: +39-06-501-703-225 (N.I.N.)
† These authors contributed equally to this work.

Simple Summary: Acute Myeloid Leukemias (AMLs) are rapidly progressive clonal neoplastic diseases. The overall 5-year survival rate is very poor: less than 5% in older patients aged over 65 years old. Elderly AML patients are often "unfit" for intensive chemotherapy, further highlighting the need of highly effective, well-tolerated new treatment options for AMLs. Growing evidence indicates that AML blasts feature a highly diverse and flexible metabolism consistent with the aggressiveness of the disease. Based on these evidences, we targeted the metabolic peculiarity and plasticity of AML cells with an association of ascorbate, which causes oxidative stress and interferes with hexokinase activity, and buformin, which completely shuts down mitochondrial contributions in ATP production. The ascorbate–buformin combination could be an innovative therapeutic option for elderly AML patients that are resistant to therapy.

Abstract: In the present study, we characterized the metabolic background of different Acute Myeloid Leukemias' (AMLs) cells and described a heterogeneous and highly flexible energetic metabolism. Using the Seahorse XF Agilent, we compared the metabolism of normal hematopoietic progenitors with that of primary AML blasts and five different AML cell lines. We assessed the efficacy and mechanism of action of the association of high doses of ascorbate, a powerful oxidant, with the metabolic inhibitor buformin, which inhibits mitochondrial complex I and completely shuts down mitochondrial contributions in ATP production. Primary blasts from seventeen AML patients, assayed for annexin V and live/dead exclusion by flow cytometry, showed an increase in the apoptotic effect using the drug combination, as compared with ascorbate alone. We show that ascorbate inhibits glycolysis through interfering with HK1/2 and GLUT1 functions in hematopoietic cells. Ascorbate combined with buformin decreases mitochondrial respiration and ATP production and downregulates glycolysis, enhancing the apoptotic effect of ascorbate in primary blasts from AMLs and sparing normal CD34+ bone marrow progenitors. In conclusion, our data have therapeutic implications especially in fragile patients since both agents have an excellent safety profile, and the data also support the clinical evaluation of ascorbate–buformin in association with different mechanism drugs for the treatment of refractory/relapsing AML patients with no other therapeutic options.

Keywords: Acute Myeloid Leukemia; Seahorse XF; metabolism; pharmacologic activity; ascorbate; buformin; OXPHOS; glycolysis; hexokinase 1/2; GLUT1

1. Introduction

Acute Myeloid Leukemias (AMLs) are rapidly progressive clonal neoplastic diseases, which derive from hematologic stem cells that have lost their homeostatic capacity [1,2]. AMLs are primarily diseases of older adults, with a median age of approximately 70 years old at diagnosis [3]. The incidence increases from 2–3 per 100,000 in young adults to 13 to 15 per 100,000 in the seventh and eighth decades of life. The overall 5-year survival rate is very poor: less than 5% in older patients aged over 65 years old [4]. Therapeutic efforts are often frustrated by AML clonal evolution and resistance to treatments, arising even in younger patients. Elderly AML patients are often "unfit" for intensive chemotherapy, further highlighting the need of highly effective, well-tolerated new treatment options for AMLs.

Growing evidence indicates that AML blasts feature a highly diverse and flexible metabolism consistent with the aggressiveness of the disease [5–7]. Aberrant enzymatic activity cooperates with mutations of tumor suppressors and oncogenes in disease progression. For example, AML cells reduce both host insulin sensitivity and secretion to increase glucose availability for malignant cells [8]. The glycolytic pathway sustains leukemia maintenance and progression. The AML bulk, stem cells and their progeny had a greater mitochondrial mass and higher rates of oxygen consumption compared to a normal hematopoietic progenitor [9]. Moreover, leukemia stem cells (LSCs) are characterized by low rates of energy metabolism and a low cellular oxidative status (termed "ROS-low"). Surprisingly, ROS-low cells are unable to utilize glycolysis when mitochondrial respiration is inhibited. Thus, the maintenance of mitochondrial function is essential for LSC survival [10]. The mitochondrial oxidative phosphorylation system (OXPHOS) is sustained by elevated amino acid metabolism in LSCs from AML [11,12]. Resistant LSCs exhibit higher mitochondrial oxygen consumption that is dependent on increased tricarboxylic acid (TCA) cycle activity and fatty acid oxidation (FAO). Importantly, at diagnosis, high and low OXPHOS AML cells coexist, while after chemotherapy, high OXPHOS cells predominantly persist and survive [13]. Clonal heterogeneity and metabolic heterogeneity are, in general, associated with the failure of anti-cancer drugs, including metabolic inhibitors [14–16]. However, the metabolic reprogramming occurring in AML hematopoietic stem cells depends on their genetic characteristics, and thus represents a promising target for treatment [17–21]. In this study, we compared the metabolic pathways underlying the different stages of differentiation of normal myeloid progenitors/precursors with that of primary blasts from six AML patients and of five AML cell lines featuring different genetic mutations commonly associated with AMLs, and diverse metabolic phenotypes. We found that AML cells have a reduced respiratory capacity and reduced glycolytic reserve than their normal cellular counterpart. Therefore, we hypothesized that resistance to therapy can be overcome by associating drugs with complemental mechanisms of action and targeting specific metabolic features of AML cells.

Ascorbic acid (vitamin C) at pharmacological concentrations has pro-oxidant [22–24] and anti-cancer activities, as reported by us and others [25–27]. Ascorbate inhibits hexokinase activity [28], which produces glucose-6-phosphate to initiate two major metabolic pathways: glycolysis and the pentose phosphate pathway. Hexokinase 1 and 2 (HK1/HK2) are also associated with the mitochondrial membrane permeability transition pore (PTP) and prevents apoptosis, thus controlling reactive oxygen species (ROS) formation [29]. Recent studies reported the capacity of ascorbate to target leukemia-initiating cells [20,21].

The oral biguanide metformin is an anti-diabetic drug that delays the gastrointestinal absorption of glucose, increases insulin sensitivity and intracellular glucose uptake and inhibits liver glucose synthesis. It induces apoptosis and inhibits tumor growth in vitro and in vivo in malignancies, including breast cancer [30–33], lung cancer [34,35], melanoma [36,37] and hepatocellular cancer [38]. Buformin (1-butylbiguanide) is an analog of metformin and is a more potent inhibitor of the mitochondrial complex I of the electron transporter chain and abolishes mitochondrial respiration. The drug inhibits tumor growth in endometrial uterine cancer [39] and is currently being tested in a trial for the treatment of diffuse large B-cell lymphoma (ClinicalTrials.gov Identifier NCT02871869).

Based on these evidences, we targeted the metabolic peculiarity and plasticity of AML cells with an association of ascorbate to induce an oxidative stress and to interfere with hexokinase activity [28] and buformin to shut down the mitochondrial contribution in ATP production. Our data support the clinical evaluation of the ascorbate–buformin combination as a treatment option for refractory/relapsing AML patients and for older and unfit patients.

2. Materials and Methods

2.1. Primary Patient Samples and Controls

Bone marrow (BM) samples were collected from 17 consecutive newly diagnosed de novo AML patients admitted at the Department of Hematology of the University of Rome Tor Vergata. All samples had at least a 70% infiltration by leukemic blasts. Normal bone marrow (NBM) and CD34+ hematopoietic progenitors, isolated from the cord blood (CB) of healthy full-term placentas, were used as controls. Written informed consent was obtained from all patients in accordance with the Declaration of Helsinki and the study was approved by the ethical committee of the University of Rome Tor Vergata. The CD34+ cells were purified from the CB and BM by positive selection using the midiMACS immunomagnetic separation system (Miltenyi Biotec, Bergisch Gladabach, Germany), according to the manufacturer's instructions. The purity of the CD34+ cells was assessed by flow cytometry using a monoclonal PE-conjugated anti-CD34 antibody and resulted in a purity of over 95% (range 92–98%). Purified human hematopoietic progenitor cells were grown in a serum-free medium: serum substitute BIT 9500 (Stem cell Technologies, Vancouver, BC, Canada). The CD34+ cells were induced into a promyelocyte (Day 7) and granulocytic differentiation (Day 13) by the addition of IL-3 (1 unit/mL), GM-CSF (0.1 ng/mL) and saturating amounts of G-CSF (500 units/mL). The morphologic and immunophenotype characterization of the cells grown under these conditions has been previously described in detail by our group [40]. Cytogenetic and molecular analyses of the AML blasts were performed as described [41] and are reported in Table 1.

Table 1. Molecular and genetic features of primary AML blasts.

N°	Age	Sex	Molecular Biology	Cytogenetic
* 1	71	F	Negative panel	46, XX
2	64	F	NPM1; FLT3-ITD (R 0.36)	NA
3	79	F	NPM1	FISH negative (chr 5, 7, 8, 11, 20)
4	61	M	Negative panel	46, XY
5	81	F	NPM1; FLT3-ITD (R 0.33)	NA
6	77	M	PLZF/RARa	46, XY, t (11; 17) (q23; q21)
7	76	F	NPM1; FLT3-ITD (R 0.22)	46, XX
8	75	F	FLT3-TKD (AR:0.5)	NA
9	74	M	Negative panel	46, XY
10	51	M	NPM1	FISH negative (chr 5, 7, 8, 11, 20)
11	69	M	Negative panel	46, XY, t (4; 16)
12	60	M	NPM1; FLT3-ITD (R 1.67)	46, XY

Table 1. *Cont.*

N°	Age	Sex	Molecular Biology	Cytogenetic
13	78	M	NPM1; FLT3-ITD (R 0.58)	NA
14	41	F	MPM1; FLT3-ITD	NA
15	53	F	Negative panel	NA
16	75	F	NPM1; FLT3-ITD (R 0.67)	46, XX
17	45	M	Negative panel	46, XX

NA: not available; Chr: chromosomes; panel of molecular biology (NPM; Nup-Can; FLT3-ITD; FLT3-D835; IDH1; IDH2; CBFb/MYH11; RUNX1/RUNX1T1); * biphenotypic (AML and LLC).

Normal bone marrow (NBM) cells and hematopoietic CD34+ progenitor cells that were isolated from the cord blood (CB) obtained from healthy full-term placentas were used as the controls.

2.2. Cell Lines and Cell Culture

U937-Mock cells (the U937 monoblastic cell line transfected with the empty Zn-inducible MT1 promoter vector) were used as the controls; U937-AETO (a zinc-inducible RUNX1/RUNX1T1 model), OCI-AML3 (an AML-M4-derived cell line carrying an NPM1 gene mutation (type A) and the DNMT3A R882C mutation) and OCI-AML2 (an AML-M4-derived cell line carrying the DNMT3A R635W mutation) were kindly provided by Emanuela Colombo, European Institute of Oncology, Milan, Italy. MV4-11 (a biphenotypic B myelomonocytic leukemia carrying the FLT3-ITD mutation and MLL/AF4 translocation) was purchased from the Leibniz Institute DSMZ-German Collection of Microorganisms and Cell Cultures (Braunschweig, Germany). The cells were cultured in an RPMI medium (Euroclone; Pero, MI, Italy), 10% fetal bovine serum (FBS) (GIBCO-BRL), 20 mM of Hepes, 100 U/mL of penicillin and 100 µg/mL of streptomycin (GIBCO-BRL). The cultures were maintained at 37 °C in a 5% CO_2 humidified incubator.

2.3. Cell Viability

A CellTiter 96® AQueous One Solution Cell Proliferation Assay was used. The AML cells were seeded in a 96-well plate at an initial density of 1×10^4 cell/well and were treated with 1 mM of ascorbate; 0.1 mM of buformin; or both for 72 h at 37 °C. Subsequently, 5 µL of the CellTiter 96® AQueous One Solution Cell Proliferation Assay (Promega; Madison, WI, USA) were added to each well and the cells were incubated for 4 h. The absorbance was read at 490 nm using a microplate reader (Thermo Scientific™ Varioskan™ Flash Multimode Reader; Waltham, MA, USA). The cell viability was assessed by comparison with the control cells treated with the vehicle alone. At least 3 independent biological replicates were performed.

A CellTiter-Glo® Luminescent Cell Viability Assay is a homogeneous method for determining the number of viable cells in a culture. It is based on the quantitation of ATP, an indicator of metabolically active cells. Briefly, the cells were plated at 2×10^4 cell/mL/well and were cultured for 72 h with or without the treatments reported above. The intracellular ATP levels were determined using the CellTiter-Glo® Substrate Assay System (Promega; Madison, WI, USA) according to the manufacturer's instructions. At least 3 independent biological replicates were performed.

2.4. Colony Formation Unit Assay

For the Colony-Forming Unit (CFU) Assay, the AML cells were seeded at 70,000 cells/mL in a Methocult 4035 medium (STEMCELL Technologies, Tukwila, WA, USA), following the manufacturer instructions, and were incubated at 37 °C at 5% pCO_2 in a humidified incubator with the addition or not of 0.1 mM of buformin and/or 1 mM of ascorbate. The healthy BM mononucleated cells were cultured as described but were seeded at a density of 20,000 cells/mL, the purified CD34+ cells at 100 cells/mL and the AML cell lines at 300 cells/mL, as recommended by the Methocult medium manufacturer instructions. The number of colonies were counted under a phase-contrast optical microscope after 8 days of culture [42].

2.5. Western Blot Analysis

Cell pellets were resuspended in a lysis buffer with 10 mM of Tris-HCl (pH 7.4), 5 mM of EDTA, 150 mM of NaCl, 1% Triton X-100, 250 µM of orthovanadate, 20 mM of β-glycerophosphate and protease inhibitors (Sigma-Aldrich, Steinheim, Germany). The lysates were centrifuged at $10,000 \times g$ for 30 min at 4 °C and the supernatants were stored at −80 °C. The protein concentration was measured by the Bradford Assay (#500–0006; Bio-Rad, München, Germany). Thirty microgram aliquots of proteins were re-suspended in a reducing Laemmli Buffer (with β-mercaptoethanol), loaded onto a 12% polyacrylamide gel and then transferred to a PVDF membrane. After blocking with 5% milk (Fluka, Sigma-Aldrich, Saint Louis, HI, USA), the membranes were incubated with primary antibodies (Table S1). Horseradish peroxidase-conjugated IgG preparations were used as secondary antibodies, and immunoreactivity was determined by the enhanced chemiluminescence (ECL) method (Amersham, Buckinghamshire, UK). The autoradiograms were exported for densitometry analysis. The protein signal intensities were measured using the Quantity One Software (Bio-Rad Laboratories, Hercules, CA, USA). The signal quantity was normalized using the unrelated protein β-actin (Cell Signaling Technology, Beverley, MA, USA) [43].

2.6. Metabolic Assays

Mitochondrial and glycolytic functions were assessed using a Seahorse Bioscience XFe96 analyzer in combination with the Seahorse Bioscience XF Cell Mito Stress Test and the Bioscience XF Cell Glycolysis Stress Test (Agilent Technologies, Santa Clara, CA, USA), respectively, as described [44]. Briefly, the extracellular acidification rate (ECAR), reflecting the conversion of glucose to lactate and resulting in a net production of protons in the extracellular medium, was measured directly using the Agilent Seahorse XF instrument. The cells were first injected with saturating concentrations of glucose (10 mM). The glucose-induced response is reported as the rate of glycolysis under basal conditions. The second injection was 2 µM of oligomycin, an ATP synthase inhibitor. Oligomycin inhibits mitochondrial ATP production and shifts the energy production to glycolysis, with the subsequent increase in ECAR revealing the maximum cellular glycolytic capacity. The final injection was 50 mM of 2-deoxy-glucose (2-DG), a glucose analog that inhibits glycolysis, confirming that the ECAR produced in the experiment was due to glycolysis. The difference between the glycolytic capacity and basal glycolysis defines the glycolytic reserve.

Mitochondrial respiration is directly measured by the oxygen consumption rate (OCR) of cells. Basal respiration represents the energetic demand of the cell under baseline conditions. Oligomycin is first injected in the assay and results in a reduction in the mitochondrial respiration or OCR. The decrease in the OCR is linked to cellular ATP production. Carbonyl cyanide-4 (trifluoromethoxy) phenylhydrazone (FCCP) is an uncoupling agent and is injected at concentrations of 1 µM following oligomycin. As a result, the electron flow through the ETC is uninhibited, and oxygen consumption reaches the maximum. This is the maximum respiration. The spare respiratory capacity, defined as the difference between maximal and basal respiration, is a measure of the ability of the cell to respond to an increased energy demand. A proton leak has its origin in the fact that no living cell converts all the energy of the proton gradient to ATP, meaning oxidative phosphorylation is incompletely 'coupled' since protons can 'leak' across the inner membrane and thus balance the gradient without ATP synthesis.

The percentage of ATP production from glycolysis and mitochondrial respiration was measured using the XF Real-Time ATP Rate Assay (Agilent Technologies). This test uses metabolic modulators (oligomycin and a mix of rotenone and antimycin A, that when serially injected, allows the calculation of the mitochondrial and glycolytic ATP production rates).

The rate of oxidation of each fuel (pyruvate, fatty acids and glutamine) was determined using the XF Mito Fuel Flex Test (Agilent Technologies).

The cells' mitochondrial dependency and flexibility for the usage of each of the fuel sources were determined by measuring the decrease in fuel oxidation (the decline in the OCR) upon addition of one or more inhibitors, including UK5099, which blocks the glucose oxidation pathway, BPTES, which blocks the glutamine oxidation pathway and Etomoxir, an inhibitor of long-chain fatty acid oxidation. Sequentially inhibiting the pathway of interest enables the calculation of how dependent the cells are on the pathway to meet the basal energy demand. Inhibiting the two alternative pathways enables the calculation of the cells' mitochondrial capacity to meet energy demands using another fuel. Fuel flexibility is calculated by subtracting the fuel dependency from the fuel capacity.

2.7. Cytofluorimetric Analysis

The markings were performed using 0.5×10^6 cells resuspended in a volume of 100 µL of current buffer (PBS + 1% FBS + 0.5% EDTA 500 mM). Cells were labeled with annexin V, which binds to the phosphatidylserine (PS) externalized on the surface of cell membranes and is used to measure early stage apoptosis, and 'Live Dead', which enters cells with damaged membranes and is used to assess the terminal stages of apoptosis. After a 15 min incubation in the dark at room temperature, the cells were washed and resuspended in 100 µL binding buffer 1×. The analysis of the samples was performed using the CytoFLEX flow cytometer (Beckman Coulter, Brea, CA, USA) equipped with three lasers. About 500,000 cells were selected for each sample based on physical size (FSC) and graininess parameters. The cells labeled with a single fluorochrome were used as controls to adjust the compensation. The data were compensated and analyzed using the FlowJo software (TreeStar, Ashland, OR, USA) [45].

2.8. Statistical Analysis

Data were analyzed using GraphPad Prism 6 (GraphPad Software Inc., San Diego, CA, USA). Statistical analyses were performed using the Student's *t*-test, Mann–Whitney test, Kruskal–Wallis one-way ANOVA and Dunn's post hoc tests or the one-way ANOVA and Tukey's multiple comparison test as indicated. Statistical significance was established at $p < 0.05$.

3. Results

3.1. Metabolic Dependence of Primary AML Blasts

To investigate the whole-substrate oxidation usage of primary AML cells, we evaluated the oxygen consumption rate (OCR) and extracellular acidification rate (ECAR) in primary blasts isolated from six AML patients (numbers 1, 5, 6, 9, 12 and 16 from Table 1) and in five human AML cell lines. The metabolic peculiarities of the leukemic cells were compared to those of normal hematopoietic precursors undergoing different stages of myeloid maturation/differentiation, as indicated by morphological and immunophenotypic changes. Primary AML blasts showed a heterogenous glucose consumption, while basal glycolysis, the glycolytic reserve and the glycolytic capacity were higher with respect to NBM but comparable to values measured in early progenitors/precursors (EP/Ps) from the CB CD34+ cells at day 13 of culture (N13, mostly granulocytic differentiated cells: CD11b 72%, CD15 80% and CD34 7%) (Figure 1a and Table 2). In line with literature reports, AML cells displayed high glucose consumption and heavily relied on it [46]. Interestingly, the EP/Ps at day 7 of culture (N7, mostly promyelocytes: CD11b Pe 16.8%, CD13 Pe 86.6%, CD14 Pe 5.1%, CD15 Pe 3.2% and CD34 Pe 45.2%) showed a higher glycolytic reserve than the AML blasts ($p = 0.02$) (Figure 1a and Table 2). Of note, at day 7 and day 13, the EP/Ps were highly proliferating cells exposed to high concentrations of growth factors, which could have affected their metabolic activities.

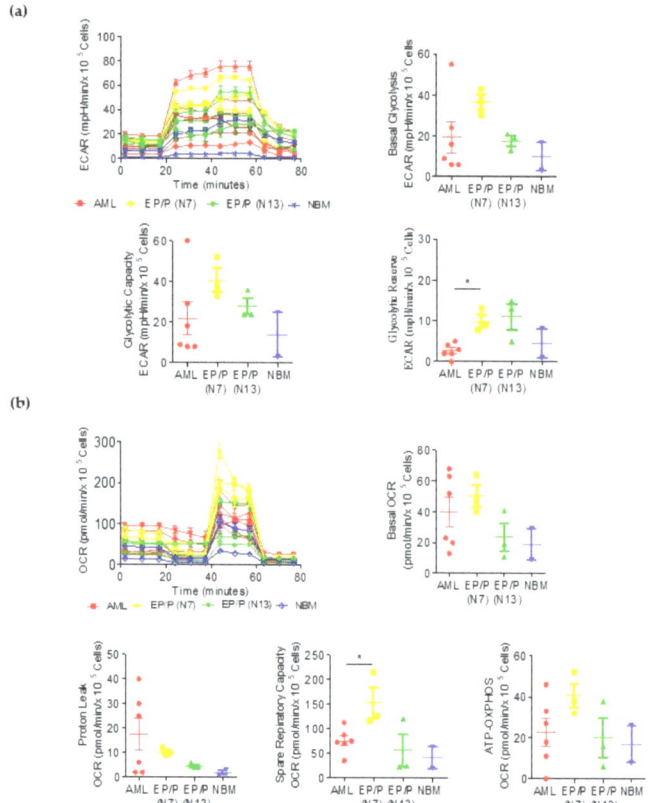

Figure 1. Metabolic characterization of primary AML blasts and early progenitors/precursors (EP/Ps) from cultured normal cord blood CD34+ cells. Metabolic characterization of primary blasts from AML patients, EP/P at day 7 (N7, mostly a promyelocyte population) and at day 13 (N13, mostly granulocytes) and in normal bone marrow (NBM). (**a**) Profile of the glycolytic activity. Histograms represent basal glycolysis, glycolytic reserve and glycolytic capacity measured using the XF Glycolytic Rate Assay. (**b**) Profile of the mitochondrial activity. Histograms represent basal respiration, spare respiratory capacity and mitochondrial ATP production measured using the XF Myto Stress Test Assay. Data are presented as mean ± SD. Statistical analyses were performed using the ANOVA, t-test and Tukey's Multiple Comparison Test; * $p \leq 0.05$.

Table 2. Glycolysis values in AML blasts and normal hematopoietic cells.

GlycolysisECAR (mpH/min/10^5 Cells)	AML	EP/P (N7)	EP/P (N13)	NBM	p-Value (AML vs. EP/P, N7)
Basal	19 ± 19	37 ± 6	18 ± 4	3 ± 0	-
Capacity	22 ± 20	41 ± 10	28 ± 7	4 ± 1	-
Reserve	3 ± 2	10 ± 3	11 ± 5	0.5 ± 0.7	0.03

ECAR (extracellular acidification rate); EP/P (early progenitors/precursors); N7 (at day 7); N13 (at day 13); NBM (normal bone marrow). Values represent the mean ± SD. Statistical significances were evaluated through Mann–Whitney test.

Regarding mitochondrial respiration, the AML blasts primary presented lower values in the spare respiratory capacity with respect to the EP/Ps (N7) ($p = 0.02$), indicating that they were more sensitive to oxidative stress than normal progenitors, as previously reported by Sriskanthadevan et al. [47]. This finding indicates that the therapeutic targeting of mitochondrial respiration can be useful in AMLs. The measurements of basal respiration and proton leaks indicated that the AML cells were distributed in two populations, one subset presenting higher values and another with lower values (Figure 1b and Table 3).

Table 3. Mitochondrial respiration values in AML blasts and normal hematopoietic cells.

Mitochondrial Respiration OCR (pmol/min/10^5 Cells)	AML	EP/P (N7)	EP/P (N13)	NBM	p-Value (AML vs. EP/P)
Basal	40 ± 24	50 ± 12	24 ± 16	9 ± 1	-
Spare Respiratory Capacity	76 ± 25	153 ± 54	56 ± 56	23 ± 4	0.02
Proton Leak	18 ± 16	10 ± 2	5 ± 1	0.5 ± 0.7	-
ATP	23 ± 16	41 ± 10	20 ± 16	8 ± 1	-

OCR (oxygen consume rate); EP/P (early progenitors/precursors); N7 (at day 7); N13 (at day 13); NBM (normal bone marrow). Values represent the mean ± SD. Statistical significances were evaluated through Mann–Whitney test.

3.2. Metabolic Dependency in AML Cell Lines

Three AML cell lines were used as metabolic models for the AMLs: OCI-AML2 (carrying the DNMT3A R635W mutation), OCI-AML3 (carrying the NPM1 gene mutation type A and the DNMT3A R882C mutation) and MV4-11 (carrying the FLT3-ITD mutation and MLL/AF4 translocation). The OCI-AML2 and OCI-AML3 cells showed higher glycolysis basal values with respect to MV4-11, the OCI-AML3 cells presented the highest levels of glycolytic capacity and glycolytic reserve (Figure 2a and Table 4) and the MV4-11 cells had greater OXPHOS values compared with the OCI-AML2 and OCI-AML3 cells (Figure 2b and Table 5).

Table 4. Glycolysis values in AML cell lines.

Glycolysis ECAR (mpH/min/10^5 Cells)	OCI-AML2	OCI-AML3	MV4-11	p-Value	p-Value
Basal	96 ± 10	104 ± 12	56 ± 5	<0.5 (Oci2 vs. MV4-11)	<0.005 (OCI3 vs. MV4-11)
Capacity	104 ± 31	146 ± 64	83 ± 10	-	<0.005 (OCI3 vs. MV4-11)
Reserve	9 ± 12	43 ± 32	27 ± 11	<0.005 (OCI2 vs. OCI3)	<0.05 (OCI2 vs. MV4-11)

ECAR (extracellular acidification rate). Values represent the mean ± SD. Statistical significances were evaluated through Kruskal–Wallis one-way ANOVA and Dunn's post hoc tests.

Table 5. Mitochondrial respiration values in AML cell lines.

Mitochondrial Respiration OCR (pmol/min/10^5 Cells)	OCI-AML2	OCI-AML3	MV4-11	p-Value	p-Value
Basal	106 ± 31	97 ± 18	160 ± 27	<0.05 MV4-11 vs. OCI3	-
Spare Respiratory Capacity	103 ± 21	180 ± 47	116 ± 15	<0.005 OCI3 vs. OCI2	-
Proton Leak	19 ± 6	22 ± 5	34 ± 4	<0.005 MV4-11 vs. OCI2	<0.05 MV4-11 vs. OCI3
ATP	87 ± 26	75 ± 14	141 ± 13	<0.05 MV4-11 vs. OCI2	<0.005 MV4-11 vs. OCI3

OCR (oxygen consume rate). Values represent the mean ± SD. Statistical significances were evaluated through Kruskal–Wallis one-way ANOVA and Dunn's post hoc tests.

Then, we analyzed the fuel used in mitochondrial respiration. The energy produced by the cells derived from the mitochondrial oxidation of glucose, glutamine and fatty acids. Dependency indicates that the cells' mitochondria were unable to compensate for the blocked pathway by oxidizing other fuels. Flexibility indicates the cells' mitochondria had the ability to compensate for the inhibited pathway by using other pathways to fuel mitochondrial respiration. The MV4-11 cells displayed a significant dependency on fatty acid oxidation (FAO) and slightly on glycolysis. OCI-AML3 strongly depended on glucose and slightly on FAs and glutamine. OCI-AML2 depended partially on glycolysis and FAs. OCI-AML3, OCI-AML2 and MV4-11 showed the highest flexibility towards all three fuels (Figure 2c, The uncropped Western blots have been shown in Figure S2). We analyzed the expression levels of two FAO key proteins, Carnitine transporter CT2 (SLC22A16) and Carnitine palmitoyl transferase I (CPT1A), and found that both of them were expressed at higher levels in the MV4-11 cells, which are highly dependent on FAs, with respect to the OCI-AML2 and OCI-AML3 cells (Figure 2d and Table 6).

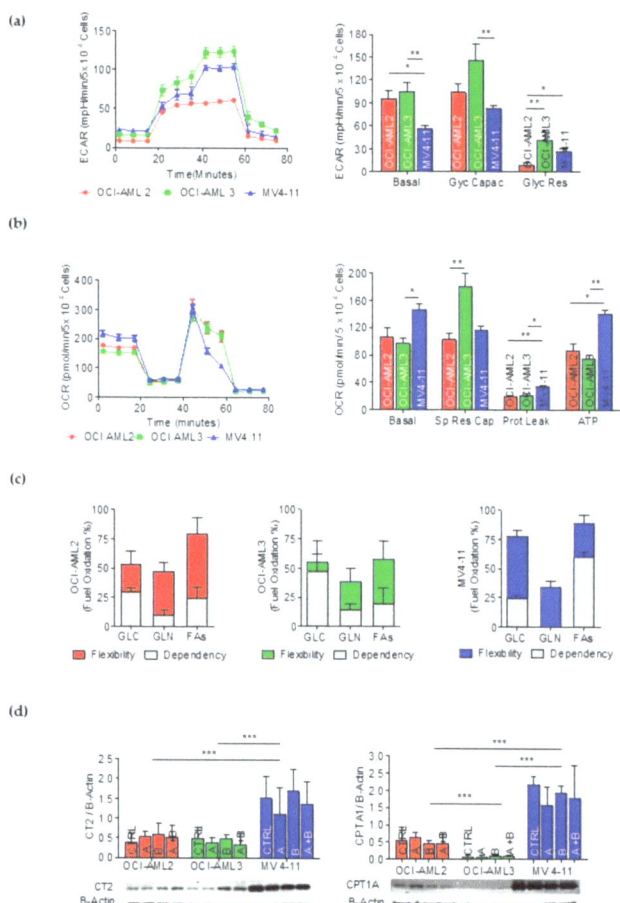

Figure 2. Metabolic characterization of OCI-AML2, OCI-AML3 and MV4-11 cell lines. (**a**) Profile of the glycolytic activity. Histograms represent basal glycolysis, glycolytic reserve and glycolytic capacity. (**b**) Profile of the mitochondrial activity. Histograms represent basal respiration, spare respiratory capacity, proton leak and mitochondrial ATP. (**c**) Evaluation of the mitochondrial fuel used (pyruvate, glutamine and FAs). Data are presented as mean ± SD. The experiments were conducted in triplicate. Statistical significances were evaluated through Kruskal–Wallis one-way ANOVA and Dunn's post hoc tests. (**d**) CT2 and CPT1A protein expression in OCI-AML2, OCI-AML3 and MV4-11 cell lines treated with 1 mM of ascorbate (A), 0.1 mM of buformin (B) or ascorbate–buformin combination (A + B). Statistical analysis by Student's *t*-test. * $p \leq 0.05$; ** $p < 0.005$; *** $p \leq 0.0005$.

Table 6. Expression levels of CT2 and CPT1A proteins in AML cell lines.

	OCI-AML2	OCI-AML3	MV4-11	*p*-Value (MV4-11 vs. Oci2)	*p*-Value (MV4-11 vs. Oci3)
CT2	0.4 ± 0.2	0.5 ± 0.3	1.5 ± 0.6	<0.0005	<0.0005
CPT1A	0.5 ± 0.4	0.1 ± 0.03	2.2 ± 0.2	<0.0005	<0.0005

Values represent the mean ± SD. Statistical significances were evaluated through Student's *t*-test.

3.3. Action of Buformin on OXPHOS Metabolism in AML Cells

Since buformin targets mitochondrial complex I [39], we evaluated the drug concentration causing 50% OXPHOS inhibition (IC50) in the AML cell lines. We treated the three AML cell lines with 0–10–50–100 µM of buformin for 24 h and evaluated the OCR at baseline and following the addition of: oligomycin-A (an ATP synthase inhibitor), to determine the amount of oxygen consumption coupled to ATP synthesis; FCCP (releases electron flow through the ETC, thus maximizing oxygen consumption) to determine the maximal respiratory capacity; and antimycin A plus rotenone (electron transporter complex III and I inhibitors) to determine the spare respiratory capacity. Our result showed that buformin inhibited the OXPHOS activity in a concentration-dependent manner, with IC50s of 49 µM for OCI-AML3, 63 µM for MV4-11 and 103 µM for OCI-AML2 (Figure 3a). These results indicate that treatment with 100µM of buformin strongly affected mitochondrial ATP production in these AML cell lines.

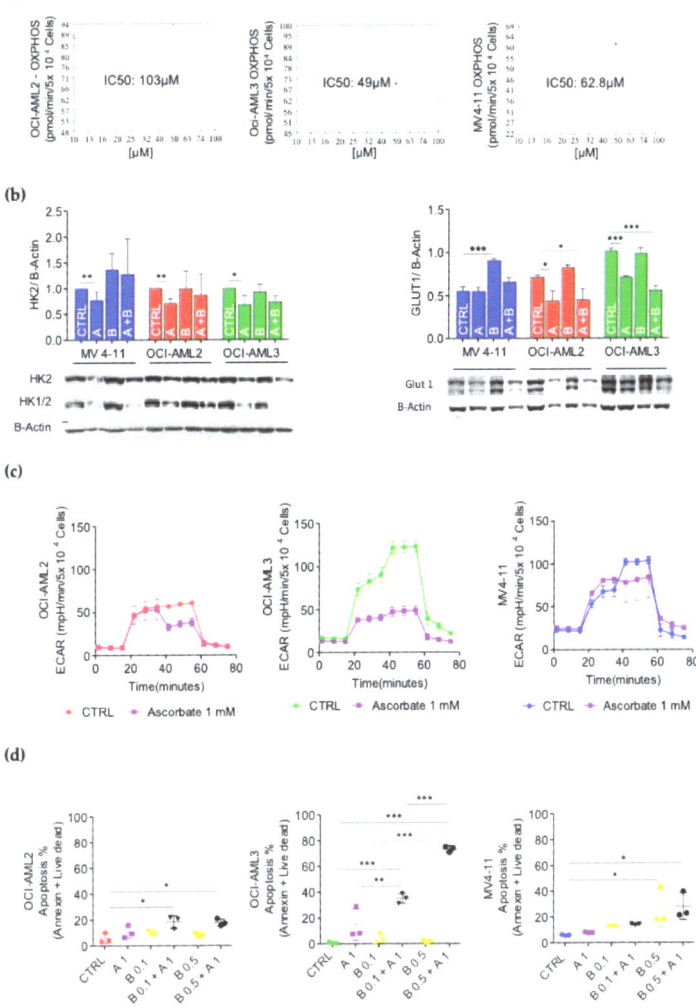

Figure 3. Metabolic effect of buformin and ascorbate in OCI-AML2, OCI-AML3 and MV4-11 cell lines. (**a**) Evaluation of OXPHOS IC50 concentration. Three independent experiments ± SD (**b**) HK2, HK1/2 and GLUT1 protein expression in OCI-AML2, OCI-AML3 and MV4-11 cell lines treated with

1 mM of ascorbate (A), 0.1 mM of buformin (B) or ascorbate–buformin combination (A + B). Statistical analysis by Student's t-test. * $p \leq 0.05$; ** $p < 0.005$; *** $p < 0.0005$. (**c**) Action of ascorbate on AML cells' glycolytic metabolism. Kinetic profile of the extracellular acidification rate (ECAR) assay. Cell lines were treated for 24 h with 1 mM of ascorbate and were evaluated by XF Glycolytic Stress Test. The experiments were performed in duplicate. (**d**) Cell death induced by 1 mM of ascorbate (A) and buformin (B) (0.1 and 0.5 mM) at 72 h by flow cytometry after annexin V + live dead staining. Data are presented as mean ± SD from three independent experiments. Statistical analysis by Student's t-test. * $p < 0.05$; ** $p < 0.005$; *** $p < 0.0005$.

3.4. Effect of Ascorbate on Glycolytic Metabolism in AML Cells

From our previous experience in treating AML cells with ascorbate, we identified the 3 mM concentration as rapidly cytotoxic due to its pro-oxidant effect [25]. To investigate the metabolic effect of the drug, in this study AML cells were treated with 1 mM of ascorbate, which significantly inhibited the expression levels of Hexokinase II (HK2), a main glycolysis-initiating enzyme in the hemopoietic system (Figure 3b) and in tumors [28]. Similar results were obtained using an antibody recognizing both Hexokinase I and HK2 (HK1/2) (Figure 3b). In addition, we investigated the effect of ascorbate on GLUT1, a transporter of glucose in hematopoietic cells [48]. We found that ascorbate significantly decreased GLUT1 expression levels in OCI-AML2 and OCI-AML3 (Figure 3c), further suggesting an effect of ascorbate on glycolysis in AML cells.

To confirm this, the XF Glycolytic Stress Test was used to determine the basal rates of glycolysis by measuring the percentage of increase in the ECAR after the addition of glucose. The glycolytic reserve is a measure of the difference in the ECAR before and after treatment with oligomycin (which inhibits ATP synthase and thereby the OXPHOS' ATP). The glycolytic reserve reflects the compensatory increase in glycolysis corresponding to the level of ATP no longer produced by the OXPHOS. It was found that 1 mM of ascorbate did not affect glycolysis in the MV4-11 and OCI-AML2 cells, whereas it lowered basal glycolysis by 1.7 folds ($p = 0.01$) and the glycolysis capacity by 1.8 folds in the OCI-AML3 cells ($p = 0.01$) (Figure 3c).

3.5. Metabolic Background Influences Apoptotic Response to Metabolic Treatments of AML Cell Lines

We then treated the OCI-AML2, OCI-AML3 and MV4-11 cell lines with ascorbate (1 mM), buformin (0.1 and 0.5 mM) and with an ascorbate–buformin combination for 72 h, measuring apoptosis with cytofluorimetric analysis. The OCI-AML3 cells showed a strong apoptotic response to the combined ascorbate–buformin treatment; buformin potentiated the ascorbate effect on apoptosis at both of the concentrations used. The MV4-11 cells were sensitive to 0.5 mM of buformin and 0.5 mM of ascorbate–buformin; the combination did not increase the apoptotic effect. In the OCI-AML2 cells, only the combination treatment significantly enhanced apoptosis (Figure 3d and Table 7). Of note that the OCI-AML3 cells, which are highly dependent on glycolysis, were the most responsive cells, whereas only modest effects were induced by these treatments in the OCI-AML2 and MV4-11 cells, presenting a lower glycolysis dependence and high fuel flexibility.

Table 7. Apoptosis effect in AML cell lines and in primary AML blasts treated with ascorbate plus buformin.

	OCI-AML2	OCI-AML3	MV4-11	AML
Ctrl	3 ± 1	3 ± 1	6 ± 1	22 ± 8
Ascorbate 1 mM	6 ± 3	22 ± 13	8 ± 1	38 ± 12
Buformin 0.1 mM	11 ± 2	10 ± 1	14 ± 1	27 ± 10
Ascorbate–buformin 0.1 mM	18 ± 5	33 ± 9	14 ± 1	51 ± 13
Buformin 0.5 mM	7 ± 4	3 ± 2	27 ± 15	49 ± 19
Ascorbate–buformin 0.5 mM	14 ± 8	72 ± 6	28 ± 10	62 ± 20

Values represent the mean ± SD.

3.6. Ascorbate Plus Buformin Combination Treatment Effectively Induces Apoptosis in Primary AML Blasts

The treatment of primary blasts from seventeen AML patients (Table 1) with ascorbate (1 mM) or buformin (0.1 and 0.5 mM) as the sole agent for 72 h induced a moderate increase in the percentage of apoptotic cells as detected by cytofluorimetric analysis (ascorbate $p < 0.05$; buformin 0.1 mM $p < 0.0005$). Remarkably, the combined ascorbate–buformin treatment significantly increased the apoptotic rate of the AML blasts. We did not observe an association with genetic alterations, probably due to the low number of samples analyzed (Figure 4a and Table 7).

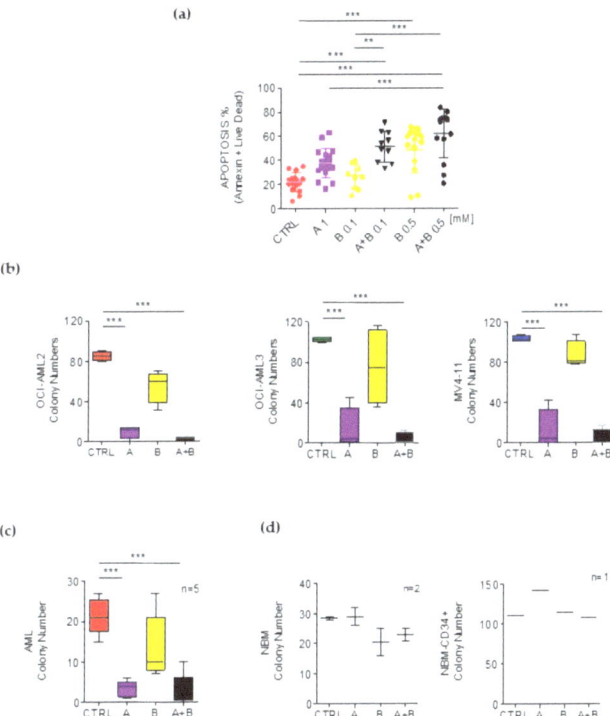

Figure 4. Effects of ascorbate and buformin on survival of AML blasts. Cells were treated with (A) ascorbate (1 mM) and (B) buformin (0.1 and 0.5 mM). (**a**) Cell death of primary blasts from AML patients evaluated by flow cytometry after annexin V + live dead staining. Statistical analysis by Student's *t*-test. ** $p \leq 0.005$; *** $p \leq 0.0005$. (**b**) Clonogenic activity of OCI-AML2, OCI-AML3 and MV4-11 cells treated in semisolid medium for 8 or 13 days. The experiments were conducted in quadruplicate. Statistical analysis by Student's *t*-test *** $p \leq 0.0005$. (**c**) Clonogenic activity of AML blasts isolated from the BM of five patients and treated in semisolid medium for 8 days. (**d**) Clonogenic activity of mononucleated cells isolated from the BM of two healthy donors (NBM) (**left**) or CD34+ cells purified from one NBM (**right**) treated in semisolid medium for 8 days. The box plots report the distribution of the number of colony-forming units. Statistical analysis by Student's *t*-test *** $p \leq 0.0005$.

Next, we studied the effect of the ascorbate, buformin and ascorbate–buformin treatments on hematopoietic colony formation. The AML cell lines treated with the ascorbate or ascorbate–buformin treatments produced a significantly lower number of colonies as compared to the cells treated with buformin or the control cells (Figure 4b and Table 8). Similar results were obtained by treating the AML primary blasts with these agents. (Figure 4c). Interestingly, the same treatments did not affect the clonogenic activity of the BM cells from healthy donors (BMC) or of the CD34+ cells purified from CB, indicating low or no toxicity of the ascorbate–buformin combination treatment on normal hematopoietic progenitors. (Figure 4d and Table 8).

Table 8. Clonogenic Assay. Colony numbers.

	Ctrl	Ascorbate 1 mM	Buformin (0.1 mM)	Ascorbate–Buformin
OCI-AML2	103 ± 3	11 ± 9	58 ± 16	2 ± 3
OCI-AML3	102 ± 2	14 ± 21	75 ± 38	4 ± 6
MV4-11	104 ± 2	13 ± 20	87 ± 14	4 ± 8
AML blasts	21 ± 5	3 ± 2	14 ± 8	3 ± 4
N-BMC	29 ± 4	29 ± 4	21 ± 6	23 ± 3
CD34+	142	142	115	109

3.7. Ascorbate Plus Buformin Inhibits Glycolysis in AML Cells

By performing the XF Glycolytic Stress Test, we observed that the ascorbate treatment decreased basal glycolysis by 1.6 times ($p < 0.01$), buformin by 2.0 times ($p < 0.001$) and the ascorbate–buformin combination by 2.1 times ($p < 0.001$) in the OCI-AML3 cells. In this AML cell line, the glycolytic capacity was reduced by 1.8 times following the ascorbate ($p < 0.01$), 3.5 times following the buformin ($p < 0.0001$) and 3.2 times after the ascorbate–buformin combination treatment ($p < 0.0001$). The glycolytic reserve was completely erased by the buformin ($p < 0.0001$) and ascorbate–buformin combinatory treatments ($p < 0.0001$) (Figure 5a and Supplementary Figure S1a). These results are in line with the high rate of apoptosis induced by these treatments in the OCI-AML3 cells (Figure 3d). The untreated MV4-11 cells showed a lower basal glycolytic rate as compared with the other cell lines. In these cells, the buformin induced an increase of 1.8 times in basal glycolysis ($p < 0.01$) and the ascorbate–buformin combination treatment of 2.4 times ($p < 0.0001$). The glycolytic capacity was enhanced by 1.7 times ($p < 0.01$) by the ascorbate–buformin treatment (Figure 5a and Supplementary Figure S1a). This event may account, at least in part, for the absence of the potentiation effect on apoptosis by the ascorbate–buformin combination treatment in the MV4-11 cells (Figure 3d). The OCI-AML2 metabolic status was not significantly affected by these treatments (Figure 5a and Supplementary Figure S1a), which is in accordance with their lower apoptotic response (Figure 3d).

In order to confirm our results and to exclude intrinsic cellular variability, we utilized U937-AETO/U937-Mock cell lines (the RUNX1/RUNX1T1 inducible system). In U937-AETO, similar to OCI-AML3, the ascorbate–buformin treatment inhibited basal glycolysis by 1.9 times ($p < 0.05$) and the glycolytic capacity by 2.3 times ($p < 0.005$), with respect to the control U937-Mock cells. The glycolytic reserve was completely erased by the buformin and ascorbate–buformin treatments ($p < 0.005$). This effect did not occur in the U937-Mock control cells (Supplementary Figure S1b). The cellular viability by the MTS assay demonstrated that the RUNX1/RUNX1T1 expression induced a higher sensitivity of the U937 cell to 1 mM of ascorbate ($p < 0.001$) (Table 9 and Supplementary Figure S1c), 0.1 mM of ascorbate–buformin ($p < 0.0001$) and 0.5 mM of ascorbate–buformin ($p < 0.0001$). These results indicated that the RUNX1/RUNX1T1 oncoprotein rendered the cells dependent on glycolytic metabolism, confirming the relationship between the inhibition of glycolysis and sensitivity to the ascorbate and ascorbate–buformin treatment in AMLs.

Table 9. Cellular Viability response to different metabolic treatments of U937-AETO/U937-Mock cell lines.

	Ctrl	Ascorbate 1 mM	Buformin (0.1 mM)	Ascorbate–Buformin 0.1	Buformin (0.5 mM)	Ascorbate–Buformin 0.5
U937-Mock	1 ± 0	0.81 ± 0.1	0.93 ± 0.06	0.97 ± 0.05	0.85 ± 0.06	0.78 ± 0.1
U937-AETO	1 ± 0	0.67 ± 0.1	0.84 ± 0.1	0.67 ± 0.1	0.80 ± 0.1	0.48 ± 0.01

Values represent the mean $\pm$ SD.

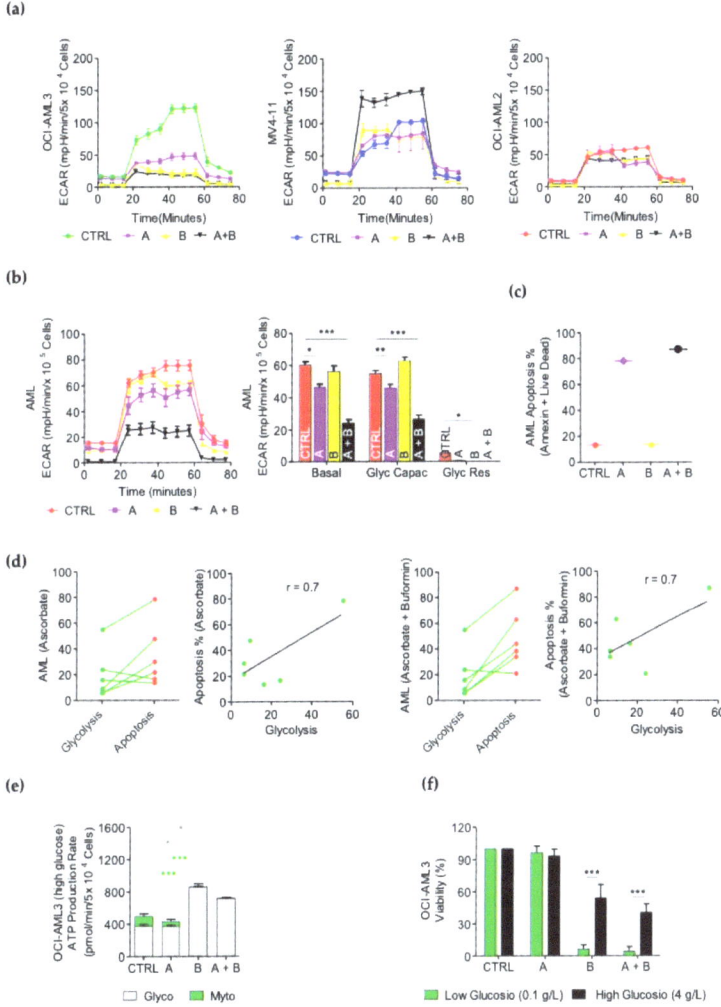

Figure 5. Glycolytic status after buformin plus ascorbate treatment in AMLs. Kinetic profile of ECAR assay in AML cells treated for 24 h with 1 mM of ascorbate (A), 0.1 mM of buformin (B) or ascorbate–buformin combination (A + B) evaluated by XF Glycolytic Stress Test. (**a**) OCI-AML3, MV4-11 and OCI-AML2. (**b**) Primary AML blasts from BM. Histograms represent basal glycolysis, glycolytic capacity (Glyc Capac) and glycolytic reserve (Glyc Res). (**c**) Cell death induced by 1 mM of ascorbate (A), 0.1 mM of buformin (B) or ascorbate–buformin combination (A + B) at 72 h in primary AML blast from the same AML patient by flow cytometry after annexin V + live dead staining. (**d**) Linear correlation between apoptosis and glycolytic levels in AML samples treated with both ascorbate or ascorbate–buformin. (**e**) XF real-time glycolytic and mitochondrial ATP production rate by the ATP Rate Assay in presence of high concentration of glucose (4 g/L) after 12 h of 1 mM of ascorbate (A), 0.1 mM of buformin (B) or ascorbate–buformin combination (A + B) in OCI-AML3 cell line. The experiments were performed in duplicate. (**f**) Cytotoxic efficacy of 1 mM of ascorbate (A), 0.1 mM of buformin (B) or ascorbate–buformin combination (A + B) using the CellTiter-Glo® Luminescent Cell Viability Assay. The cells were cultured at low (0.1 g/L) or high (4 g/L) concentrations of glucose. Three independent experiments were performed in triplicate. Data are presented as mean ± SD. Statistical analysis by Student's t-test. * $p < 0.05$; ** $p < 0.005$; *** $p < 0.0005$.

Interestingly, the primary blasts from an AML patient (N°15, Table 1) with a high dependence on glycolysis in the basal conditions showed, as all the AML cell lines analyzed, OXPHOS inhibition after treatment with buformin or with the ascorbate–buformin combination (Supplementary Figure S1d). To note in these cells, the ascorbate–buformin combination decreased basal glycolysis by two times and the glycolytic capacity by 2.5 times (Figure 5b). Those cells resulted highly sensitive to the induction of apoptosis by the ascorbate and ascorbate–buformin treatments (Figure 5c), further confirming that these treatments are mostly effective in cells that are highly dependent on glycolysis. Important analyzing the six samples for metabolic and apoptotic values we found a positive correlation between apoptosis and glycolytic levels in the AML blast treated with both the ascorbate and ascorbate–buformin treatments (Pearson's coefficient r = 0.7) (p = 0.1) (Figure 5d); even if these results are not significant, which would probably be due to the low number of samples, there is a clear trend in line with our previous results.

3.8. Resistance to Ascorbate–Buformin Combined Treatment Depends on Metabolic Plasticity of AML Cells

To characterize the metabolic background of resistance to these treatments, we evaluated the effect of 1 mM of ascorbate, 0.1 mM of buformin and the ascorbate–buformin combination on the metabolic behavior of the OCI-AML2, OCI-AML3 and MV4-11 cell lines. The OXPHOS was inhibited by the buformin and by the ascorbate–buformin combination in all the three cell lines (Figure 3a and Supplementary Figure S1e). As pointed out before, glycolysis was affected differently in the cell lines. The OCI-AML2 cells did not show significant variations, the OCI-AML3 cells showed inhibition and the MV4-11 cells showed increased glycolysis (Figure 5a and Supplementary Figure S1a). This suggests that glycolytic behavior is the discriminant between the response and resistance to the treatment, in line with the higher sensitivity observed in the glycolysis-dependent OCI-AML3 cells. Conversely, the OCI-AML2 cells and the more flexible MV4-11 cells, which did not rely upon glycolysis in the basal conditions, escaped the ascorbic–buformin treatment, probably switching to glycolytic metabolism. Since these treatments induced differential effects on glycolysis, we evaluated the changes in the total ATP production rate and the fractional contribution of the individual pathways to the bioenergetics demands.

In these AML cell lines. We simultaneously measured, in real time, ATP production from the two major key energetic pathways, glycolysis and mitochondrial respiration, using Agilent Seahorse Extracellular Flux analysis. A decrease of approximately 95% in mitochondrial ATP production rates after treatment with 0.1 mM of buformin was measurable in all the three AML cell lines after 12 h. Importantly, the OCI-AML2 and MV4-11 cell lines totally compensated the lower ATP production levels by increasing the glycolytic ATP production (Supplementary Figure S1f).

Conversely, the OCI-AML3 cells could not efficiently switch metabolism and the energetic state of the cells decreased in line with the major sensitivity observed (Supplementary Figure S1f). By adding a high concentration of glucose (4 g/L), the OCI-AML3 cells compensated for the ATP production (Figure 5d), confirming their glycolytic dependence.

The cellular viability, measured by the CellTiter-Glo Assay on the OCI-AML3 cells at low (0.1 g/L) or high (4 g/L) glucose concentrations, increased at high concentrations of glucose, buformin (p < 0.0001) and ascorbate–buformin (p < 0.0001) (Figure 5e), confirming that the inability of the AML cells to switch to glycolysis is relevant for the induction of apoptosis after ascorbate–buformin treatment.

4. Discussion

AML's phenotypic landscape is characterized by high heterogeneity, clonal evolution and considerable dynamics of genetic and epigenetic events over the course of the disease [1,4,49,50]. Data from clonal evolution studies suggest that the genes commonly involved in epigenetic regulation (i.e., DNMT3A, ASXL1, IDH2 and TET2) are deregulated in pre-leukemic hematopoietic stem cells [2,51]. Such pre-leukemic stem cells are capable of multilineage differentiation, can survive chemotherapy and expand during disease remission. Most of the time, chemotherapy only provides a selective pressure for the expansion of resistant subclones, which vary in their genomic and metabolic phenotypes, and AMLs often relapse [11,50,52–54].

To study the efficacy of a metabolic-oriented synergic treatment, we endeavored to define the metabolic landscape and capacity to compensate after the treatment of different AML cells.

We used three cell lines as metabolic models of AMLs. The MV4-11 cells had greater basal OXPHOS values, whereas OCI-AML2 and OCI-AML3 had greater basal glycolysis values. The MV4-11 cells displayed a significant dependency on fatty acid (FA) oxidation fuel and slightly on pyruvate. OCI-AML3 had a strong dependency on glucose fuel and slightly on FAs. OCI-AML2 depended partially on pyruvate and FAs. All these AML cell lines showed high flexibility towards all three fuels. We confirmed the result obtained in the AML cell lines in the primary blasts from AML patients, presenting diverse metabolic backgrounds. Our findings suggest different sensitivities of AML blasts to metabolic therapies, and, in our opinion, acknowledge them as reliable models to foresee the effects of ascorbate–buformin combination therapy in AML patients. Previous studies demonstrated that metformin inhibits the molecular reduction of oxygen in hepatocytes and leukemia cell lines [55,56]. Buformin is chemically related to metformin but is more active and has never been tested in leukemia. Therefore, given its inhibitory effect on complex I, which completely shuts down mitochondrial contributions in ATP production, we addressed its effect on AML cells in combination with ascorbate.

Studies have shown that ascorbate (vitamin C), at pharmacological doses, targets many of the mechanisms that cancer cells utilize for their survival and growth, including redox imbalances and oxygen-sensing regulations [57]. In addition, ascorbate treatment re-establishes TET2 function in AML blasts that present decreased TET2 activity in vitro and in vivo [20,58–60]. Altered TET2 function in AMLs can result from heterozygous TET2 mutations and in mutations in IDH1, IDH2 and WT1 [61,62]. Zhao et al. found that ascorbate plus decitabine prior to aclarubicin and cytarabine (A-DCAG) significantly increased the chance of clinical remission after the first induction therapy and extended the median overall survival by 6 months, compared to DCAG alone in AML patients who were over 60 years old [63].

Here, we show that ascorbate inhibits glycolysis by interfering with HK1/2 and GLUT1 functions in hematopoietic cells. The inhibition of HK1/2 and GLUT1 in highly glycolytic OCI-AML3 cells by ascorbate, with the disrupting effect of buformin on the oxygen mitochondrial chain, ultimately leads to an 'energy crisis' and cell death. OCI-AML2 and MV4-11 cells, which in basal conditions do not rely upon the glycolysis pathway, switch metabolism and, in part, escape cytotoxicity. Overall, these results suggest that glycolytic behavior is the discriminant between the response and resistance to ascorbate–buformin treatment. This evidence is in line with the higher sensitivity observed in the U937 cells, following the RUNX/RUNX1T1 expression, which turned dependent on glycolysis and were more sensitive to the ascorbate–buformin treatment than the U937-Mock cells. In addition, we observed a positive correlation between the ascorbate treatment and basal glycolytic levels in the six AML samples analyzed. Although it will be necessary to confirm these results in a larger number of AML patient samples, those data clearly depict an effect of ascorbate on glycolysis. Our data contribute to elucidating the targets and mechanisms by which ascorbate and buformin exerts anti-cancer effects. Further insight will be essential for identifying predictive biomarkers for patient stratification and for developing potent combination strategies that lead to durable disease remissions.

Since the efficacy of a treatment should be measured as the capacity of inhibiting the growth of leukemia-initiating cells, by performing clonogenic assays, we demonstrated that an ascorbate–buformin combination treatment induces a drastic reduction in the number of colonies as compared to the untreated AML cell lines and primary blasts from AML patients. The efficiency of the vitamin c treatment in inhibiting leukemic colony formation might also depend on its previously reported ability to restore TET2 function, which drives DNA hypomethylation, by enhancing 5 hmC formations and thereby suppressing leukemic colony formation and the leukemic progression of primary human leukemia patient-derived xenografts (PDXs) [20,60]. Of note that this effect was achieved with low or no toxicity in normal BMC and CD34+ cells from healthy donors, as expected from the higher spare respiratory capacity and high glycolytic reserve of hematopoietic precursors. Overall, our findings indicate that ascorbate–buformin is a suitable therapy to be used, in association with drugs targeting different mechanisms, in fragile patients.

5. Conclusions

In conclusion, our data have therapeutic implications especially in fragile patients since both agents have an excellent safety profile, and they support the clinical evaluation of ascorbate–buformin for the treatment of refractory/relapsing AML patients with no other therapeutic options. Since buformin potentiates the effect of ascorbate without adding toxicity, the combination treatment could be associated to other targeted therapies in randomized clinical trials to gauge their utility in the clinic.

Supplementary Materials: The following supporting information can be downloaded at: https://www.mdpi.com/article/10.3390/cancers14102565/s1, Figure S1: Metabolic effect of buformin (B) and ascorbate (A) in AML cells; Figure S2: Original Western blot images. Table S1. List of primary antibodies used.

Author Contributions: C.B. and G.C. co-wrote the manuscript, carried out the experiments and analyzed the results; A.Z. and S.T. performed the W blot and Q-RT-PCR experiments; P.N., T.O. and M.D. characterized and collected the samples from the AML patients; M.S. provided the cord blood samples; E.P. carried out the differentiation experiments of the CD34+ progenitor cells; G.G. and D.F.A. carried out the cytofluorimetric analysis; E.A., U.T., C.N. and L.B. critically reviewed the manuscript and amended the final report; N.I.N. and M.T.V. contributed to the study design, analyzed the experiments and co-wrote the manuscript. All authors have read and agreed to the published version of the manuscript.

Funding: This research was funded by AIRC 5 × 1000 call "Metastatic disease: the key unmet need in oncology" to MYNERVA project, #21267 (MYeloid NEoplasms Research Venture AIRC. A detailed description of the MYNERVA project is available at http://www.progettoagimm.it, accessed on 2 April 2022) to MTV, by PRIN 2017WXR7ZT_004 to MTV, by grant from the Ministero della Salute, Rome, Italy (Finalizzata 2018, NET-2018-12365935, Personalized medicine program on myeloid neoplasms: characterization of the patient's genome for clinical decision making and systematic collection of real world data to improve quality of health care) to MTV and by PRIN 2017WWB99Z to C.N.

Institutional Review Board Statement: This study was conducted in accordance with the Declaration of Helsinki and was approved by the Ethics Committee of Policlinico Tor Vergata (study protocol AIRC-MYNERVA code 171/19 and date of approval, 8 February 2013).

Informed Consent Statement: Informed consent was obtained from all subjects involved in the study.

Data Availability Statement: Not applicable.

Conflicts of Interest: The authors declare no conflict of interest.

References

1. Welch, J.S.; Ley, T.J.; Link, D.C.; Miller, C.A.; Larson, D.E.; Koboldt, D.C.; Wartman, L.D.; Lamprecht, T.L.; Liu, F.; Xia, J.; et al. The Origin and Evolution of Mutations in Acute Myeloid Leukemia. *Cell* **2012**, *150*, 264–278. [CrossRef]
2. Shlush, L.I.; Zandi, S.; Mitchell, A.; Chen, W.C.; Brandwein, J.M.; Gupta, V.; Kennedy, J.A.; Schimmer, A.D.; Schuh, A.C.; Yee, K.W.; et al. Identification of pre-leukaemic haematopoietic stem cells in acute leukaemia. *Nature* **2014**, *506*, 328–333. [CrossRef]
3. Estey, E.; Döhner, H. Acute myeloid leukaemia. *Lancet* **2006**, *368*, 1894–1907. [CrossRef]
4. Döhner, H.; Weisdorf, D.J.; Bloomfield, C.D. Acute Myeloid Leukemia. *N. Engl. J. Med.* **2015**, *373*, 1136–1152. [CrossRef]
5. Kreitz, J.; Schönfeld, C.; Seibert, M.; Stolp, V.; Alshamleh, I.; Oellerich, T.; Steffen, B.; Schwalbe, H.; Schnütgen, F.; Kurrle, N.; et al. Metabolic Plasticity of Acute Myeloid Leukemia. *Cells* **2019**, *8*, 805. [CrossRef]
6. Rashkovan, M.; Ferrando, A. Metabolic dependencies and vulnerabilities in leukemia. *Genes Dev.* **2019**, *33*, 1460–1474. [CrossRef]

7. Noguera, N.I.; Hasan, S.K.; Ammatuna, E.; Venditti, A. Editorial: Metabolic Rewiring in Leukemias. *Front. Oncol.* **2021**, *11*, 775167. [CrossRef]
8. Ye, H.; Adane, B.; Khan, N.; Alexeev, E.; Nusbacher, N.; Minhajuddin, M.; Stevens, B.M.; Winters, A.C.; Lin, X.; Ashton, J.M.; et al. Subversion of Systemic Glucose Metabolism as a Mechanism to Support the Growth of Leukemia Cells. *Cancer Cell* **2018**, *34*, 659–673.e6. [CrossRef]
9. Škrtić, M.; Sriskanthadevan, S.; Jhas, B.; Gebbia, M.; Wang, X.; Wang, Z.; Hurren, R.; Jitkova, Y.; Gronda, M.; Maclean, N.; et al. Inhibition of Mitochondrial Translation as a Therapeutic Strategy for Human Acute Myeloid Leukemia. *Cancer Cell* **2011**, *20*, 674–688. [CrossRef]
10. Lagadinou, E.D.; Sach, A.; Callahan, K.; Rossi, R.M.; Neering, S.J.; Minhajuddin, M.; Ashton, J.M.; Pei, S.; Grose, V.; O'Dwyer, K.M.; et al. BCL-2 Inhibition Targets Oxidative Phosphorylation and Selectively Eradicates Quiescent Human Leukemia Stem Cells. *Cell Stem Cell* **2013**, *12*, 329–341. [CrossRef]
11. Jones, C.L.; Stevens, B.M.; D'Alessandro, A.; Reisz, J.A.; Culp-Hill, R.; Nemkov, T.; Pei, S.; Khan, N.; Adane, B.; Ye, H.; et al. Inhibition of Amino Acid Metabolism Selectively Targets Human Leukemia Stem Cells. *Cancer Cell* **2018**, *34*, 724–740.e4. [CrossRef]
12. Jones, C.L.; Stevens, B.M.; D'Alessandro, A.; Culp-Hill, R.; Reisz, J.A.; Pei, S.; Gustafson, A.; Khan, N.; DeGregori, J.; Pollyea, D.A.; et al. Cysteine depletion targets leukemia stem cells through inhibition of electron transport complex II. *Blood* **2019**, *134*, 389–394. [CrossRef]
13. Farge, T.; Saland, E.; De Toni, F.; Aroua, N.; Hosseini, M.; Perry, R.; Bosc, C.; Sugita, M.; Stuani, L.; Fraisse, M.; et al. Chemotherapy-Resistant Human Acute Myeloid Leukemia Cells Are Not Enriched for Leukemic Stem Cells but Require Oxidative Metabolism. *Cancer Discov.* **2017**, *7*, 716–735. [CrossRef]
14. Yoshida, G.J. Metabolic reprogramming: The emerging concept and associated therapeutic strategies. *J. Exp. Clin. Cancer Res.* **2015**, *34*, 111. [CrossRef]
15. Kang, S.-R.; Song, H.-C.; Byun, B.H.; Oh, J.-R.; Kim, H.-S.; Hong, S.-P.; Kwon, S.Y.; Chong, A.; Kim, J.; Cho, S.-G.; et al. Intratumoral Metabolic Heterogeneity for Prediction of Disease Progression After Concurrent Chemoradiotherapy in Patients with Inoperable Stage III Non-Small-Cell Lung Cancer. *Nucl. Med. Mol. Imaging* **2014**, *48*, 16–25. [CrossRef]
16. Yoshida, G.J. Emerging roles of Myc in stem cell biology and novel tumor therapies. *J. Exp. Clin. Cancer Res.* **2018**, *37*, 1. [CrossRef]
17. Intlekofer, A.M.; Finley, L.W.S. Metabolic signatures of cancer cells and stem cells. *Nat. Metab.* **2019**, *1*, 177–188. [CrossRef]
18. Zhang, J.; Nuebel, E.; Daley, G.Q.; Koehler, C.M.; Teitell, M.A. Metabolic Regulation in Pluripotent Stem Cells during Reprogramming and Self-Renewal. *Cell Stem Cell* **2012**, *11*, 589–595. [CrossRef]
19. Presti, C.L.; Fauvelle, F.; Jacob, M.-C.; Mondet, J.; Mossuz, P. The metabolic reprogramming in acute myeloid leukemia patients depends on their genotype and is a prognostic marker. *Blood Adv.* **2021**, *5*, 156–166. [CrossRef]
20. Cimmino, L.; Dolgalev, I.; Wang, Y.; Yoshimi, A.; Martin, G.H.; Wang, J.; Ng, V.; Xia, B.; Witkowski, M.T.; Mitchell-Flack, M.; et al. Restoration of TET2 Function Blocks Aberrant Self-Renewal and Leukemia Progression. *Cell* **2017**, *170*, 1079–1095.e20. [CrossRef]
21. Smith-Díaz, C.C.; Magon, N.J.; McKenzie, J.L.; Hampton, M.B.; Vissers, M.C.M.; Das, A.B. Ascorbate Inhibits Proliferation and Promotes Myeloid Differentiation in TP53-Mutant Leukemia. *Front. Oncol.* **2021**, *11*, 709543. [CrossRef]
22. Chen, Q.; Espey, M.G.; Sun, A.Y.; Lee, J.-H.; Krishna, M.C.; Shacter, E.; Choyke, P.L.; Pooput, C.; Kirk, K.L.; Buettner, G.R.; et al. Ascorbate in pharmacologic concentrations selectively generates ascorbate radical and hydrogen peroxide in extracellular fluid in vivo. *Proc. Natl. Acad. Sci. USA* **2007**, *104*, 8749–8754. [CrossRef]
23. Granger, M.; Eck, P. Dietary Vitamin C in Human Health. *Adv. Food Nutr. Res.* **2018**, *83*, 281–310. [CrossRef]
24. Mastrangelo, D.; Massai, L.; Fioritoni, G.; Coco, F.L.; Noguera, N.; Testa, U. High Doses of Vitamin C and Leukemia: In Vitro Update. In *Myeloid Leukemia*; Lasfar, A., Ed.; IntechOpen: London, UK, 2018.
25. Noguera, N.I.; Pelosi, E.; Angelini, D.F.; Piredda, M.L.; Guerrera, G.; Piras, E.; Battistini, L.; Massai, L.; Berardi, A.; Catalano, G.; et al. High-dose ascorbate and arsenic trioxide selectively kill acute myeloid leukemia and acute promyelocytic leukemia blasts in vitro. *Oncotarget* **2017**, *8*, 32550–32565. [CrossRef]
26. Cameron, E.; Pauling, L. Supplemental ascorbate in the supportive treatment of cancer: Prolongation of survival times in terminal human cancer. *Proc. Natl. Acad. Sci. USA* **1976**, *73*, 3685–3689. [CrossRef]
27. Mastrangelo, D.; Massai, L.; Coco, F.L.; Noguera, N.I.; Borgia, L.; Fioritoni, G.; Berardi, A.C.; Iacone, A.; Muscettola, M.; Pelosi, E.; et al. Cytotoxic effects of high concentrations of sodium ascorbate on human myeloid cell lines. *Ann. Hematol.* **2015**, *94*, 1807–1816. [CrossRef]
28. Fiorani, M.; De Sanctis, R.; Scarlatti, F.; Vallorani, L.; De Bellis, R.; Serafini, G.; Bianchi, M.; Stocchi, V. Dehydroascorbic acid irreversibly inhibits hexokinase activity. *Mol. Cell. Biochem.* **2000**, *209*, 145–153. [CrossRef]
29. Heneberg, P. Redox Regulation of Hexokinases. *Antioxid. Redox Signal.* **2019**, *30*, 415–442. [CrossRef]
30. Zakikhani, M.; Dowling, R.; Fantus, I.G.; Sonenberg, N.; Pollak, M. Metformin Is an AMP Kinase–Dependent Growth Inhibitor for Breast Cancer Cells. *Cancer Res.* **2006**, *66*, 10269–10273. [CrossRef]
31. Wahdan-Alaswad, R.S.; Cochrane, D.R.; Spoelstra, N.S.; Howe, E.N.; Edgerton, S.M.; Anderson, S.M.; Thor, A.D.; Richer, J.K. Metformin-Induced Killing of Triple-Negative Breast Cancer Cells Is Mediated by Reduction in Fatty Acid Synthase via miRNA-193b. *Horm. Cancer* **2014**, *5*, 374–389. [CrossRef]
32. Queiroz, E.A.I.F.; Puukila, S.; Eichler, R.; Sampaio, S.C.; Forsyth, H.L.; Lees, S.J.; Barbosa, A.M.; Dekker, R.F.H.; Fortes, Z.B.; Khaper, N. Metformin Induces Apoptosis and Cell Cycle Arrest Mediated by Oxidative Stress, AMPK and FOXO3a in MCF-7 Breast Cancer Cells. *PLoS ONE* **2014**, *9*, e98207. [CrossRef]

33. Orecchioni, S.; Reggiani, F.; Talarico, G.; Mancuso, P.; Calleri, A.; Gregato, G.; Labanca, V.; Noonan, D.M.; Dallaglio, K.; Albini, A.; et al. The biguanides metformin and phenformin inhibit angiogenesis, local and metastatic growth of breast cancer by targeting both neoplastic and microenvironment cells. *Int. J. Cancer* **2015**, *136*, E534–E544. [CrossRef]
34. Memmott, R.M.; Mercado, J.R.; Maier, C.R.; Kawabata, S.; Fox, S.D.; Dennis, P.A. Metformin Prevents Tobacco Carcinogen–Induced Lung Tumorigenesis. *Cancer Prev. Res.* **2010**, *3*, 1066–1076. [CrossRef]
35. Guo, Q.; Liu, Z.; Jiang, L.; Liu, M.; Ma, J.; Yang, C.; Han, L.; Nan, K.; Liang, X. Metformin inhibits growth of human non-small cell lung cancer cells via liver kinase B-1-independent activation of adenosine monophosphate-activated protein kinase. *Mol. Med. Rep.* **2016**, *13*, 2590–2596. [CrossRef]
36. Tomic, T.; Botton, T.; Cerezo, M.; Robert, G.; Luciano, F.; Puissant, A.; Gounon, P.; Allegra, M.; Bertolotto, C.; Bereder, J.-M.; et al. Metformin inhibits melanoma development through autophagy and apoptosis mechanisms. *Cell Death Dis.* **2011**, *2*, e199. [CrossRef]
37. Janjetovic, K.; Harhaji-Trajkovic, L.; Misirkic-Marjanovic, M.; Vucicevic, L.; Stevanovic, D.; Zogovic, N.; Sumarac-Dumanovic, M.; Micic, D.; Trajkovic, V. In vitro and in vivo anti-melanoma action of metformin. *Eur. J. Pharmacol.* **2011**, *668*, 373–382. [CrossRef]
38. Bhat, M.; Yanagiya, A.; Graber, T.; Razumilava, N.; Bronk, S.; Zammit, D.; Zhao, Y.; Zakaria, C.; Metrakos, P.; Pollak, M.; et al. Metformin requires 4E-BPs to induce apoptosis and repress translation of Mcl-1 in hepatocellular carcinoma cells. *Oncotarget* **2017**, *8*, 50542–50556. [CrossRef]
39. Kilgore, J.; Jackson, A.L.; Clark, L.H.; Guo, H.; Zhang, L.; Jones, H.M.; Gilliam, T.P.; Gehrig, P.A.; Zhou, C.; Bae-Jump, V.L. Buformin exhibits anti-proliferative and anti-invasive effects in endometrial cancer cells. *Am. J. Transl. Res.* **2016**, *8*, 2705–2715.
40. Careccia, S.; Mainardi, S.; Pelosi, A.; Gurtner, A.; Diverio, D.; Riccioni, R.; Testa, U.; Pelosi, E.; Piaggio, G.; Sacchi, A.; et al. A restricted signature of miRNAs distinguishes APL blasts from normal promyelocytes. *Oncogene* **2009**, *28*, 4034–4040. [CrossRef]
41. Banella, C.; Ginevrino, M.; Catalano, G.; Fabiani, E.; Falconi, G.; Divona, M.; Curzi, P.; Panetta, P.; Voso, M.T.; Noguera, N.I. Absence of FGFR3–TACC3 rearrangement in hematological malignancies with numerical chromosomal alteration. *Hematol. Oncol. Stem Cell Ther.* **2021**, *14*, 163–168. [CrossRef]
42. Masciarelli, S.; Capuano, E.; Ottone, T.; Divona, M.; De Panfilis, S.; Banella, C.; Noguera, N.I.; Picardi, A.; Fontemaggi, G.; Blandino, G.; et al. Retinoic acid and arsenic trioxide sensitize acute promyelocytic leukemia cells to ER stress. *Leukemia* **2018**, *32*, 285–294. [CrossRef]
43. Noguera, N.I.; Piredda, M.L.; Taulli, R.; Catalano, G.; Angelini, G.; Gaur, G.; Nervi, C.; Voso, M.T.; Lunardi, A.; Pandolfi, P.P.; et al. PML/RARa inhibits PTEN expression in hematopoietic cells by competing with PU.1 transcriptional activity. *Oncotarget* **2016**, *7*, 66386–66397. [CrossRef]
44. Quattrocchi, A.; Maiorca, C.; Billi, M.; Tomassini, S.; De Marinis, E.; Cenfra, N.; Equitani, F.; Gentile, M.; Ceccherelli, A.; Banella, C.; et al. Genetic lesions disrupting calreticulin 3′-untranslated region in JAK2 mutation-negative polycythemia vera. *Am. J. Hematol.* **2020**, *95*, E263–E267. [CrossRef]
45. Banella, C.; Catalano, G.; Travaglini, S.; Divona, M.; Masciarelli, S.; Guerrera, G.; Fazi, F.; Lo-Coco, F.; Voso, M.T.; Noguera, N.I. PML/RARa Interferes with NRF2 Transcriptional Activity Increasing the Sensitivity to Ascorbate of Acute Promyelocytic Leukemia Cells. *Cancers* **2019**, *12*, 95. [CrossRef]
46. Cunningham, I.; Kohno, B. 18 FDG-PET/CT: 21st century approach to leukemic tumors in 124 cases. *Am. J. Hematol.* **2016**, *91*, 379–384. [CrossRef]
47. Sriskanthadevan, S.; Jeyaraju, D.V.; Chung, T.E.; Prabha, S.; Xu, W.; Skrtic, M.; Jhas, B.; Hurren, R.; Gronda, M.; Wang, X.; et al. AML cells have low spare reserve capacity in their respiratory chain that renders them susceptible to oxidative metabolic stress. *Blood* **2015**, *125*, 2120–2130. [CrossRef]
48. Sarrazy, V.; Viaud, M.; Westerterp, M.; Ivanov, S.; Giorgetti-Peraldi, S.; Guinamard, R.; Gautier, E.L.; Thorp, E.B.; De Vivo, D.C.; Yvan-Charvet, L. Disruption of Glut1 in Hematopoietic Stem Cells Prevents Myelopoiesis and Enhanced Glucose Flux in Atheromatous Plaques of ApoE(-/-) Mice. *Circ. Res.* **2016**, *118*, 1062–1077. [CrossRef]
49. Ley, T.J.; Miller, C.; Ding, L.; Raphael, B.J.; Mungall, A.J.; Robertson, A.; Hoadley, K.; Triche, T.J.; Laird, P.W.; Baty, J.D.; et al. Genomic and epigenomic landscapes of adult de novo acute myeloid leukemia. *N. Engl. J. Med.* **2013**, *368*, 2059–2074. [CrossRef]
50. Ding, L.; Ley, T.J.; Larson, D.E.; Miller, C.A.; Koboldt, D.C.; Welch, J.S.; Ritchey, J.K.; Young, M.A.; Lamprecht, T.L.; McLellan, M.D.; et al. Clonal evolution in relapsed acute myeloid leukaemia revealed by whole-genome sequencing. *Nature* **2012**, *481*, 506–510. [CrossRef]
51. Seton-Rogers, S. Leukaemia: A pre-leukaemic reservoir. *Nat. Rev. Cancer* **2014**, *14*, 212. [CrossRef]
52. Jongen-Lavrencic, M.; Grob, T.; Hanekamp, D.; Kavelaars, F.G.; Al Hinai, A.; Zeilemaker, A.; Erpelinck-Verschueren, C.A.J.; Gradowska, P.L.; Meijer, R.; Cloos, J.; et al. Molecular Minimal Residual Disease in Acute Myeloid Leukemia. *N. Engl. J. Med.* **2018**, *378*, 1189–1199. [CrossRef]
53. Shlush, L.I.; Mitchell, A.; Heisler, L.; Abelson, S.; Ng, S.W.K.; Trotman-Grant, A.; Medeiros, J.J.F.; Rao-Bhatia, A.; Jaciw-Zurakowsky, I.; Marke, R.; et al. Tracing the origins of relapse in acute myeloid leukaemia to stem cells. *Nature* **2017**, *547*, 104–108. [CrossRef] [PubMed]
54. Ye, H.; Adane, B.; Khan, N.; Sullivan, T.; Minhajuddin, M.; Gasparetto, M.; Stevens, B.; Pei, S.; Balys, M.; Ashton, J.M.; et al. Leukemic Stem Cells Evade Chemotherapy by Metabolic Adaptation to an Adipose Tissue Niche. *Cell Stem Cell* **2016**, *19*, 23–37. [CrossRef] [PubMed]

55. Foretz, M.; Hébrard, S.; Leclerc, J.; Zarrinpashneh, E.; Soty, M.; Mithieux, G.; Sakamoto, K.; Andreelli, F.; Viollet, B. Metformin inhibits hepatic gluconeogenesis in mice independently of the LKB1/AMPK pathway via a decrease in hepatic energy state. *J. Clin. Investig.* **2010**, *120*, 2355–2369. [CrossRef]
56. Scotland, S.; Saland, E.; Skuli, N.; De Toni, F.; Boutzen, H.; Micklow, E.; Sénégas, I.; Peyraud, R.; Peyriga, L.; Theodoro, F.; et al. Mitochondrial energetic and AKT status mediate metabolic effects and apoptosis of metformin in human leukemic cells. *Leukemia* **2013**, *27*, 2129–2138. [CrossRef]
57. Ngo, B.; Van Riper, J.M.; Cantley, L.C.; Yun, J. Targeting cancer vulnerabilities with high-dose vitamin C. *Nat. Rev. Cancer* **2019**, *19*, 271–282. [CrossRef]
58. Young, J.I.; Züchner, S.; Wang, G. Regulation of the Epigenome by Vitamin C. *Annu. Rev. Nutr.* **2015**, *35*, 545–564. [CrossRef]
59. Blaschke, K.; Ebata, K.T.; Karimi, M.M.; Zepeda-Martínez, J.A.; Goyal, P.; Mahapatra, S.; Tam, A.; Laird, D.J.; Hirst, M.; Rao, A.; et al. Vitamin C induces Tet-dependent DNA demethylation and a blastocyst-like state in ES cells. *Nature* **2013**, *500*, 222–226. [CrossRef]
60. Agathocleous, M.; Meacham, C.E.; Burgess, R.J.; Piskounova, E.; Zhao, Z.; Crane, G.M.; Cowin, B.L.; Bruner, E.; Murphy, M.M.; Chen, W.; et al. Ascorbate regulates haematopoietic stem cell function and leukaemogenesis. *Nature* **2017**, *549*, 476–481. [CrossRef]
61. Figueroa, M.E.; Abdel-Wahab, O.; Lu, C.; Ward, P.S.; Patel, J.; Shih, A.; Li, Y.; Bhagwat, N.; VasanthaKumar, A.; Fernandez, H.F.; et al. Leukemic IDH1 and IDH2 Mutations Result in a Hypermethylation Phenotype, Disrupt TET2 Function, and Impair Hematopoietic Differentiation. *Cancer Cell* **2010**, *18*, 553–567. [CrossRef]
62. Rampal, R.; Akalin, A.; Madzo, J.; Vasanthakumar, A.; Pronier, E.; Patel, J.; Li, Y.; Ahn, J.; Abdel-Wahab, O.; Shih, A.; et al. DNA Hydroxymethylation Profiling Reveals that WT1 Mutations Result in Loss of TET2 Function in Acute Myeloid Leukemia. *Cell Rep.* **2014**, *9*, 1841–1855. [CrossRef] [PubMed]
63. Zhao, H.; Zhu, H.; Huang, J.; Zhu, Y.; Hong, M.; Zhu, H.; Zhang, J.; Li, S.; Yang, L.; Lian, Y.; et al. The synergy of Vitamin C with decitabine activates TET2 in leukemic cells and significantly improves overall survival in elderly patients with acute myeloid leukemia. *Leuk. Res.* **2018**, *66*, 1–7. [CrossRef] [PubMed]

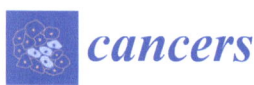

Review

How Warburg-Associated Lactic Acidosis Rewires Cancer Cell Energy Metabolism to Resist Glucose Deprivation

Zoé Daverio [1], Aneta Balcerczyk [2], Gilles J. P. Rautureau [3,†] and Baptiste Panthu [1,*,†]

[1] Laboratoire CarMeN, Institut National de la Santé et de la Recherche Médicale U1060, Université Claude Bernard Lyon 1, 69100 Lyon, France
[2] Department of Oncobiology and Epigenetics, Faculty of Biology and Environmental Protection, University of Lodz, 90-236 Lodz, Poland
[3] Institut de Chimie et Biochimie Moléculaires et Supramoléculaires, Université Claude Bernard Lyon 1, 69622 Lyon, France
* Correspondence: baptiste.panthu@univ-lyon1.fr
† These authors contributed equally to this study.

Simple Summary: Lactic acidosis is a prominent feature of the tumour microenvironment and a key player in cancer metabolism. This review is aimed at combining the mechanisms through which lactic acidosis alters the metabolism of cancer cells, and determining how this effect could bring valuable contribution to the current understanding of the metabolism of whole tumours. This work also highlights the therapeutic perspectives that advances in lactic acidosis understanding open up.

Abstract: Lactic acidosis, a hallmark of solid tumour microenvironment, originates from lactate hyperproduction and its co-secretion with protons by cancer cells displaying the Warburg effect. Long considered a side effect of cancer metabolism, lactic acidosis is now known to play a major role in tumour physiology, aggressiveness and treatment efficiency. Growing evidence shows that it promotes cancer cell resistance to glucose deprivation, a common feature of tumours. Here we review the current understanding of how extracellular lactate and acidosis, acting as a combination of enzymatic inhibitors, signal, and nutrient, switch cancer cell metabolism from the Warburg effect to an oxidative metabolic phenotype, which allows cancer cells to withstand glucose deprivation, and makes lactic acidosis a promising anticancer target. We also discuss how the evidence about lactic acidosis' effect could be integrated in the understanding of the whole-tumour metabolism and what perspectives it opens up for future research.

Keywords: lactic acidosis; glucose deprivation; tumour heterogeneity; metabolic symbiosis; Warburg effect

1. Introduction

Lactic acidosis is a hallmark of the tumour microenvironment, one that has been shown to promote cancer resistance to chemotherapy [1]. It results from the intensive secretion of lactate and protons in the presence of glucose by cells displaying the Warburg effect, a characteristic anomaly of proliferating, and, particularly, cancer cells. Cells harbouring the Warburg effect perform high-rate glycolysis, lactic fermentation, and co-excretion of lactate and protons [2]. This enables them to proliferate at a high rate in the presence of glucose, which they consume avidly. However, the rapid consumption of glucose leads to its exhaustion, and an energetic dead-end and paradox. Interestingly, lactic acidosis has been shown to help cancer cells withstand glucose deprivation [3]. In media conditioned with high lactate concentration and acidity, cancer cell lines avoid apoptosis and survive 10 times longer in the absence of glucose. Further studies have demonstrated that cancer cells resist glucose starvation by reprogramming their metabolism [4,5]. In this review, we focus on the essential literature addressing how lactic acidosis affects energy metabolism

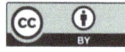

and preserves homeostasis in glucose-deprived cancer cells, and what therapeutic prospects it opens up. We then discuss how this effect at the cellular scale could help understand the metabolism of whole tumours.

2. Defining the Experimental Conditions of the Presented Studies

In this work, we review a series of studies relevant to address how lactic acidosis helps cells resist glucose deficiency. These studies are performed in varying conditions (Table 1). In order to clarify the various experimental conditions, we emphasise the following definitions [3]. "Lactosis" refers to an in vitro condition in which extracellular lactate concentration exceeds 15 mM. It must be noted that most presented studies were performed with culture media containing 10% foetal bovine serum, which brings ~1.5 mM lactate to the medium [6]. At pH 6.7, >15 mM added lactate helps cancer cells resist glucose deprivation [3]. "Acidosis" refers to an extracellular pH of 5.8–6.7. Under pH 6.7 normal cells suffer from acidosis, and tumour pH can drop down to 5.8 [4]. "Lactic acidosis" refers to the combination of both lactosis and acidosis. Lactic acidosis and acidosis are frequently encountered in tumours [7]. Both originate from the co-secretion of lactate and protons, and acidosis is also caused by the mitochondrial production of CO_2 and its dissociation into HCO_3^- and H^+ [8]. Lactosis is a condition virtually absent in vivo, but one that can be achieved easily in vitro to study the effect of lactate independently from acidification by adding buffered sodium lactate to the medium.

"Glucose deprivation" or "depletion" refers to conditions where glucose is scarce, but not necessarily absent from the milieu. Intratumoral glucose concentration can drop to 0.1–0.4 mM, while its level in healthy tissues is ~1 mM [9]. In vitro studies recreate glucose deprivation with culture media that contain, initially, up to 3 mM glucose, the amount that cancer cells typically deplete in one day [3,6].

Table 1. The presented studies addressing lactic acidosis' impact on cell energy metabolism are performed under various conditions. For each reference, the tested cell line or cancer type and medium conditions (glucose concentration, lactate concentration, and pH) are specified. When unspecified, the pH value was assumed to equal 7.4.

Reference	Glucose Concentration (mM)	Lactate Concentration (mM)	pH	Cell Lines or Tumour Origin
[3]	3	20	6.7	4T1, Bcap37, RKO, SGC7901
[10]	Unspecified	25	6 to 6.7	HMEC, DU145, SiHa, WiDr
[4]	10	10	6.5	MCF-7, MDA-MB-468, MDA-MB-231, SkBr3
[11]	5 and 25	5 to 30	6.7	U251 and glioblastoma
[12]	Unspecified	10 or 20	7.4	A549, H1299
[13]	10	5 to 30	7.4	A549, H1299
[14]	Unspecified	10 or 30	7.4	SiHa and mouse xenograft
[5]	6	25	6.5	4T1, Bcap37, HeLa, A549
[15]	Unspecified	4 to 40	5 to 8	MCF7, T47D
[16]	Unspecified	5 or 10	7.4	A549, H1299, BEAS-2B
[17]	10	3 to 40	6.2	A549, A427, MCF7, MRC5
[18]	Unspecified	0	6.5	A549, H1299, MRC5
[19]	5	10	7.4	SiHa, HeLa
[20]	10	10 or 25	6.7	MCF-7, ZR-75-1, T47D, MDA-MB-231, MDA-MB-157
[21]	5.6	10 or 20	6.7	LS174T, HCT116, MCT4
[22]	Unspecified	20	7.4	MCF7
[23]	Unspecified	10	7.4	MDA-MB-231
[24]	0	28	6.2	A549, A427
[25]	Unspecified	20	7.4	U87-MG, A172, U251
[1]	Unspecified	20	7.4	92.1
[26]	0	10	7.4	MDA436 and mouse xenograft
[27]	10	2 to 20	7.4	Human myeloid cell lines

Table 1. *Cont.*

Reference	Glucose Concentration (mM)	Lactate Concentration (mM)	pH	Cell Lines or Tumour Origin
[28]	0.175	4	7.4	glioma stem cells
[29]	2.5 or 25	10	7.4	Colo205, Ls174T, Mosers, HT29
[30]	1 to 2.5	25	7.4	MCF-7
[31]	Unspecified	20	7.4	Huh-7, Hep3B
[32]	0	20	6.8	A549
[33]	0	20	6.7	4T1, HeLa, NCI–H460
[34]	Unspecified	0	6.5	PANC-1, SW1990
[35]	Unspecified	12	6.8	PaTu-8902, HeLa, HepG2, HDF

3. Lactic Acidosis Seen by Cancer Research: A Brief History

In the 2000s, cancer research took a renewed interest in the Warburg effect, a hallmark of cancer discovered a century ago [2,36,37]. As a consequence, views on lactic acidosis changed drastically.

Acidosis had been known to promote tumour aggressiveness by exerting a selective pressure. Some cancer cells had been shown to survive acidosis by maintaining an alkaline intracellular pH, while other cells—cancerous or healthy—underwent hydrolysis and death [38–40]. The proliferation of those selected cells, which are more resistant to unfavourable environments, had been known to increase tumour malignancy [41,42]. As for lactate, it had been considered more of a by-product of glycolysis until the 1980s, when its use as a nutrient in non-cancerous tissues was discovered [43,44]. The role of extracellular lactate in cancer was investigated only later, in the 2000s [45,46], when it was found to correlate with tumour malignancy [47–50]. Two explanations for this were initially proposed. First, lactate promotes relaxation of the tissue surrounding the tumour, which would make room for its development and metastasis [48]. Second, lactate makes the cellular environment hostile, as does acidosis [38], which promotes angiogenesis [47].

The metabolic importance of extracellular lactate and lactic acidosis was first evidenced in 2008. Lactic acidosis was shown to alter the expression of metabolism genes [10] and, more importantly, lactate was proven to be, per se, a key source of energy for cancer cells [51]. In 2009, the term "reverse Warburg effect" was first used to describe cancer cells not showing the Warburg effect, but instead inducing it in neighbouring stromal fibroblasts and consuming the lactate produced by them [52]. These discoveries reappraised the paradigm of the Warburg effect, showing that it wasn't compulsory in cancer since lactate could be metabolised rather than only produced. Following these works, in 2012, Wu et al., demonstrated that lactic acidosis allows cells to avoid glucose starvation [3]. Lactic acidosis rescues glucose-deprived cancer cells, but importantly, acidosis or lactosis alone have much more limited effects. After this pioneering work, lactic acidosis was further shown to reprogram cell metabolism [5]. Nowadays, extracellular lactate and acidosis are viewed as central players in cancer cell metabolism [53–55].

4. Lactic Acidosis' Effect on Energy Metabolism

Lactic acidosis was shown to impact numerous aspects of energy metabolism. We focus here on nutrient import, glycolysis, the tricarboxylic acid (TCA) cycle, oxidative phosphorylation (OxPhos), and pathways generating reduced coenzymes (Figure 1).

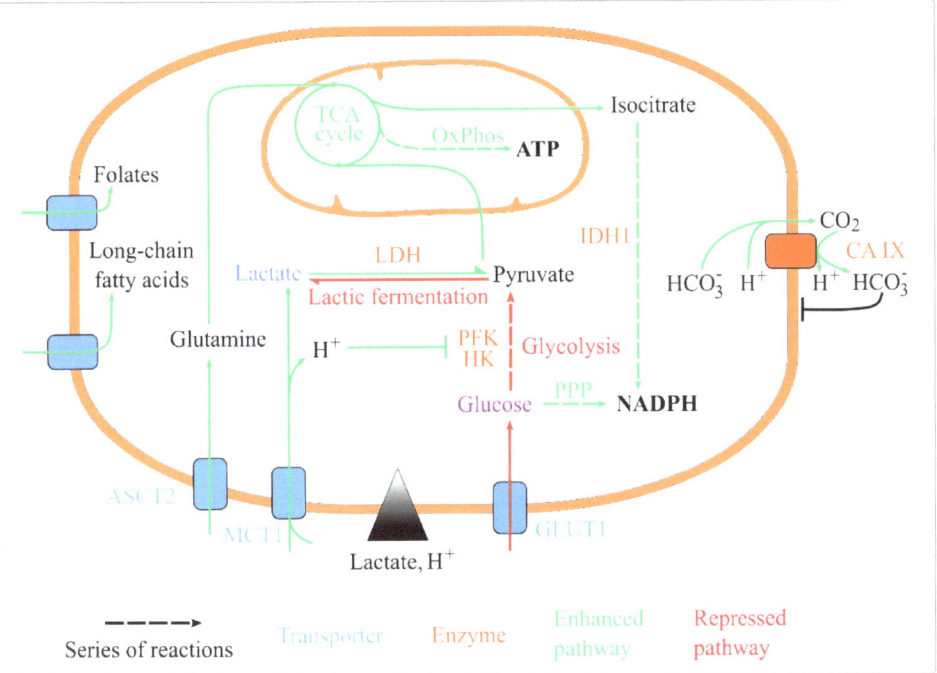

Figure 1. Lactic acidosis rewires energy metabolism and maintains cellular homeostasis. Lactic acidosis enhances the uptake of folate, long-chain fatty acids, glutamine, and lactate. It represses glucose import, glycolysis (by inhibiting HK and PFK, its rate-limiting enzymes) and lactic fermentation. It enhances lactate conversion to pyruvate, routing of pyruvate and glutamine towards the TCA cycle, ATP generation by OxPhos, and coenzyme reduction by IDH1 and the oxidative PPP. It also upregulates CA IX expression, which basifies intracellular pH. Abbreviations: ASCT2: Alanine, Serine, Cysteine Transporter 2; CA IX: carbonate anhydrase 1; GLUT1: glucose transporter 1; HK: hexokinase; IDH1: isocitrate dehydrogenase 1; MCT1: monocarboxylate transporter 1; OxPhos: oxidative phosphorylation; PFK1: phosphofructokinase 1; PPP: pentose phosphate pathway; TCA: tricarboxylic acid.

4.1. Lactic Acidosis and Exchanges at the Plasma Membrane

In glucose deprivation, the capacity of cancer cells to uptake and metabolise alternative nutrients is key to their survival [56]. Extracellular acidosis and lactosis were shown to increase such capacity.

4.1.1. Acidosis Sustains the Activity of Proton-Nutrient Symporters

Extracellular acidosis has a direct impact on exchanges at the plasma membrane [57]. In healthy tissues, protons are more concentrated inside the cell than outside. In tumours, the contrary is true [58,59]. Extracellular acidosis inverts the transmembrane proton gradient in tumour cells, which may positively impact proton-nutrient symports. Of interest, lactate is imported in cancer cells via the monocarboxylate transporters (MCTs) [51]. Since MCTs co-transport lactate with a proton, lactate import should be sensitive to the proton gradient and facilitated under acidosis. This mechanism is expected to explain why cancer cells respond differently to lactosis and lactic acidosis [3], since a rise in extracellular lactate only increases intracellular lactate levels in acidic conditions [60]. The co-transport of extracellular lactate and protons probably underlies the synergy of their effects on intracellular metabolism (Figure 1).

Of note, protons are also co-imported with several other nutrients, such as Fe^{2+}, folates, amino acids and peptides. Brown & Ganapathy suggested that acidosis may affect their uptake (Figure 1), but this hypothesis remains to be confirmed [61].

4.1.2. Lactate and Acidosis Indirectly Enhance Nutrient Uptake

Extracellular lactic acidosis indirectly promotes the uptake of several nutrients (Figure 1). The import of lactate itself is increased in lactic acidosis, in part due to MCT1 overexpression [11], which is a response to an extracellular lactate signal [62] that is potentiated by extracellular acidity [12]. Extracellular lactate induces MCT1 and MCT4 via the G-protein-coupled receptor 81 (GPR81) transduction pathway [62]. In acidosis, extracellular lactate can also induce GPR81 expression [12,13]. Extracellular lactate signal enhancing MCT-mediated lactate import is necessary to cancer cell survival in absence of glucose, glutamine and pyruvate [62]. This supports the idea that 'lactate induces its own metabolism', which doesn't exclude other regulations of MCT expression [63].

Glutamine uptake is increased by extracellular lactate or acidosis, as both conditions increase the expression of the glutamine transporter ASCT2 (alanine, serine and cysteine transporter 2) [14,64]. Fatty acid uptake is enhanced by acidosis [65], and folate import is intensified by 10 mM extracellular lactic acid [15].

Finally, and importantly, lactic acidosis seems to minimise glucose uptake, but not in all cell lines and cancers. Lactic acidosis decreases glucose uptake in various cell lines [5], as lactate in lung cancer cell lines [16]. On the opposite, 10 mM lactate has no effect on glucose uptake in the T47D breast cancer cell line [15]. The expression of the glucose transporters GLUT1 and GLUT4 are decreased by 2 mM lactate and acidosis in lung and breast cancer cell lines [17], and by acidosis in cervix, pharynx and colon cancer cell lines [64] but not in lung cancer cell lines [18].

4.1.3. Lactic Acidosis and pH Homeostasis

Cell exposure to lactic acidosis is associated with a drop in intracellular pH from 7.3 to ~6.9 [5]. Behind this acidification, several probable effects may be discerned. On the one hand, as discussed earlier, acidosis enhances proton-nutrient co-import, which could contribute to cellular acidification. On the other hand, lactate as a signal can mitigate the drop in pH by favouring alkalinization. A level of 10 mM extracellular lactate induces Carbonic Anhydrase IX (CA IX) [19], a transmembrane enzyme supporting proton export and a key regulator of cell pH [66] (Figure 1).

4.2. Lactic Acidosis, Glycolysis, and Lactic Fermentation

Unlike cells showing the Warburg effect, in which glycolysis and lactate dehydrogenase (LDH)-catalysed lactic fermentation are known to be hyperactive, cells exposed to lactic acidosis show a reduction in these pathways' activity.

In glucose abundance, acidosis and lactic acidosis lower glucose consumption and lactate secretion [4,5,20], which indicates that glycolysis and lactic fermentation are downregulated. More interestingly, lactic acidosis decreases cancer cell dependency on glucose catabolism [1]. Thus, in glucose sufficiency, lactic acidosis minimises glucose catabolism activity and its importance in cell survival (Figure 1).

Glycolysis and lactic fermentation are likely downregulated at the level of both gene expression and enzyme activity. The expression of glycolysis enzymes is reduced by lactic acidosis in breast cancer cell lines [10], and by extracellular lactate in lung cancer cell lines [16], but it is maintained by extracellular lactate in breast cancer cell lines [21,22]. The activity of glycolysis enzymes, especially the rate-limiting hexokinase and phosphofructokinase [67], is directly decreased by intracellular acidification [4] (Figure 1). In line, intracellular acidification has been predicted in silico to hinder the Warburg effect [68]. Intracellular lactate accumulation, in parallel, directly inhibits lactic fermentation [5] (Figure 1). The interconversion of lactate and pyruvate through LDH follows the mass action law, therefore a rise in lactate concentration inhibits its production from pyruvate and favours the reverse reaction. This thermodynamic effect leads to a complete stop of lactic fermentation at ~25 mM intracellular lactate [5]. This concentration is within the range resulting from lactic acidosis.

4.3. Lactic Acidosis and Mitochondrial Catabolism

4.3.1. Lactic Acidosis Intensifies Mitochondrial Catabolism

Lactic acidosis enhances mitochondrial metabolic activity, in particular the TCA cycle and OxPhos. Both lactic acidosis and lactosis enhance mitochondrial biogenesis [23,24] and the expression of the enzymes of the TCA cycle and OxPhos [11,25], which potentiates mitochondrial catabolism and ATP production. The reactivation of those pathways allows the maintenance of the cellular ATP concentration in glucose deprivation and increases resistance to starvation [11].

4.3.2. Lactic Acidosis Shapes TCA Cycle Alternative Fueling

In addition to glucose-derived pyruvate, the TCA cycle can be supplied with various substrates. This flexibility is particularly true of cancer cells [69]. In challenging nutritional contexts such as glucose deprivation, the TCA cycle of cancer cells can be sustained by alternative nutrients. Lactate and glutamine are its main substrate suppliers after glucose [70]. The use of both is promoted by lactic acidosis.

The pyruvate generated from lactate can directly sustain the TCA cycle [26–31,71] (Figure 1). This pathway depends on upstream lactate import by MCTs, whose enhancement in lactic acidosis is discussed in Section 4.1.2. In line, extracellular lactate increases the mitochondrial membrane potential, and hence ATP production efficiency in OxPhos [21,72], and could even be necessary to pro-tumoural cell proliferation [32]. In more detail, the routing of lactate to mitochondria is debated. In the classical view, lactate is converted to pyruvate in the cytosol, then pyruvate is shuttled to mitochondria [73,74]. In addition to this classical way, Brooks et al. proposed an alternative model in which lactate would be shuttled to mitochondria via the mitochondrial lactate oxidation complex (mLOC), that includes MCT1 [75]. The controversy raised by this model has been well-reviewed in [76,77], that summarized the evidence for and against it in non-cancer cells. In cancer cells supplied with sufficient glucose, lactate's contribution to the TCA cycle over glucose remains under debate: some studies suggest that lactate shuttled to mitochondria is preferred [71], while others question this [78]. Either way, under glucose deprivation, we can hypothesise that lactate's contribution to the TCA cycle is of significant importance.

Glutamine is a major nutrient for cancer cells. It undergoes oxidative glutaminolysis in mitochondria, where it is processed by glutaminase 1 or 2 (GLS1/2) and then glutamate dehydrogenase 1 (GDH1) to sustain the TCA cycle. Lactic acidosis [20], acidosis [20,64], and lactate [14] upregulate GLS1 and GLS2 and stimulate oxidative glutaminolysis. Lactic acidosis, however, doesn't necessarily promote glutamine consumption compared to lactosis [23]. In summary, either extracellular lactate, acidosis or lactic acidosis enhance glutamine utilisation by inducing glutaminase expression (Figure 1).

4.4. Lactic Acidosis and Redox Homeostasis

Cell survival requires redox homeostasis, i.e., controlled levels of reactive oxygen species (ROS) and redox coenzymes. The former lead to cell death when they accumulate, and the latter support the entire metabolism and cellular antioxidant defences.

Particularly, a high $NADPH/NADP^+$ ratio kinetically favours anabolic reactions and helps keep ROS levels low. In cancer cells this ratio is abnormally high and sustains hyperactive anabolism [70]. High NADPH levels are supported by the oxidation of nutrients, such as lactate and glutamine via the TCA cycle and then oxidation of glutamine- and lactate-derived malate and isocitrate by the malic enzyme 1 (ME1) and Isocitrate Dehydrogenase 1 (IDH1), and mainly glucose via the pentose phosphate pathway (PPP). Redox homeostasis in cancer cells is therefore particularly sensitive to nutritional stress such as glucose deprivation.

In this condition, lactic acidosis helps stabilise the NADPH/NADP$^+$ ratio at ~50% of its level in glucose sufficiency [3]. Likely, the gatekeepers of the NADPH/NADP$^+$ ratio in glucose abundance have reduced efficiency under glucose deprivation and lactic acidosis, whereas new control mechanisms gain importance. On the one hand, glutamine use via ME1 is not necessary to the maintenance of the NADPH/NADP$^+$ ratio under lactic acidosis [33]. Glutamine would indeed be completely degraded in mitochondrial catabolism instead of sustaining ME1 activity [20]. On the other hand, the glucose directed away from glycolysis towards the PPP would prevail more in NADPH/NADP$^+$ maintenance under lactic acidosis. Lactic acidosis [20] and acidosis [34] respectively increase the expression and activity of glucose-6-phosphate dehydrogenase (G6PD), the first enzyme of the PPP, and lactic acidosis makes G6PD activity necessary to NADPH/NADP$^+$ ratio maintenance and cell survival [20] in glucose sufficiency. However in glucose deprivation, the PPP alone cannot maintain redox balance [33]. Alternatively, lactate would become a key player in NADPH/NADP$^+$ ratio maintenance, via the TCA cycle [35], and IDH1 [33].

Whether, in glucose abundance, such reprogramming strengthens cell defences against ROS level increase is uncertain. Acidosis increases ROS levels [35] and cell sensitivity to oxidative stress, but cell adaptation to acidosis decreases them [34]. Lactate import through MCT1 is key to maintain low ROS levels [79]. Lactic acidosis was found to either increase ROS levels, as does acidosis [20], or to rescue acidosis' negative effect [35]. At any rate, in glucose deprivation, lactic acidosis mainly prevents increased ROS levels by providing IDH1 with its substrate [33].

A high NADH/NAD$^+$ ratio supports ATP production. Lactic acidosis impact on the NADH/NAD$^+$ ratio has not been directly investigated. However lactate use by the TCA cycle increases the NADH/NAD$^+$ ratio in glucose deprivation [30]. This increase could contribute to the inhibition of glycolysis by lactic acidosis: a high NADH/NAD$^+$ ratio would inhibit glycolysis according to the mass action law. Yet this hypothesis remains to be tested.

4.5. Section Summary

In the energy metabolism of cancer cells, acidosis and extracellular lactate act as enzymatic inhibitors, and lactate as a signal and a nutrient. They mostly curb glycolysis and lactic fermentation and enhance the TCA cycle and OxPhos (Figure 1). Acidification and lactate accumulation in the tumour microenvironment would promote and sustain an oxidative phenotype, which is fitter than the fermenting phenotype in glucose deprivation, an adverse nutritional context that is common in tumours.

5. Therapeutic Strategies Targeting Lactic Acidosis

Nowadays, lactic acidosis *per se* is targeted in therapies directed against cancer. Of note, it is also a major target in the treatment of type 2 diabetes [80,81]. Neutralising acidosis in tumours has been proposed as a way to restore sensitivity of cancer cells to glucose starvation and increase the efficacy of regular treatments. The proof of principle of this approach has been established by combining transarterial chemoembolization (TACE) with the infusion of bicarbonate, a basifying agent that turns neoplastic lactic acidosis into lactosis [82,83]. Compared to TACE alone, TILA-TACE (Targeting-Intratumoural-Lactic-Acidosis TACE) presented a very significantly enhanced anticancer activity for patients with hepatocellular carcinoma. The mechanisms underlying this activity have been evaluated in detail by Ying et al. [84].

Modulating extracellular lactate availability in tumours by nanomedicine is another promising therapeutic strategy. The delivery by nanoparticles of a cocktail of lactate oxidases and catalases to colon carcinoma cells in vitro suppresses tumoural lactosis and stops cell proliferation [85]. The delivery by nanoparticles of a glucose catalase combined with a MCT1 inhibitor, that together prevent the use of both glucose and lactate by tumour cells, inhibits the proliferation of SiHa cell line xenografts in mice [86]. Conversely, lactate-loaded nanoparticles induce an overload of lactate and cytotoxicity in orthotopic glioblastoma models, although only in normoxic conditions and not in hypoxia [87].

Understanding the effects of lactic acidosis also helps reappraise the potential of already-existing targets. In particular, the lactate transporter MCT1 was formerly targeted to inhibit lactate secretion in cells showing the Warburg effect, and is now targeted to hamper lactate uptake [27,88–91]. Similarly the strategies targeting LDH isoforms were aimed historically at inhibiting lactate production from pyruvate. The LDHA isoform, that has a higher affinity for pyruvate than for lactate and catalyses preferentially lactate production, is a historical target that still attracts much attention [92]. However, with the discovery of lactic acidosis effect, the LDHB isoform that catalyses preferentially the conversion of lactate to pyruvate now rises as an alternative target [32].

6. Implications of Lactic Acidosis in the Whole-Tumour Metabolism

Deciphering how lactic acidosis impacts cancer cells enlightens important aspects of the metabolism of the whole tumour, and raises new perspectives to complement its understanding.

From the belief that cancer cells have a unique metabolic signature, i.e., the Warburg effect, research has progressively recognized intratumoural heterogeneity as the metabolic hallmark of cancer [55]. The main metabolic heterogeneity in tumours is now suggested to be mitochondrial activity [93,94], that is promoted and sustained by lactic acidosis. To describe this heterogeneity, tumours have traditionally been modelled as the coexistence of two metabolic populations: oxidative cells relying on OxPhos and fermenting cells showing the Warburg effect and relying on glycolysis and lactic fermentation [17,28,51,91,95,96]. Oxidative cells would be located in normoxic regions, in perivascular compartments [7,11,97], and fermenting cells in hypoxic regions farther from blood vessels [11,51,97] (Figure 2). Each population would thrive on different energy sources, fermenting cells glucose and oxidative ones lactate, and lactate would be transferred from fermenting to oxidative cells [95]. This model is supported by the coexistence in tumours of cells overexpressing MCT4, a preferential lactate exporter, and cells overexpressing MCT1, a preferential lactate importer [11,51,95,98]. Interestingly, a possible lactate transport via gap junctions has been evidenced recently [99–101]. This lactate transfer supports the idea of a metabolic symbiosis between both populations within tumours [17,28,46,51,61,91,95,96,101–103]. In this model, a central question is how the metabolic phenotypes of both populations are determined [46]. Hypoxia is thought to be the major promoter of the fermenting phenotype [102,104]. Lactic acidosis, according to the evidence presented in this work, is likely the promoter of the oxidative phenotype [5,11].

However this hypothetical scenario raises a paradox: the oxidative phenotype, that derives from lactic acidosis, i.e., from the fermenting phenotype that is promoted by hypoxia, cannot thrive in hypoxic conditions. Two hypotheses could solve this paradox. In the first hypothesis, fermenting cells would induce the oxidative phenotype in their neighbours, located in better-perfused regions. However lactic acidosis intensity, maximal around secretory cells, decreases with the distance [51,105], which raises the question of the minimal level of lactic acidosis necessary to promote the oxidative phenotype. In the second hypothesis, lactic acidosis would feedback the Warburg effect in fermenting cells by switching them to an oxidative phenotype, which questions the minimal oxygen level necessary for the oxidative phenotype to survive. A possible answer to this question is that in the meantime, lactic acidosis could promote angiogenesis [38,47,61]. This questions the timeline of lactic acidosis action, in the promotion of both oxidative phenotype and angiogenesis. A third perspective to answer the paradox is to address how, earlier, hypoxia and lactic acidosis may interplay in the promotion of metabolic phenotypes, which has caught little attention until now [18,20,23,106].

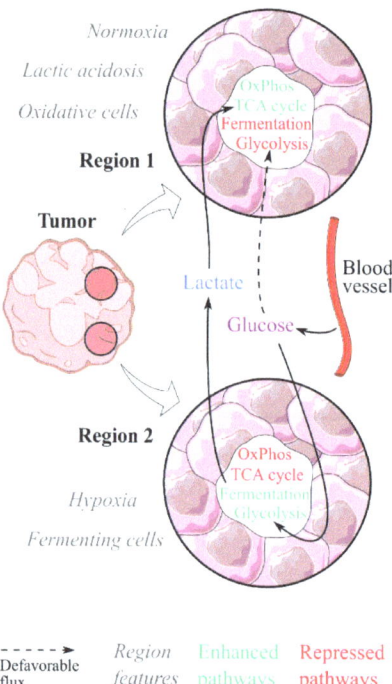

Figure 2. Lactic acidosis would contribute to a metabolic symbiosis between fermenting and oxidative cells within tumours. In this model, two populations coexist in tumours: fermenting cells in hypoxic regions, and oxidative cells in normoxic regions where lactic acidosis would exert its effect. Fermenting cells would consume the glucose spared by oxidative cells and generate the lactate fueling them, both being in a metabolic symbiosis. Lactic acidosis promotes the switch from a fermenting to an oxidative phenotype.

7. Conclusions

Lactic acidosis associated with tumour progression allows cancer cells to survive in unfavourable environments. In the last decade, the influence of neoplastic lactic acidosis on the energy metabolism of cancer cells has been deciphered. Lactic reduces glycolysis and lactic fermentation, stimulates the TCA cycle and OxPhos, and promotes the use of alternative nutrients. All in all, it contributes to cell resistance to glucose deprivation. Cancelling lactic acidosis' effect is therefore a relevant anticancer strategy that restores cancer cell sensitivity to glucose deprivation, a common feature of the tumour microenvironment. In the future, clarifying how lactic acidosis action is integrated in the whole-tumour metabolism would be of high interest.

Author Contributions: Writing—original draft preparation, Z.D.; writing—review and editing, Z.D., A.B., G.J.P.R. and B.P.; supervision, G.J.P.R. and B.P.; funding acquisition, G.J.P.R. and B.P. All authors have read and agreed to the published version of the manuscript.

Funding: Financial support from ITMO Cancer of Aviesan within the framework of the 2021–2030 Cancer Control Strategy, on funds administered by Inserm.

Conflicts of Interest: The authors declare no conflict of interest.

References

1. Barnes, E.M.E.; Xu, Y.; Benito, A.; Herendi, L.; Siskos, A.P.; Aboagye, E.O.; Nijhuis, A.; Keun, H.C. Lactic acidosis induces resistance to the pan-Akt inhibitor uprosertib in colon cancer cells. *Br. J. Cancer* **2020**, *122*, 1298–1308. [CrossRef] [PubMed]
2. Warburg, O. The Metabolism of Carcinoma Cells. *J. Cancer Res.* **1925**, *9*, 148–163. [CrossRef]

3. Wu, H.; Ding, Z.; Hu, D.; Sun, F.; Dai, C.; Xie, J.; Hu, X. Central role of lactic acidosis in cancer cell resistance to glucose deprivation-induced cell death. *J. Pathol.* **2012**, *227*, 189–199. [CrossRef] [PubMed]
4. Gao, J.; Guo, Z.; Cheng, J.; Sun, B.; Yang, J.; Li, H.; Wu, S.; Dong, F.; Yan, X. Differential metabolic responses in breast cancer cell lines to acidosis and lactic acidosis revealed by stable isotope assisted metabolomics. *Sci. Rep.* **2020**, *10*, 21967. [CrossRef]
5. Xie, J.; Wu, H.; Dai, C.; Pan, Q.; Ding, Z.; Hu, D.; Ji, B.; Luo, Y.; Hu, X. Beyond Warburg effect—Dual metabolic nature of cancer cells. *Sci. Rep.* **2015**, *4*, 4927. [CrossRef]
6. Lefevre, C.; Panthu, B.; Naville, D.; Guibert, S.; Pinteur, C.; Elena-Herrmann, B.; Vidal, H.; Rautureau, G.J.P.; Mey, A. Metabolic Phenotyping of Adipose-Derived Stem Cells Reveals a Unique Signature and Intrinsic Differences between Fat Pads. *Stem Cells Int.* **2019**, *2019*, e9323864. [CrossRef]
7. Grasmann, G.; Mondal, A.; Leithner, K. Flexibility and Adaptation of Cancer Cells in a Heterogenous Metabolic Microenvironment. *Int. J. Mol. Sci.* **2021**, *22*, 1476. [CrossRef]
8. Corbet, C.; Feron, O. Tumour acidosis: From the passenger to the driver's seat. *Nat. Rev. Cancer* **2017**, *17*, 577–593. [CrossRef]
9. Hirayama, A.; Kami, K.; Sugimoto, M.; Kami, K.; Sugimoto, M.; Sugawara, M.; Toki, N.; Onozuka, H.; Kinoshita, T.; Saito, N.; et al. Quantitative Metabolome Profiling of Colon and Stomach Cancer Microenvironment by Capillary Electrophoresis Time-of-Flight Mass Spectrometry. *Cancer Res.* **2009**, *69*, 4918–4925. [CrossRef]
10. Chen, J.L.-Y.; Lucas, J.E.; Schroeder, T.; Mori, S.; Wu, J.; Nevins, J.; Dewhirst, M.; West, M.; Chi, J.-T. The genomic analysis of lactic acidosis and acidosis response in human cancers. *PLoS Genet.* **2008**, *4*, e1000293. [CrossRef]
11. Duan, K.; Liu, Z.J.; Hu, S.Q.; Liu, Z.-J.; Hu, S.-Q.; Huo, H.-Y.; Xu, Z.-R.; Ruan, J.-F.; Sun, Y.; Dai, L.-P.; et al. Lactic acid induces lactate transport and glycolysis/OXPHOS interconversion in glioblastoma. *Biochem. Biophys. Res. Commun.* **2018**, *503*, 888–894. [CrossRef] [PubMed]
12. Li, X.; Zhang, Z.; Zhang, Y.; Cao, Y.; Wei, H.; Wu, Z. Upregulation of lactate-inducible snail protein suppresses oncogene-mediated senescence through p16INK4a inactivation. *J. Exp. Clin. Cancer Res.* **2018**, *37*, 39. [CrossRef] [PubMed]
13. Xie, Q.; Zhu, Z.; He, Y.; Zhang, Z.; Zhang, Y.; Wang, Y.; Luo, J.; Peng, T.; Cheng, F.; Gao, J.; et al. A lactate-induced Snail/STAT3 pathway drives GPR81 expression in lung cancer cells. *Biochim. Biophys. Acta BBA-Mol. Basis Dis.* **2020**, *1866*, 165576. [CrossRef] [PubMed]
14. Pérez-Escuredo, J.; Dadhich, R.K.; Dhup, S.; Cacace, A.; Van Hée, V.F.; De Saedeleer, C.J.; Sboarina, M.; Rodriguez, F.; Fontenille, M.-J.; Brisson, L.; et al. Lactate promotes glutamine uptake and metabolism in oxidative cancer cells. *Cell Cycle* **2015**, *15*, 72–83. [CrossRef]
15. Guedes, M.; Araújo, J.R.; Correia-Branco, A.; Gregório, I.; Martel, F.; Keating, E. Modulation of the uptake of critical nutrients by breast cancer cells by lactate: Impact on cell survival, proliferation and migration. *Exp. Cell Res.* **2016**, *341*, 111–122. [CrossRef]
16. Jiang, J.; Huang, D.; Jiang, Y.; Hou, J.; Tian, M.; Li, J.; Sun, L.; Zhang, Y.; Zhang, T.; Li, Z.; et al. Lactate Modulates Cellular Metabolism through Histone Lactylation-Mediated Gene Expression in Non-Small Cell Lung Cancer. *Front. Oncol.* **2021**, *11*, 647559. [CrossRef]
17. Prado-Garcia, H.; Campa-Higareda, A.; Romero-Garcia, S. Lactic Acidosis in the Presence of Glucose Diminishes Warburg Effect in Lung Adenocarcinoma Cells. *Front. Oncol.* **2020**, *10*, 807. [CrossRef]
18. Giatromanolaki, A.; Liousia, M.; Arelaki, S.; Kalamida, D.; Pouliliou, S.; Mitrakas, A.; Tsolou, A.; Sivridis, E.; Koukourakis, M. Differential effect of hypoxia and acidity on lung cancer cell and fibroblast metabolism. *Biochem. Cell Biol.* **2017**, *95*, 428–436. [CrossRef]
19. Panisova, E.; Kery, M.; Sedlakova, O.; Brisson, L.; Debreova, M.; Sboarina, M.; Sonveaux, P.; Pastorekova, S.; Svastova, E. Lactate stimulates CA IX expression in normoxic cancer cells. *Oncotarget* **2017**, *8*, 77819–77835. [CrossRef]
20. Lamonte, G.; Tang, X.; Chen, J.L.-Y.; Wu, J.; Ding, C.-K.C.; Keenan, M.M.; Sangokoya, C.; Kung, H.-N.; Ilkayeva, O.; Boros, L.G.; et al. Acidosis induces reprogramming of cellular metabolism to mitigate oxidative stress. *Cancer Metab.* **2013**, *1*, 23. [CrossRef]
21. Jin, L.; Guo, Y.; Chen, J.; Wen, Z.; Jiang, Y.; Qian, J. Lactate receptor HCAR1 regulates cell growth, metastasis and maintenance of cancer-specific energy metabolism in breast cancer cells. *Mol. Med. Rep.* **2022**, *26*, 268. [CrossRef] [PubMed]
22. Ishihara, S.; Hata, K.; Hirose, K.; Okui, T.; Toyosawa, S.; Uzawa, N.; Nishimura, R.; Yoneda, T. The lactate sensor GPR81 regulates glycolysis and tumor growth of breast cancer. *Sci. Rep.* **2022**, *12*, 6261. [CrossRef]
23. Romero-Garcia, S.; Prado-Garcia, H.; Valencia-Camargo, A.D.; Alvarez-Pulido, A. Lactic Acidosis Promotes Mitochondrial Biogenesis in Lung Adenocarcinoma Cells, Supporting Proliferation Under Normoxia or Survival Under Hypoxia. *Front. Oncol.* **2019**, *9*, 1053. [CrossRef] [PubMed]
24. Longhitano, L.; Vicario, N.; Tibullo, D.; Giallongo, C.; Broggi, G.; Caltabiano, R.; Barbagallo, G.M.V.; Altieri, R.; Baghini, M.; Di Rosa, M.; et al. Lactate Induces the Expressions of MCT1 and HCAR1 to Promote Tumor Growth and Progression in Glioblastoma. *Front. Oncol.* **2022**, *12*, 871798. [CrossRef] [PubMed]
25. Longhitano, L.; Giallongo, S.; Orlando, L.; Broggi, G.; Longo, A.; Russo, A.; Caltabiano, R.; Giallongo, C.; Barbagallo, I.; Di Rosa, M.; et al. Lactate Rewrites the Metabolic Reprogramming of Uveal Melanoma Cells and Induces Quiescence Phenotype. *Int. J. Mol. Sci.* **2022**, *24*, 24. [CrossRef]
26. Park, S.; Chang, C.Y.; Safi, R.; Liu, X.; Baldi, R.; Jasper, J.S.; Anderson, G.R.; Liu, T.; Rathmell, J.C.; Dewhirst, M.W.; et al. ERRα-Regulated Lactate Metabolism Contributes to Resistance to Targeted Therapies in Breast Cancer. *Cell. Rep.* **2016**, *15*, 323–335. [CrossRef]

27. Erdem, A.; Marin, S.; Pereira-Martins, D.A.; Geugien, M.; Cunningham, A.; Pruis, M.G.; Weinhäuser, I.; Gerding, A.; Bakker, B.M.; Wierenga, A.T.J.; et al. Inhibition of the succinyl dehydrogenase complex in acute myeloid leukemia leads to a lactate-fuelled respiratory metabolic vulnerability. *Nat. Commun.* **2022**, *13*, 2013. [CrossRef]
28. Minami, N.; Tanaka, K.; Sasayama, T.; Kohmura, E.; Saya, H.; Sampetrean, O. Lactate Reprograms Energy and Lipid Metabolism in Glucose-Deprived Oxidative Glioma Stem Cells. *Metabolites* **2021**, *11*, 325. [CrossRef]
29. Montal, E.D.; Bhalla, K.; Dewi, R.E.; Ruiz, C.F.; Haley, J.A.; Ropell, A.E.; Gordon, C.; Girnun, G.D.; Haley, J.D. Inhibition of phosphoenolpyruvate carboxykinase blocks lactate utilization and impairs tumor growth in colorectal cancer. *Cancer Metab.* **2019**, *7*, 8. [CrossRef]
30. Otto, A.M.; Hintermair, J.; Janzon, C. NADH-linked metabolic plasticity of MCF-7 breast cancer cells surviving in a nutrient-deprived microenvironment. *J. Cell. Biochem.* **2015**, *116*, 822–835. [CrossRef] [PubMed]
31. Zhao, Y.; Li, M.; Yao, X.; Fei, Y.; Lin, Z.; Li, Z.; Cai, K.; Zhao, Y.; Luo, Z. HCAR1/MCT1 Regulates Tumor Ferroptosis through the Lactate-Mediated AMPK-SCD1 Activity and Its Therapeutic Implications. *Cell Rep.* **2020**, *33*, 108487. [CrossRef]
32. Deng, H.; Gao, Y.; Trappetti, V.; Hertig, D.; Karatkevich, D.; Losmanova, T.; Urzi, C.; Ge, H.; Geest, G.A.; Bruggmann, R.; et al. Targeting lactate dehydrogenase B-dependent mitochondrial metabolism affects tumor initiating cells and inhibits tumorigenesis of non-small cell lung cancer by inducing mtDNA damage. *Cell. Mol. Life Sci.* **2022**, *79*, 445. [CrossRef]
33. Ying, M.; You, D.; Zhu, X.; Cai, L.; Zeng, S.; Hu, X. Lactate and glutamine support NADPH generation in cancer cells under glucose deprived conditions. *Redox Biol.* **2021**, *46*, 102065. [CrossRef]
34. Chen, S.; Ning, B.; Song, J.; Yang, Z.; Zhou, L.; Chen, Z.; Mao, L.; Liu, H.; Wang, Q.; He, S.; et al. Enhanced pentose phosphate pathway activity promotes pancreatic ductal adenocarcinoma progression via activating YAP/MMP1 axis under chronic acidosis. *Int. J. Biol. Sci.* **2022**, *18*, 2304–2316. [CrossRef]
35. Koncošová, M.; Vrzáčková, N.; Křížová, I.; Tomášová, P.; Rimpelová, S.; Dvořák, A.; Vítek, L.; Rumlová, M.; Ruml, T.; Zelenka, J. Inhibition of Mitochondrial Metabolism Leads to Selective Eradication of Cells Adapted to Acidic Microenvironment. *Int. J. Mol. Sci.* **2021**, *22*, 10790. [CrossRef] [PubMed]
36. Koppenol, W.H.; Bounds, P.L.; Dang, C.V. Otto Warburg's contributions to current concepts of cancer metabolism. *Nat. Rev. Cancer* **2011**, *11*, 325–337. [CrossRef] [PubMed]
37. Urbano, A.M. Otto Warburg: The journey towards the seminal discovery of tumor cell bioenergetic reprogramming. *Biochim. Biophys. Acta BBA-Mol. Basis Dis.* **2021**, *1867*, 165965. [CrossRef] [PubMed]
38. Gatenby, R.A.; Gillies, R.J. Why do cancers have high aerobic glycolysis? *Nat. Rev. Cancer* **2004**, *4*, 891–899. [CrossRef]
39. Laconi, E. The evolving concept of tumor microenvironments. *BioEssays* **2007**, *29*, 738–744. [CrossRef]
40. Gatenby, R.A.; Gillies, R.J. A microenvironmental model of carcinogenesis. *Nat. Rev. Cancer* **2008**, *8*, 56–61. [CrossRef]
41. Damaghi, M.; Tafreshi, N.K.; Lloyd, M.C.; Sprung, R.; Estrella, V.; Wojtkowiak, J.W.; Morse, D.L.; Koomen, J.M.; Bui, M.M.; Gatenby, R.A.; et al. Chronic acidosis in the tumour microenvironment selects for overexpression of LAMP2 in the plasma membrane. *Nat. Commun.* **2015**, *6*, 8752. [CrossRef] [PubMed]
42. Damaghi, M.; Gillies, R.J. Lysosomal protein relocation as an adaptation mechanism to extracellular acidosis. *Cell Cycle* **2016**, *15*, 1659–1660. [CrossRef]
43. Ferguson, B.S.; Rogatzki, M.J.; Goodwin, M.L.; Kane, D.A.; Rightmire, Z.; Gladden, L.B. Lactate metabolism: Historical context, prior misinterpretations, and current understanding. *Eur. J. Appl. Physiol.* **2018**, *118*, 691–728. [CrossRef] [PubMed]
44. Cori, C.F. The Glucose-Lactic Acid Cycle and Gluconeogenesis. In *Current Topics in Cellular Regulation*; Elsevier: Amsterdam, The Netherlands, 1981; Volume 18, pp. 377–387. [CrossRef]
45. Vaupel, P.; Kallinowski, F.; Okunieff, P. Blood Flow, Oxygen and Nutrient Supply, and Metabolic Microenvironment of Human Tumors: A Review. *Cancer Res.* **1989**, *18*, 6449–6465.
46. Nakajima, E.C.; Van Houten, B. Metabolic symbiosis in cancer: Refocusing the Warburg lens. *Mol. Carcinog.* **2013**, *52*, 329–337. [CrossRef]
47. Walenta, S.; Wetterling, M.; Lehrke, M.; Schwickert, G.; Sundfør, K.; Rofstad, E.K.; Mueller-Klieser, W. High Lactate Levels Predict Likelihood of Metastases, Tumor Recurrence, and Restricted Patient Survival in Human Cervical Cancers. *Cancer Res.* **2000**, *60*, 916–921.
48. Stern, R.; Shuster, S.; Neudecker, B.A.; Formby, B. Lactate stimulates fibroblast expression of hyaluronan and CD44: The Warburg effect revisited. *Exp. Cell Res.* **2002**, *276*, 24–31. [CrossRef]
49. Fantin, V.R.; St-Pierre, J.; Leder, P. Attenuation of LDH-A expression uncovers a link between glycolysis, mitochondrial physiology, and tumor maintenance. *Cancer Cell* **2006**, *9*, 425–434. [CrossRef]
50. Christofk, H.R.; Vander Heiden, M.G.; Harris, M.H.; Ramanathan, A.; Gerszten, R.E.; Wei, R.; Fleming, M.D.; Schreiber, S.L.; Cantley, L.C. The M2 splice isoform of pyruvate kinase is important for cancer metabolism and tumour growth. *Nature* **2008**, *452*, 230–233. [CrossRef]
51. Sonveaux, P.; Végran, F.; Schroeder, T.; Vegran, F.; Schroeder, T.; Wergin, M.C.; Verrax, J.; Rabbani, Z.N.; De Saedeleer, C.J.; Kennedy, K.M.; et al. Targeting lactate-fueled respiration selectively kills hypoxic tumor cells in mice. *J. Clin. Investig.* **2008**, *118*, 3930–3942. [CrossRef]
52. Pavlides, S.; Whitaker-Menezes, D.; Castello-Cros, R.; Flomenberg, N.; Witkiewicz, A.K.; Frank, P.G.; Casimiro, M.C.; Wang, C.; Fortina, P.; Addya, S.; et al. The reverse Warburg effect: Aerobic glycolysis in cancer associated fibroblasts and the tumor stroma. *Cell Cycle* **2009**, *8*, 3984–4001. [CrossRef] [PubMed]

53. Yang, Z.; Yan, C.; Ma, J.; Peng, P.; Ren, X.; Cai, S.; Shen, X.; Wu, Y.; Zhang, S.; Wang, X.; et al. Lactylome analysis suggests lactylation-dependent mechanisms of metabolic adaptation in hepatocellular carcinoma. *Nat. Metab.* **2023**, *5*, 61–79. [CrossRef]
54. Zhang, C.; Quinones, A.; Le, A. Metabolic reservoir cycles in cancer. *Semin. Cancer Biol.* **2022**, *86*, 180–188. [CrossRef] [PubMed]
55. Jacquet, P.; Stéphanou, A. Searching for the Metabolic Signature of Cancer: A Review from Warburg's Time to Now. *Biomolecules* **2022**, *12*, 1412. [CrossRef] [PubMed]
56. Papalazarou, V.; Maddocks, O.D.K. Supply and demand: Cellular nutrient uptake and exchange in cancer. *Mol. Cell* **2021**, *81*, 3731–3748. [CrossRef] [PubMed]
57. Elingaard-Larsen, L.O.; Rolver, M.G.; Sørensen, E.E.; Pedersen, S.F. How Reciprocal Interactions between the Tumor Microenvironment and Ion Transport Proteins Drive Cancer Progression. In *From Malignant Transformation to Metastasis*; Stock, C., Pardo, L.A., Eds.; Reviews of Physiology, Biochemistry and Pharmacology; Springer: Cham, Switzerland, 2020; Volume 182, pp. 1–38. [CrossRef]
58. Gillies, R.J.; Raghunand, N.; Karczmar, G.S.; Bhujwalla, Z.M. MRI of the tumor microenvironment. *J. Magn. Reson. Imaging* **2002**, *16*, 430–450. [CrossRef] [PubMed]
59. Gallagher, F.A.; Kettunen, M.I.; Day, S.E.; Hu, D.-E.; Ardenkjær-Larsen, J.H.; Zandt, R.I.; Jensen, P.R.; Karlsson, M.; Golman, K.; Lerche, M.H.; et al. Magnetic resonance imaging of pH in vivo using hyperpolarized 13C-labelled bicarbonate. *Nature* **2008**, *453*, 940–943. [CrossRef]
60. Hu, X.; Chao, M.; Wu, H. Central role of lactate and proton in cancer cell resistance to glucose deprivation and its clinical translation. *Signal Transduct. Target Ther.* **2017**, *2*, 16047. [CrossRef]
61. Brown, T.P.; Ganapathy, V. Lactate/GPR81 signaling and proton motive force in cancer: Role in angiogenesis, immune escape, nutrition, and Warburg phenomenon. *Pharmacol. Ther.* **2020**, *206*, 107451. [CrossRef]
62. Roland, C.L.; Arumugam, T.; Deng, D.; Liu, S.H.; Philip, B.; Gomez, S.; Burns, W.R.; Ramachandran, V.; Wang, H.; Cruz-Monserrate, Z.; et al. Cell surface lactate receptor GPR81 is crucial for cancer cell survival. *Cancer Res.* **2014**, *74*, 5301–5310. [CrossRef]
63. Payen, V.L.; Mina, E.; Van Hée, V.F.; Porporato, P.E.; Sonveaux, P. Monocarboxylate transporters in cancer. *Mol. Metab.* **2020**, *33*, 48–66. [CrossRef] [PubMed]
64. Corbet, C.; Draoui, N.; Polet, F.; Pinto, A.; Drozak, X.; Riant, O.; Feron, O. The SIRT1/HIF2α axis drives reductive glutamine metabolism under chronic acidosis and alters tumor response to therapy. *Cancer Res.* **2014**, *74*, 5507–5519. [CrossRef] [PubMed]
65. Corbet, C.; Bastien, E.; de Jesus, J.P.S.; Dierge, E.; Martherus, R.; Linden, C.V.; Doix, B.; Degavre, C.; Guilbaud, C.; Petit, L.; et al. TGFβ2-induced formation of lipid droplets supports acidosis-driven EMT and the metastatic spreading of cancer cells. *Nat. Commun.* **2020**, *11*, 454. [CrossRef] [PubMed]
66. Queen, A.; Bhutto, H.N.; Yousuf, M.; Syed, M.A.; Hassan, I. Carbonic anhydrase IX: A tumor acidification switch in heterogeneity and chemokine regulation. *Semin. Cancer Biol.* **2022**, *86*, 899–913. [CrossRef] [PubMed]
67. Xie, J.; Dai, C.; Hu, X. Evidence That Does Not Support Pyruvate Kinase M2 (PKM2)-catalyzed Reaction as a Rate-limiting Step in Cancer Cell Glycolysis. *J. Biol. Chem.* **2016**, *291*, 8987–8999. [CrossRef] [PubMed]
68. Persi, E.; Duran-Frigola, M.; Damaghi, M.; Roush, W.R.; Aloy, P.; Cleveland, J.L.; Gillies, R.J.; Ruppin, E. Systems analysis of intracellular pH vulnerabilities for cancer therapy. *Nat. Commun.* **2018**, *9*, 2997. [CrossRef]
69. Corbet, C.; Feron, O. Cancer cell metabolism and mitochondria: Nutrient plasticity for TCA cycle fueling. *Biochim. Biophys. Acta BBA-Rev. Cancer* **2017**, *1868*, 7–15. [CrossRef]
70. Inigo, M.; Deja, S.; Burgess, S.C. Ins and Outs of the TCA Cycle: The Central Role of Anaplerosis. *Annu. Rev. Nutr.* **2021**, *41*, 19–47. [CrossRef] [PubMed]
71. Faubert, B.; Li, K.Y.; Cai, L.; Hensley, C.T.; Kim, J.; Zacharias, L.G.; Yang, C.; Do, Q.N.; Doucette, S.; Burguete, D.; et al. Lactate metabolism in human lung tumors. *Cell* **2017**, *171*, 358–371. [CrossRef]
72. Chen, L.B. Mitochondrial Membrane Potential in Living Cells. *Annu. Rev. Cell Biol.* **1988**, *4*, 155–181. [CrossRef]
73. Herzig, S.; Raemy, E.; Montessuit, S.; Veuthey, J.-L.; Zamboni, N.; Westermann, B.; Kunji, E.R.S.; Martinou, J.-C. Identification and functional expression of the mitochondrial pyruvate carrier. *Science* **2012**, *337*, 93–96. [CrossRef] [PubMed]
74. Bricker, D.K.; Taylor, E.B.; Schell, J.C.; Orsak, T.; Boutron, A.; Chen, Y.-C.; Cox, J.E.; Cardon, C.M.; Van Vranken, J.G.; Dephoure, N.; et al. A Mitochondrial Pyruvate Carrier Required for Pyruvate Uptake in Yeast, Drosophila, and Humans. *Science* **2012**, *337*, 96–100. [CrossRef] [PubMed]
75. Hashimoto, T.; Hussien, R.; Brooks, G.A. Colocalization of MCT1, CD147, and LDH in mitochondrial inner membrane of L6 muscle cells: Evidence of a mitochondrial lactate oxidation complex. *Am. J. Physiol. Endocrinol. Metab.* **2006**, *290*, E1237–E1244. [CrossRef] [PubMed]
76. Brooks, G.A. The Science and Translation of Lactate Shuttle Theory. *Cell Metab.* **2018**, *27*, 757–785. [CrossRef] [PubMed]
77. Li, X.; Yang, Y.; Zhang, B.; Lin, X.; Fu, X.; An, Y.; Zou, Y.; Wang, J.-X.; Wang, Z.; Yu, T. Lactate metabolism in human health and disease. *Signal Transduct. Target Ther.* **2022**, *7*, 305. [CrossRef]
78. Ying, M.; Guo, C.; Hu, X. The quantitative relationship between isotopic and net contributions of lactate and glucose to the tricarboxylic acid (TCA) cycle. *J. Biol. Chem.* **2019**, *294*, 9615–9630. [CrossRef]
79. Tasdogan, A.; Faubert, B.; Ramesh, V.; Ubellacker, J.M.; Shen, B.; Solmonson, A.; Murphy, M.M.; Gu, Z.; Gu, W.; Martin, M.; et al. Metabolic heterogeneity confers differences in melanoma metastatic potential. *Nature* **2020**, *577*, 115. [CrossRef] [PubMed]

80. Aoi, W.; Hosogi, S.; Niisato, N.; Yokoyama, N.; Hayata, H.; Miyazaki, H.; Kusuzaki, K.; Fukuda, T.; Fukui, M.; Nakamura, N.; et al. Improvement of insulin resistance, blood pressure and interstitial pH in early developmental stage of insulin resistance in OLETF rats by intake of propolis extracts. *Biochem. Biophys. Res. Commun.* **2013**, *432*, 650–653. [CrossRef] [PubMed]
81. Gillies, R.J.; Pilot, C.; Marunaka, Y.; Fais, S. Targeting Acidity in Cancer and Diabetes. *Biochim. Biophys. Acta Rev. Cancer.* **2019**, *1871*, 273–280. [CrossRef]
82. Chao, M.; Wu, H.; Jin, K.; Li, B.; Wu, J.; Zhang, G.; Yang, G.; Hu, X. A nonrandomized cohort and a randomized study of local control of large hepatocarcinoma by targeting intratumoral lactic acidosis. *eLife* **2016**, *5*, e15691. [CrossRef] [PubMed]
83. Dong, Q.; Zhou, C.; Ren, H.; Zhang, Z.; Cheng, F.; Xiong, Z.; Chen, C.; Yang, J.; Gao, J.; Zhang, Y.; et al. Lactate-induced MRP1 expression contributes to metabolism-based etoposide resistance in non-small cell lung cancer cells. *Cell Commun. Signal* **2020**, *18*, 167. [CrossRef] [PubMed]
84. Ying, C.; Jin, C.; Zeng, S.; Chao, M.; Hu, X. Alkalization of cellular pH leads to cancer cell death by disrupting autophagy and mitochondrial function. *Oncogene* **2022**, *41*, 3886–3897. [CrossRef] [PubMed]
85. Choi, H.; Yeo, M.; Kang, Y.; Kim, H.J.; Park, S.G.; Jang, E.; Park, S.H.; Kim, E.; Kang, S. Lactate oxidase/catalase-displaying nanoparticles efficiently consume lactate in the tumor microenvironment to effectively suppress tumor growth. *J. Nanobiotechnol.* **2023**, *21*, 5. [CrossRef] [PubMed]
86. Yu, J.; Wei, Z.; Li, Q.; Wan, F.; Chao, Z.; Zhang, X.; Lin, L.; Meng, H.; Tian, L. Advanced Cancer Starvation Therapy by Simultaneous Deprivation of Lactate and Glucose Using a MOF Nanoplatform. *Adv. Sci.* **2021**, *8*, e2101467. [CrossRef] [PubMed]
87. Chavarria, V.; Ortiz-Islas, E.; Salazar, A.; la Cruz, V.P.-D.; Espinosa-Bonilla, A.; Figueroa, R.; Ortíz-Plata, A.; Sotelo, J.; Sánchez-García, F.J.; Pineda, B. Lactate-Loaded Nanoparticles Induce Glioma Cytotoxicity and Increase the Survival of Rats Bearing Malignant Glioma Brain Tumor. *Pharmaceutics* **2022**, *14*, 327. [CrossRef] [PubMed]
88. Guan, X.; Rodriguez-Cruz, V.; Morris, M.E. Cellular Uptake of MCT1 Inhibitors AR-C155858 and AZD3965 and Their Effects on MCT-Mediated Transport of L-Lactate in Murine 4T1 Breast Tumor Cancer Cells. *AAPS J.* **2019**, *21*, 13. [CrossRef]
89. Beloueche-Babari, M.; Galobart, T.C.; Delgado-Goni, T.; Wantuch, S.; Parkes, H.G.; Tandy, D.; Harker, J.A.; Leach, M.O. Monocarboxylate transporter 1 blockade with AZD3965 inhibits lipid biosynthesis and increases tumour immune cell infiltration. *Br. J. Cancer* **2020**, *122*, 895–903. [CrossRef]
90. Ma, R.; Li, X.; Gong, S.; Ge, X.; Zhu, T.; Ge, X.; Weng, L.; Tao, Q.; Guo, J. Dual Roles of Lactate in EGFR-TKI-Resistant Lung Cancer by Targeting GPR81 and MCT1. *J. Oncol.* **2022**, *2022*, 3425841. [CrossRef]
91. Pisarsky, L.; Bill, R.; Fagiani, E.; Dimeloe, S.; Goosen, R.W.; Hagmann, J.; Hess, C.; Christofori, G. Targeting Metabolic Symbiosis to Overcome Resistance to Anti-Angiogenic Therapy. *Cell Rep.* **2016**, *15*, 1161–1174. [CrossRef]
92. Sharma, D.; Singh, M.; Rani, R. Role of LDH in tumor glycolysis: Regulation of LDHA by small molecules for cancer therapeutics. *Semin. Cancer Biol.* **2022**, *87*, 184–195. [CrossRef]
93. Xiao, Z.; Dai, Z.; Locasale, J.W. Metabolic landscape of the tumor microenvironment at single cell resolution. *Nat. Commun.* **2019**, *10*, 3763. [CrossRef] [PubMed]
94. Li, W.; Wang, J. Uncovering the Underlying Mechanisms of Cancer Metabolism through the Landscapes and Probability Flux Quantifications. *IScience* **2020**, *23*, 101002. [CrossRef] [PubMed]
95. Curry, J.M.; Tuluc, M.; Whitaker-Menezes, D.; Ames, J.A.; Anantharaman, A.; Butera, A.; Leiby, B.; Cognetti, D.; Sotgia, F.; Lisanti, M.P.; et al. Cancer metabolism, stemness and tumor recurrence. *Cell Cycle* **2013**, *12*, 1371–1384. [CrossRef] [PubMed]
96. Phipps, C.; Molavian, H.; Kohandel, M. A microscale mathematical model for metabolic symbiosis: Investigating the effects of metabolic inhibition on ATP turnover in tumors. *J. Theor. Biol.* **2015**, *366*, 103–114. [CrossRef]
97. Hensley, C.T.; Faubert, B.; Yuan, Q.; Lev-Cohain, N.; Jin, E.; Kim, J.; Jiang, L.; Ko, B.; Skelton, R.; Loudat, L.; et al. Metabolic Heterogeneity in Human Lung Tumors. *Cell* **2016**, *164*, 681–694. [CrossRef]
98. Pereira-Nunes, A.; Afonso, J.; Granja, S.; Baltazar, F. Lactate and Lactate Transporters as Key Players in the Maintenance of the Warburg Effect. *Adv. Exp. Med. Biol.* **2020**, *1219*, 51–74. [CrossRef]
99. Swietach, P.; Monterisi, S. A Barter Economy in Tumors: Exchanging Metabolites through Gap Junctions. *Cancers* **2019**, *11*, 117. [CrossRef]
100. Dovmark, T.H.; Saccomano, M.; Hulikova, A.; Alves, F.; Swietach, P. Connexin-43 channels are a pathway for discharging lactate from glycolytic pancreatic ductal adenocarcinoma cells. *Oncogene* **2017**, *36*, 4538–4550. [CrossRef]
101. Zhou, M.; Zheng, M.; Zhou, X.; Tian, S.; Yang, X.; Ning, Y.; Li, Y.; Zhang, S. The roles of connexins and gap junctions in the progression of cancer. *Cell Commun. Signal* **2023**, *21*, 8. [CrossRef]
102. Guillaumond, F.; Leca, J.; Olivares, O.; Lavaut, M.-N.; Vidal, N.; Berthezène, P.; Dusetti, N.J.; Loncle, C.; Calvo, E.; Turrini, O.; et al. Strengthened glycolysis under hypoxia supports tumor symbiosis and hexosamine biosynthesis in pancreatic adenocarcinoma. *Proc. Natl. Acad. Sci. USA* **2013**, *110*, 3919–3924. [CrossRef]
103. Martinez, C.A.; Scafoglio, C. Heterogeneity of Glucose Transport in Lung Cancer. *Biomolecules* **2020**, *10*, 868. [CrossRef]
104. Shibao, S.; Minami, N.; Koike, N.; Fukui, N.; Yoshida, K.; Saya, H.; Sampetrean, O. Metabolic heterogeneity and plasticity of glioma stem cells in a mouse glioblastoma model. *Neuro-Oncology* **2018**, *20*, 343–354. [CrossRef] [PubMed]

105. Kubelt, C.; Peters, S.; Ahmeti, H.; Huhndorf, M.; Huber, L.; Cohrs, G.; Hövener, J.-B.; Jansen, O.; Synowitz, M.; Held-Feindt, J. Intratumoral Distribution of Lactate and the Monocarboxylate Transporters 1 and 4 in Human Glioblastoma Multiforme and Their Relationships to Tumor Progression-Associated Markers. *Int. J. Mol. Sci.* **2020**, *21*, 6254. [CrossRef] [PubMed]
106. Tang, X.; Lucas, J.E.; Chen, J.L.-Y.; LaMonte, G.; Wu, J.; Wang, M.C.; Koumenis, C.; Chi, J.-T. Functional interaction between responses to lactic acidosis and hypoxia regulates genomic transcriptional outputs. *Cancer Res.* **2012**, *72*, 491–502. [CrossRef] [PubMed]

Disclaimer/Publisher's Note: The statements, opinions and data contained in all publications are solely those of the individual author(s) and contributor(s) and not of MDPI and/or the editor(s). MDPI and/or the editor(s) disclaim responsibility for any injury to people or property resulting from any ideas, methods, instructions or products referred to in the content.

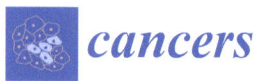

Review

Amino Acids in Cancer and Cachexia: An Integrated View

Maurizio Ragni [1], Claudia Fornelli [2], Enzo Nisoli [1,*] and Fabio Penna [2,*]

[1] Center for Study and Research on Obesity, Department of Biomedical Technology and Translational Medicine, University of Milan, 20129 Milan, Italy
[2] Department of Clinical and Biological Sciences, University of Torino, 10125 Turin, Italy
* Correspondence: enzo.nisoli@unimi.it (E.N.); fabio.penna@unito.it (F.P.)

Simple Summary: Cancer metabolism is an emerging field of investigation aimed at identifying cancer cell vulnerabilities in order to define novel anti-cancer therapeutic approaches based on interventions that modulate the availability of specific nutrients. Amino acids (AAs) are used by cancer cells as both building blocks for protein synthesis required for rapid tumor growth and as sources of energy. The current review aims to describe the most relevant alterations of AA metabolism that could be targeted by either AA deprivation or AA supplementation to limit tumor growth. In parallel, the reader will understand how AA availability mainly relies on and impacts cancer-host metabolism, eventually leading to a wasting paraneoplastic syndrome called cachexia. The above-mentioned AA-based interventions are here discussed also in view of their impact on the tumor host, in an attempt to provide a broader view that can improve our understanding of the patient outcome.

Abstract: Rapid tumor growth requires elevated biosynthetic activity, supported by metabolic rewiring occurring both intrinsically in cancer cells and extrinsically in the cancer host. The Warburg effect is one such example, burning glucose to produce a continuous flux of biomass substrates in cancer cells at the cost of energy wasting metabolic cycles in the host to maintain stable glycemia. Amino acid (AA) metabolism is profoundly altered in cancer cells, which use AAs for energy production and for supporting cell proliferation. The peculiarities in cancer AA metabolism allow the identification of specific vulnerabilities as targets of anti-cancer treatments. In the current review, specific approaches targeting AAs in terms of either deprivation or supplementation are discussed. Although based on opposed strategies, both show, in vitro and in vivo, positive effects. Any AA-targeted intervention will inevitably impact the cancer host, who frequently already has cachexia. Cancer cachexia is a wasting syndrome, also due to malnutrition, that compromises the effectiveness of anti-cancer drugs and eventually causes the patient's death. AA deprivation may exacerbate malnutrition and cachexia, while AA supplementation may improve the nutritional status, counteract cachexia, and predispose the patient to a more effective anti-cancer treatment. Here is provided an attempt to describe the AA-based therapeutic approaches that integrate currently distant points of view on cancer-centered and host-centered research, providing a glimpse of several potential investigations that approach cachexia as a unique cancer disease.

Keywords: amino acid; cancer metabolism; cachexia; nutrition; supplement

1. Introduction

Cancer metabolism is a broad and emerging field of study at the frontier of cancer discovery, aimed at understanding tumorigenesis, tumor progression, and disorders of cell metabolism, as well as for designing new prospective therapies [1]. The dysregulation of metabolic circuitries occurs at several levels beyond cancer cells, affecting tumor stroma, the immune system, and eventually the whole host, resulting in uncontrolled tumor growth, immunoescape, and cachexia, respectively. Understanding the cellular tissue and systemic metabolic alterations will likely uncover, on the one side, exploitable metabolic vulnerabilities for reducing tumor growth and improving anti-tumor therapies, and on the other side, specific nutrient host deficiencies which, upon supplementation, will counteract cachexia and support a more effective fight against the cancer. The objective of the current review is to focus on amino acid (AA) metabolism in both cancer cells and the tumor host in order to highlight potential AA-based therapeutic approaches that integrate the currently distant points of view on cancer-centered and host-centered research.

1.1. Impact of AAs on Cancer Metabolism and Mitochondrial Function

The elevated biosynthetic activity of cancer cells is supported by several strategies aimed at increasing growth. Oncogenic mutations allow tumor cells to sustain angiogenesis, evade apoptosis, enable constitutive proliferation signaling by tyrosine kinase receptors, and to escape from growth suppression signaling [2]. Moreover, profound metabolic alterations also confer to cancers the ability to optimize substrate utilization; one typical example of metabolic reprogramming is the Warburg effect (aerobic glycolysis), the observation that cancer cells convert glucose to lactate even in an oxygen-rich environment, dates back to almost 100 years ago [3]. The Warburg effect is not exclusive to cancer cells, but also occurs in normal, non-cancerous, rapidly dividing cells, such as activated macrophages and lymphocytes, haematopoietic stem and progenitor cells, or during angiogenesis, and this confirms the growth advantage conferred by this metabolic adaptation [4]. Initially ascribed to defective mitochondria, this apparently inefficient metabolic reprogramming is now hypothesized to have the aim, rather than ATP production, of maximizing carbon delivery to the cell's anabolic pathway for the synthesis of biomass. In both living organisms and in culture, cells in fact rarely experience shortages of glucose, which is always kept at high/constant levels in the culture medium or bloodstream; this means that proliferating cells do not have a real need to maximize ATP synthesis from glucose [5]. Therefore, by engaging glucose into aerobic glycolysis, cancer cells avoid its complete catabolism to ATP in mitochondria; this spares glucose carbon that can be used for generating acetyl-Coa, glycolytic intermediates, and ribose for the synthesis of fatty acids, non-essential amino acids (NEAA), and nucleotides, respectively [6]. Since the major part of these pathways require functional mitochondria, this implies that, in proliferating cancer cells, mitochondria are not dysfunctional; however, as a consequence of aerobic glycolysis, they are rather used as a biosynthetic organelle for the synthesis of glucose-derived lipid and NEAA, instead of ATP. Furthermore, cancer cells are also able to efficiently utilize mitochondria for directing other cell substrates for macromolecule synthesis and, in this process, amino acids (AA) play a pivotal role [7]. The role of AAs as constituents of proteins and/or signaling molecules involved in the regulation of macroautophagy, the process of endosomal/lysosomal recycling of cellular components, or as activators of biosynthetic cell pathways through mammalian target of rapamycin (mTOR), has been the subject of many other comprehensive reviews [8–10]. However, AAs show an intimate connection with mitochondrial function. One such example is glutamine (Gln), which, together with glucose, is the main molecule utilized by the majority of mammalian cells in culture.

1.2. Cancer Mitochondria Support Biosynthesis of Macromolecules through Glutamine-Dependent Anaplerosis

Since the early discovery that HeLa cells consume Gln from 10 to 100 orders of magnitude more than other amino acids [11], and that Gln is used as a major source of cell energy, rather than for incorporation into proteins [12], the observation that transformed cells display a high rate of Gln consumption has been confirmed in several other cancer cell types, such as glioblastoma, ovarian, pancreatic, and breast cancer [13–16]. Through mitochondrial glutaminolysis, Gln is utilized to provide both carbon and nitrogen for anabolic reactions; in particular, through the process of anaplerosis, which leads to the replenishment of the pools of metabolic intermediates of the tricarboxylic acid cycle (TCA) in times of high energy requirements [17], Gln is a major carbon source for the synthesis of proteins, nucleotides, and lipids. In this pathway, Gln is first converted into glutamate (Glu) via mitochondrial glutaminase (GLS), and then glutamate dehydrogenase (GDH) convert glutamate into α-ketoglutarate (α-KG); alternatively, a second pathway of conversion of Glu in α-KG involves the activity of both mitochondrial and cytosolic transaminases such as aspartate transaminase (AST), alanine transaminase (ALT), or phosphoserine transaminase (PSAT). The routing of glutamate to the dehydrogenation or to the transamination pathway depend on the metabolic status of the cell and has important metabolic consequences; although the prevalence of transamination over dehydrogenation has been positively correlated with proliferation rate [18] and glucose levels, both pathways enable the optimization of amino acid uptake and consumption with growth and biomass production, with transamination being prevalent in times of glucose abundance, while the glutamate dehydrogenation pathway has been shown to be induced during glucose shortages, thus enabling cell survival [19,20]. Furthermore, sequential glutaminase and glutamate dehydrogenase reactions produce ammonia (NH_3) and ammonium (NH_4^+), respectively, which is considered a cell toxic by-product which requires scavenging through urea; however, ammonia is also a major diffusible autophagy inducer [21], which could therefore help cancer cells increase fitness by eliminating damaged and potentially toxic macromolecules and organelles. Moreover, in breast cancer, extracellular ammonia synthesized in the liver can be recycled by tumor cells through reductive amination by GDH to form glutamate which is then used for macromolecule biosynthesis [22], and Gln-derived ammonia can also promote sterol regulatory element binding protein (SREBP) mediated lipogenesis and support tumor growth [23]. A graphical representation of the above-described metabolic scenario is provided in Figure 1. Glutamate transamination, on the contrary, does not produce ammonia, but generates the NEAAs aspartate (Asp), alanine (Ala), and serine (Ser) which, together with α-KG, serve as anaplerotic substrates in the TCA cycle, thus promoting biosynthesis. In this process, Oxaloacetate (Oaa) produced by α-KG from glutaminolysis condenses with pyruvate-derived Acetyl-CoA to produce citrate at the citrate synthase step; citrate is then not committed to the isocitrate dehydrogenase step (which is instead involved in reductive carboxylation—see below), but is instead exported to cytosol where ATP-citrate lyase reforms Acetyl-CoA, which is then used for malonyl-Coa synthesis and de novo lipogenesis. Glutaminolysis flux also generates reduced nicotinamide adenine dinucleotide (NADH) and reduced nicotinamide adenine dinucleotide phosphate (NADPH), as reducing equivalents for the electron transport chain (ETC) and both redox balance and lipogenesis, respectively. Beyond glutaminolysis, which is considered as the oxidative branch of Gln metabolism, the alternate metabolic fate of Gln is through the reductive carboxylation pathway, which involves the engaging of α-KG in a "reverse" mitochondrial TCA cycle through NADPH-dependent isocitrate dehydrogenases 1 and 2 (IDH1 and IDH2) and therefore producing citrate for lipid biosynthesis [24–26]. This pathway seems to be predominant in cancer subjected to hypoxia, displaying constitutive hypoxia-inducible factor 1 alpha (HIF1α) activation, or have defective mitochondria [27,28] and has been confirmed to occur also in vivo [28,29].

1.3. Mitochondrial Electron Transport Chain and AA Metabolism

Beyond the evidence coming from glutamine/glutamate metabolism, several other studies clearly demonstrate that the function of mitochondria in sustaining cell proliferation goes beyond the simple ATP synthesis, and that biomass production and macromolecule synthesis depend on to the strict connection and crosslink between mitochondrial activity and AA metabolism. A striking example on how mitochondrial function and AA metabolism are reciprocally intertwined comes from two studies which show that the most essential function of the ETC in proliferating cells is to provide electron acceptors to support Asp biosynthesis which, in turn, is required for the synthesis of purine and pyrimidines [30,31]. By recycling NAD^+, ETC provides oxidized cofactor for malate dehydrogenase 2 (MDH2) which, in turn, produces Oaa that is used by mitochondrial aspartate transaminase (GOT2) for the synthesis of Asp. However, when ETC is dysfunctional, the ratio $NAD^+/NADH$ decreases, and Asp synthesis is switched to the reductive carboxylation of Gln to citrate which, through ATP-citrate lyase, produces Oaa to drive Asp synthesis. This suggests that, in proliferating cells, the high NAD$^+$/NADH ratio maintained by mitochondrial respiration is essentially used for Asp/nucleotide synthesis, rather than for ensuring constant TCA cycle/OXPHOS function. Treatment of acute myeloid leukemia (AML) cells with IACS-010759, a complex I inhibitor, reduced cell viability, decreased NAD$^+$/NADH ratio, and, among AAs, exclusively reduced Asp levels while increasing Gln utilization, thus confirming that the interconnection between mitochondrial activity, redox state, and Asp synthesis is extended to cancer cells [32]. This relationship has also been recently confirmed in vivo; treatment of mouse neuroblastoma xenografts with IACS-010759 affected ETC activity, redox state and Asp metabolism, as well as activation of reductive carboxylation of Gln. In addition, treatment of xenografted mice with metformin, a commercial available antidiabetic drug and complex I inhibitor, dose-dependently inhibited tumor growth, together with a decrease in intratumor NAD$^+$/NADH ratio and Asp levels [33,34]. The evidence of reprogramming of the cancer mitochondrial function to support Asp synthesis for survival comes not only from studies based on pharmacological inhibition of complex I, but also from genetic disruption of ETC components, which resemble mitochondrial alterations in tumors; inactivating mutations of mitochondrial succinate dehydrogenase (SDH) are frequent in cancers and increase susceptibility to the development of different tumors and, as such, SDH has tumor suppressor functions. Immortalized kidney mouse cells deficient in SDH become addicted to extracellular pyruvate for proliferation, which, through carboxylation to Oaa, is diverted to Asp synthesis. Notably, SDH ablation in absence of pyruvate also decreased the NAD$^+$/NADH ratio, thus confirming that, in cancer cells, mitochondrial function is strictly connected to Asp biosynthesis through the modulation of its redox state [35]. Moreover, a very recent paper revealed a close relationship between ETC, redox state, and Gln utilization for biomass production: in 143B cells, respiration inhibited by both mitochondrial DNA (mtDNA) depletion of parental ϱ0 cells and chemical ETC inhibition, the reduced mitochondrial NAD+/NADH ratio reversed mitochondrial GOT2 as well as succinate and malate dehydrogenases to promote mitochondrial oxidation of NADH to NAD+; this, in turn, enabled GDH-dependent Gln anaplerosis to support cell proliferation [36]. Beyond Asp, mitochondrial NAD$^+$ regeneration has been shown to be essential also for the synthesis of Ser, which is another carbon source for the production of nucleotides; in fact, withdrawal of Ser from culture medium increased sensitivity of melanoma cell lines to the anti-proliferative effects of both rotenone or metformin; furthermore, Ser deprivation depleted cells of purine nucleotides and rotenone treatment further increased their depletion [37]. Alteration of Ser synthesis also occurs in response to cells depleted of mtDNA; this causes bioenergetic failure and induction of activating transcription factor 4 (ATF4), a master transcription factor which regulates cell response to AA starvation during the integrated stress response (ISR) [38]. mtDNA depleted cells display increased Ser synthesis and decreased Ser consumption, thus reflecting elevated reliance on serine for survival [39]. Ser, together with glycine (Gly), is also involved in one-carbon (1C) metabolism, a process shared by both mitochondria and cytosol which, through the folate cycle, leads to the production of 1C methyl units for several biochemical pathways such as purine and pyrimidine biosynthesis, and synthesis of methionine (Met), as well as providing the moiety for methylation reactions for epigenetic control of gene expression [40]. Being a central hub for a plethora of anabolic pathways, cancer cells can therefore become reliant on generation of 1C units from both Gly and Ser. Ser can be converted to Gly by the cytosolic or mitochondrial serine hydroxymethyltransferase SHMT1 and SHMT2, respectively, with the transfer of Ser-derived 1C unit to tetrahydrofolate (THF), generating methylene-THF which, in turn, is required for purine and pyrimidine biosynthesis. As a result, cancer cells have been shown to both avidly consume extracellular Ser and also to strongly depend on endogenous Ser synthesis, displaying an elevated Ser flux [41–44]. Ser can be synthesized from the glycolytic intermediate 3-phosphoglycerate (3-PG) through the enzyme phosphoglycerate dehydrogenase (PHGDH), which is in a genomic locus of copy number gain in both breast cancer and melanoma, and whose protein levels are increased in 70% of estrogen receptor (ER)-negative breast cancers [42,44]. The overexpression of

PHGDH in tumors allows elevated rates of de novo Ser biosynthesis which, as a result, increases the biosynthesis and metabolic pathways associated with the folate pool, amino acid, lipids, and redox regulation [44]. However, in tumors, this metabolic adaptation requires a diminished flux of pyruvate toward mitochondrial oxidation, thus redirecting upstream glycolytic intermediates, such as 3-PG, to Ser and Gly synthesis; in many cancer cells, this is accomplished by preferential expression of the M2 isoform of pyruvate kinase (PKM2), which displays lower kinase activity compared to PKM1, thus promoting the accumulation 3-PG and other glycolytic intermediates which are precursors for biosynthesis of Ser, as well as nucleotides, amino acids, and lipids required for proliferation [45]. Notably, Ser is an allosteric activator of PKM2, and this allows cancer cells to rapidly increase Ser biosynthesis in response to its environmental shortage since, when Ser levels fall, the decrease in PKM2 activity allows more glucose-derived carbon to be diverted into serine biosynthesis [46]. Although Ser can be synthesized by both SHMT1 and SHMT2, the mitochondrial isoform is strongly upregulated in cancers and has been shown to have a stronger impact on cancer metabolism [42,47]. Mitochondrial 5,10-methylenetetrahydrofolate production by SHMT2 provides methyl groups for mitochondrial tRNA modification, which are required for proper mitochondrial translation and function [48,49]. Furthermore, SHMT2 is required for complex I assembly, and mice deficient in SHMT2 display embryonic lethality and defective mitochondrial respiration [50,51].

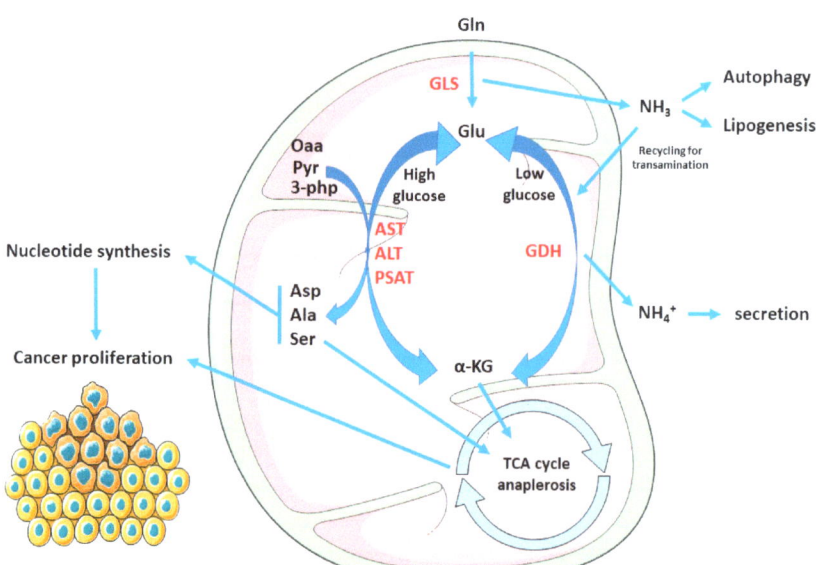

Figure 1. Rewiring of the metabolic fate of AAs in cancers: Gln- derived Glu yield α-kg through both transamination or dehydrogenation, by means of AST, ALT, PSAT, or GDH, respectively. The first pathway prevails in conditions of glucose abundance, resulting in production of the NEAAs Asp, Ala, and Ser, and enabling proliferation. Asp is used in nucleotide synthesis while α-kg, Ala, and Ser can feed the TCA cycle. On the other hand, GDH is activated during glucose scarcity or cell quiescence, supporting cell survival and stress resistance. Furthermore, GLS-derived ammonia in cancer can stimulate autophagy, lipogenesis, or being re-incorporated to Glu synthesis, which can be re-routed for transamination and biomass production. Abbreviations: Gln, glutamine; Glu, glutamate; Asp, aspartate; Ala, alanine; Ser, serine; GDH, glutamate dehydrogenase; GLS, glutaminase. AST, aspartate transaminase; ALT, alanine transaminase; PSAT, phosphoserine transaminase; Oaa, oxaloacetate; Pyr, pyruvate; 3-Php, 3-phosphohydroxypyruvate; α-KG, alpha-ketoglutarate.

1.4. Targeting AA Metabolism as Anti-Cancer Strategy

The data herein reported indicate that the connection between AA metabolism and cancer mitochondrial function goes beyond the well-known role of AAs as mitochondrial substrates and can also explain why tumors are dependent on some AAs. Notably, this addiction also includes AAs usually classified as non-essential such as Gln, Ser, and Asp, therefore implying that the mitochondrial reprogramming of cancer metabolism also redefines and crosses the distinction between essential and non-essential AAs. This AA dependency highlights a metabolic vulnerability, which could be exploited for a highly specific anticancer therapy aimed to starve or deplete cancer cells of selected amino acids, or to block crucial AA metabolic pathways [52].

GLN Glutaminase inhibition has been long proposed as a main cancer therapeutic target, and several Glnase inhibitors have been developed, of which the most studied are 6-diazo-5-oxo-L-norleucine (DON), bis-2-(5-phenyl acetamido-1,2,4-thiadiazol-2-yl) ethyl sulfide (BPTES), and CB-839; however, since glutaminolysis is not an exclusive feature of cancer cells (see above), low specificity/high toxicity concerns and poor solubility issues have limited their employment in clinic, and only CB-839 (Telaglenastat) has since been entered in a clinical trial and is currently in phase II [53].

ASN Asparagine (Asn) depletion by means of the bacterial enzyme asparaginase (ASNase) is presently the only approved anticancer treatment based on an AA-depleting approach and has been long used as an anticancer strategy, especially toward pediatric acute lymphoblastic leukemia (ALL) [54,55]. Contrary to most cells, leukemia cells express low levels of asparagine synthetase (ASNS), which render them highly dependent on Asn, thus making ASNase treatment effective [56]. Although several toxic side effects have also been also reported, the majority of them are manageable, but ASNase is almost exclusively used only in ALL [57].

ARG Inhibition of cancer cell proliferation by means of arginase (ARGase) treatment was reported almost 70 years ago [58]; since then, the depletion of Arginine (Arg) through ARGase or arginine deiminase (ADI) administration has been constantly explored as an anticancer therapy, also supported by the finding of absent or low expression of argininosuccinate synthetase (ASS1) in several tumors, especially those associated with chemoresistance and poor clinical outcome, such as hepatocellular carcinoma (HCC), melanoma, mesothelioma, pancreatic cancer, prostate cancer, renal cell carcinoma, sarcoma, and small cell lung cancer [59–62], which result in Arg dependence. While Arg-deprived, non-cancer cells undergo quiescence and cycle arrest at G0/G1 phase, cancer cells starved for Arg continue instead to DNA synthesis, leading to unbalanced growth and ultimately to cell death [63]. Currently, ARGase, as a PEGylated derivative, is employed in clinical trials for the treatment of HCC, melanoma, prostate adenocarcinoma, and pediatric acute myeloid leukemia (AML), while trials with PEGylated ADI are ongoing for the treatment of small cell lung cancer, melanoma, AML, HCC, and mesothelioma [64].

SER, GLY The importance of targeting Ser, Gly, and Met metabolic pathways, which are strictly interconnected to folate 1C metabolism, is highlighted by the long-known use of antifolate drugs as chemoterapics [65]; methotrexate (MTX), the most used antifolate, deplete cells of tetrahydrofolate and is routinely used for the treatment of multiple cancers. However, MTX treatment has some concerns of toxicity [66]. Since, in tumors, the majority of 1C units derive from Ser, many efforts to develop inhibitors of Ser biosynthesis to inhibit cancer 1C metabolism, alone or in combination with other antifolates, have been put forward [67]. Pyrazolopyran, an herbicide compound, which was originally shown to inhibit plant SHMT, has been shown to inhibit human SHMT1 and to induce cell death in lung cancer cells [68]. An optimized pyrazolopyran derivative, by targeting both SHMT1 and SHMT2, blocked proliferation of colon, pancreatic, and several B-Cell derived malignancies, which displayed different grades of sensitivity according to their proficiency in folate metabolism and glycine uptake, thus confirming amino acid vulnerability as a key target for anti-cancer drug development. Furthermore, incubation of many cancer cells in medium lacking Ser/Gly greatly increased the sensitivity of the cells to the PHGDH inhibitor PH755, while PH755 treatment in vivo to xenografted mice significantly potentiated the anti-cancer response of dietary serine/glycine restriction, thus underscoring the effectiveness of a combined dietary and chemotherapeutic approach [69].

2. Amino Acid Supplementation as Anticancer Therapy: Targeting Multiple and Complex Metabolic Networks

The majority of anticancer strategies aimed at targeting the AA metabolism and/or the AA dependency of tumor cells are based on AA starvation; less is known about AA supplementation which has also shown to be beneficial [70]. Dietary starvation of a single AA is not a simple task and strategies to limit Gln, Asp, or Ser/Gly intake had a limited positive response due to compensatory metabolic mechanisms [71,72]; clinically speaking, nutritional enrichment of selected AAs is certainly a more accessible objective. Supplementation of branched-chain amino acids (BCAA) is long-known to have favorable effects in patients with hepatocellular carcinoma [73–76] and is recommended to cirrhotic patients according to the guidelines of the American Association for the Study of Liver Diseases (AASLD) and the European Association for the Study of the Liver (EASL) [70]. Despite its well-known role in fueling cancer proliferation, Gln supplementation, by both increasing its dietary content and supplementation in drinking water, blocked melanoma growth in mice by affecting the epigenetic marks of oncogenic gene expression [77]. Furthermore, dietary supplementation of histidine (His) by enhancing its catabolic flux and depleting tumor cells of tetrahydrofolate, which is also a major target of MTX, increased the sensitivity of leukemia xenografts to MTX chemotherapy [78]. Moreover, a more recent report showed that an AA-defined diet enriched in EAAs decreased tumor growth in mice [79]. Mechanistically, dietary enrichment of EAAs activated BCAA catabolism, inhibited glycolysis and mTOR signaling and induced cancer cell apoptosis through a ATF4-mediated ER stress response, which derived from an intracellular Glu shortage. These results suggest that supplementation of AAs can lead to inhibition of cancer cell proliferation through multiple mechanisms.

The finding that supplementation of EAA can lead to a decrease in levels of other AAs [79] highlights the complexity of intracellular AA metabolic pathways, which are known to be closely linked to each other, showing reciprocal cross-talk, sharing many metabolic intermediates, and also responding with different cues in a strong context-dependent manner [52]. A deep analysis of human metabolic networks showed that AAs are strongly interconnected within specific groups: Gly, Ser, Ala, and Thr; cysteine (Cys) and Met; valine (Val), leucine, and isoleucine (Ile) display the most interconnected pathways [80]. Furthermore, AAs are connected to 39 different cellular processes; notably, these include not only well-characterized AA pathways such as protein synthesis, biomass production and membrane transport, but also specific metabolic pathways like fatty acid oxidation, metabolism of glutathione, nicotinamide adenine dinucleotide, and sphingolipids [80]. Within these, AAs share about 1139 metabolites which are involved in AA metabolism, both directly and indirectly, through interactions with other downstream pathways. Among the top metabolites linked to AA metabolism, NADPH, ATP, NADP$^+$, ADP, and NAD$^+$ play a pivotal role in regulating other core cellular metabolic pathways: this indicates a ubiquitous role for AA in the control of cell metabolism [80]. According to their multifaceted role in cell physiology, many key regulators of cancer AA signaling show a double-face nature; the two isoforms of Glnase, GLS1 and GLS2, are usually over- and under-expressed in cancers, with GLS2 considered as a tumor suppressor, in opposition to the established role of GLS1 as a pro-oncogenic gene [53,81]. Consistently, the PI3K/Akt pathway and mTORC2, two main regulators of cell growth and proliferation, have been shown to be inhibited by exogenously supplemented BCAA [82]. It is noteworthy that, through systems biology analysis, these pleiotropic functions of AAs and their different connections to cell metabolites have been recently shown to have the potential to be exploited for the treatment of multifactorial diseases [80,83]. The intricate and non-univocal impact of either starving or supplementing AAs in cancer cells is summarized in Figure 2.

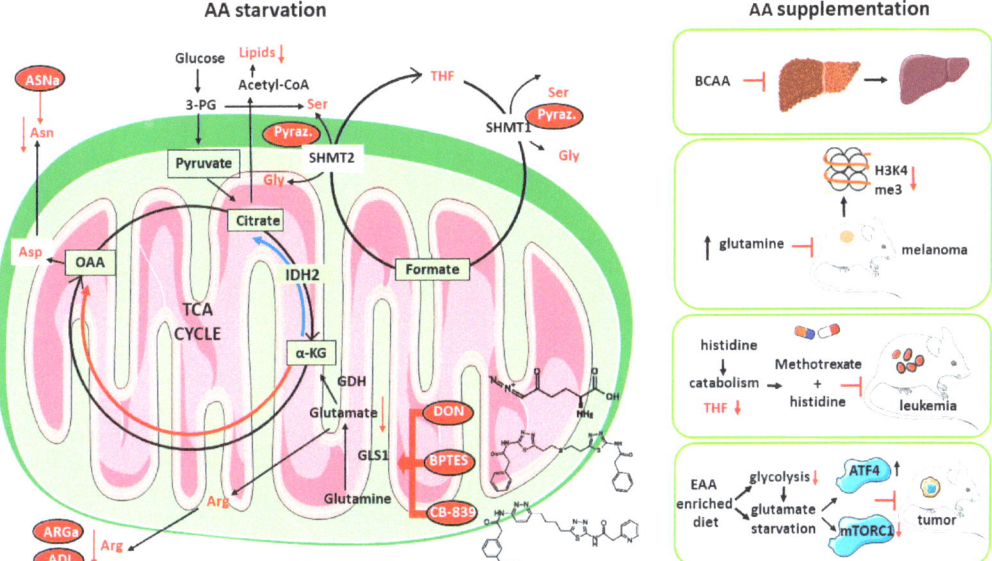

Figure 2. Both amino acid starvation (**left**) and supplementation (**right**) are valuable anti-cancer strategies. (**Left**) panel: mitochondrial glutamine consumption in cancer feeds TCA cycle in both oxidative (red) and reductive (blue) directions which, by providing carbon source for the synthesis of precursors, increases cancer biomass. Interfering with glutaminase (GLS1) activity with the inhibitors DON, BPTES, or CB-839 leads to the depletion of key anabolic intermediates such as lipids and aminoacids. Anti-cancer enzymatic approaches through asparaginase (ASNase), arginase (ARGase), or arginine deaminase (ADI) also lead to the decrease in blood levels of indispensable tumor AAs. Furthermore, interfering with serine or glycine metabolism with the dual SHMT1/SHMT2 inhibitor pyralozopyran also results in depletion of tetrahydrofolate (THF), a key metabolite essential for cancer growth. (**Right**) panel: BCAA supplementation is beneficial in cirrhotic patients, while diet with high gln content blocks melanoma xenografts in mice by reprogramming the tumor epigenetic control of gene expression. Histidine supplementation, by increasing His catabolism and depleting THF, increases methotrexate sensitivity in leukemia-bearing mice, while an EAA-enriched diet impairs tumor growth in mice by inhibiting glycolysis and mTORC1 signaling by means of an EAA-induced ATF4 activation through shortage of glutamate. Abbreviations: 3-PG, 3-phosphoglycerate; IDH2, isocitrate dehydrogenase 2; SHMT1/SHMT2, serine hydroxymethyltransferase $\frac{1}{2}$; GDH, glutamate dehydrogenase; α-KG, alpha-ketoglutarate; ATF4, activating transcription factor 4; mTORC1, mammalian target of rapamycin complex1; H3K4me3, lysine-methylated histone 3; pyraz, pyrazolopyran. The icons used were obtained at: https://smart.servier.com/ (accessed on 10 November 2022).

Cancer is a complex disease. Beyond being influenced by genetic, physiological, and environmental factors, it also has, especially in advanced stages, several outcomes for the whole organism, which are the result of a network of metabolic alterations which involve different organs' dysfunctions. As such, an effective therapeutic strategy aimed at targeting the multiple complications of cancer will require a comprehensive approach. By engaging and targeting different and complex metabolic pathways, AA-based approaches are therefore supposed to impinge more effectively on the multiple dysfunctions developing in the different tissues affected by cancer complications. Cachexia, which lead to weakness, muscle atrophy, systemic inflammation and weight loss can be considered as a paradigm of the complex multifactorial condition associated with cancer [3] and is therefore particularly suitable for nutritional and dietary AA-based approaches.

2.1. Cancer-Induced Cachexia

Cancer cachexia is a complex multiorgan syndrome that affects more than half of all cancer patients (50–80%) and is the direct cause for about 20% of cancer deaths [84,85]. It is characterized by involuntary loss of body weight and adipose tissue that cannot be fully restored by conventional nutritional support, as well by systemic inflammation, anorexia, asthenia, fatigue, metabolic alterations, and muscle wasting, resulting in progressive functional impairment [86,87]. These changes induce detrimental effects on the immune system, increasing susceptibility to infections or other complications, affecting the efficacy and the tolerance to chemotherapy and surgery and, finally, impacting on a patient's quality of life [87,88]. Furthermore, 30 to 90% of cancer patients show malnutrition, characterized by reduced appetite, calorie intake, and changes in taste, accompanied by malabsorption, maldigestion and dysmetabolism, and diminished food intake. This condition may be exacerbated by antineoplastic treatment-related side effects which act on the intestinal epithelium of the host and are responsible for nausea and vomiting (see previous chapter) [89].

Sarcopenia is a gradual and progressive decline in skeletal muscle mass and functional capacity, considered as an age-associated syndrome but also occurring earlier in life in association with chronic diseases, including cancer [90]. Loss of skeletal muscle mass and strength are considered the main clinical criteria for the diagnosis of sarcopenia. The occurrence of the syndrome is confirmed by different techniques including dual-energy X-ray absorptiometry (DXA), computerized tomography (CT), and magnetic resonance imaging (MRI), together with the evaluation of walking speed and handgrip strength, but the absence of standardized evaluation methods in clinical practice could make it difficult to discriminate sarcopenic from non-sarcopenic individuals [86,91]. Moreover, sarcopenia is often associated with other underlying clinical conditions that affect muscle wasting including frailty, cachexia, and sarcopenic obesity, increasing the risk of adverse health-related outcomes such as physical disability, postoperative infections, hospitalization, and institutionalization, resulting in poor quality of life and mortality [86,91–93].

Cancer cachexia is associated with metabolic alterations. In particular, patients show a simultaneous hyper-metabolism, hyper-catabolism, and hypo-anabolism, resulting in a decrease in biomolecule synthesis and a concomitant increased degradation, aggravating the weight loss and causing impaired energy metabolism [85]. For these reasons, cachexia could be considered as an 'energy wasting' disorder in which the homeostatic control of energy intake and expenditure is lost and depends on the type of tumor and its stage [84,85]. Impaired protein turnover is a general hallmark of the energy waste typical of cancer cachexia, both in patients and in experimental models. In fact, there is an activated muscle proteolysis, accompanied by hypo-anabolism and mitochondrial alterations (impaired biogenesis, dynamics, and degradation) [94]. In cancer cachexia, AAs captured by the tumor and other metabolically active tissues such as the liver are obtained from lean tissues, in particular the skeletal muscle, thanks to the activation of two main proteolytic systems, namely the proteasome and the autophagic-lysosomal pathway induced by inflammation-dependent transcription factors, such as FoxO1/3 and NF-κB [95]. Previous studies demonstrated in the muscle of tumor-bearing animals and in cancer patients a hyper-activation of the autophagic system, inflammation and increased reactive oxygen species (ROS) [96,97]. The pro-oxidant species damage the mitochondria, leading to further ROS production and stimulating mitophagy, affecting mitochondrial abundance in the muscle [96–99]. Since mitochondria represent the main producers of energy required for contraction, alterations of their homeostasis impair muscle function [97]. In parallel, it was reported that antioxidant enzymes, such as superoxide dismutase (SOD), catalase, and glutathione peroxidase (GPx), are up-regulated in the muscle of tumor-bearing animals in the attempt to counteract the oxidative insult, albeit not enough to maintain the redox balance, while others reported a down-regulation of the same enzymes, further promoting oxidative stress [99].

So far, although several drugs are being tested in clinical trials; none of them proved effective enough to be used in common practice. Most of the compounds tested in cancer patients so far are based on orexigenic and anabolic compounds [100,101], the former aimed at reversing anorexia and increasing the food intake, the latter at stimulating the signaling pathways controlling muscle protein synthesis and at repressing the signals activating muscle protein catabolism. The current research aims to reverse muscle wasting, targeting several aspects of the syndrome, i.e., reducing energy expenditure, fatigue, anorexia, and systemic inflammation, improving the patient's quality of life and physical state. Beyond this, one of the goals is to understand how the molecular alterations underlying muscle wasting impinge on metabolic and oxidative capacity and mitochondrial function, impairing muscle metabolism and not only muscle mass [102].

One fundamental prerequisite for making any anti-cachexia therapeutic intervention effective is to avoid the occurrence of malnutrition. The European Society for Clinical Nutrition and Metabolism (ESPEN) releases continuously updated guidelines on the management of cancer patients from the nutritional standpoint [103]. The best way to increase protein and energy intake is by food, but unfortunately this is not always possible and or sufficient [104]; appetite stimulants or dietary supplement hardly restore an optimal nutritional status and only partially reduce fat and skeletal muscle loss. AAs, as building blocks of proteins, represent for mammals the only source of nitrogen and the main component of skeletal muscle mass and, as described above, are also used as TCA cycle intermediates for producing ATP [105]. AAs are involved in the regulation of key physiological pathways in the body and their homeostasis is altered in various pathological conditions characterized by mitochondrial dysfunction and oxidative stress [105]. According to the ESPEN, a protein intake lower than 1 g protein/kg/day, not reaching a daily energy request of 25 kcal/Kg, and a nitrogen optimal uptake from protein between 1.2 and 2 g/kg/day is associated with decreased physical function and an increased risk of mortality [89,100,106]. Circulating AA levels are altered in cancer patients due to tumor demand of AAs, especially essential amino acids (EAAs), Gln, Gly, and Asp [89]. In particular, variations in plasma AAs were found in cancer patients depending on the occurrence of metabolic alterations, metastasis, anorexia, malnutrition, and weight loss; for these reasons, plasma AAs were considered as biomarkers for diagnosis and screening of cancer and a potential therapeutic target for improving protein synthesis and consequently muscle wasting [89,105]. More specifically, high levels of circulating AAs were described in breast cancer, while low levels were found in patients with gastric and colorectal cancers, as well as decreased levels of Arg in pancreatic and lung cancers [89].

2.2. Nutritional (AA-Based) Anti-Cachexia Supportive Interventions

In line with the commonly described AA shortage, many studies exploited the possibility of supplementing single AAs or mixtures of essential AAs as a therapeutic strategy in conditions characterized by oxidative stress, catabolic state, or altered energy balance, such as sarcopenia, sepsis, cardiac and metabolic diseases. Various compounds were studied, such as β-hydroxy-β-methylbutyrate (HMB), Gly, Leu, Arg, Gln, or AA mixtures [89,107,108]. A detailed description of the potential for each compound against cancer cachexia follows and is summarized in Figure 3. The ample evidence of AA efficacy in preclinical animal models of cachexia, however, does not align with a corresponding abundance of clinical trials in cancer patients, where most of the AAs tested were provided along with anti-inflammatory and antioxidant mixtures, not allowing for the discrimination of the AA contribution.

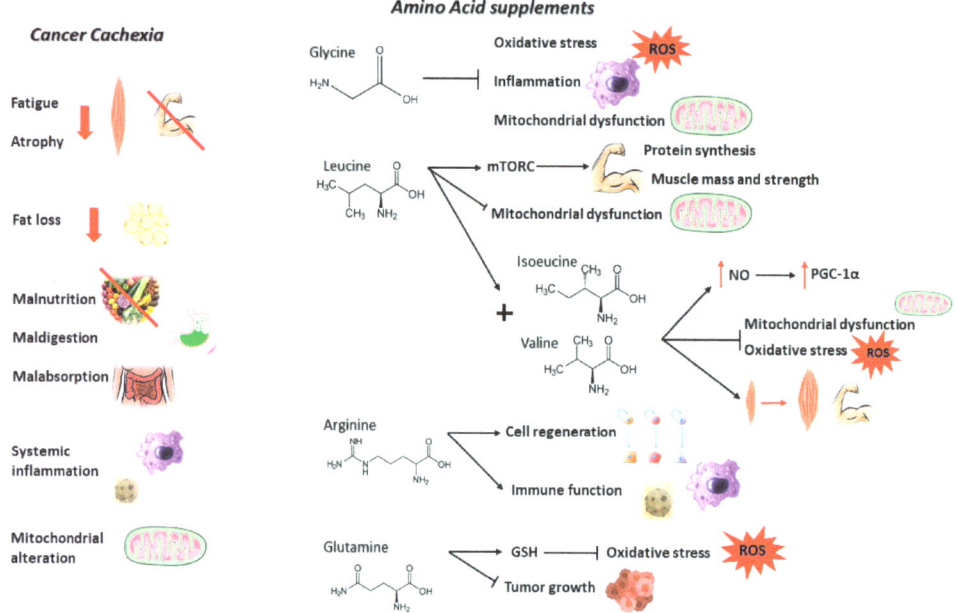

Figure 3. Main alterations underlying cancer cachexia (**left**) and the impact of specific AA supplementation in counteracting such manifestation or promoting beneficial anti-tumor effects (**right**). A detailed description of the anti-cachexia action is provided in the following text. The icons used were obtained at: https://smart.servier.com/ (accessed on 10 November 2022).

2.3. HMB

HMB is an endogenous product of Leu metabolism normally present in foods such as avocado, grapefruit, and catfish. It derives from Leu oxidation into ketoisocaproate, 95% of which is metabolized into Coenzyme A and the remaining 5% is converted into HMB [106]. Many supplementations that involve HMB alone or in combination with other AAs (Arg and Gln) were tested, and found to be safe and well tolerated in cancer patients [107,108]. In particular, HMB has been proposed to be effective in reducing inflammation and muscle proteolysis, and in stimulating protein synthesis through mechanistic target of rapamycin (mTOR) complex 1 (mTORC1), with beneficial effects in the maintenance of muscle mass and function in the elderly [86,89,91,105,108]. Many parameters were reported to be improved, including skeletal muscle mass, postoperative hospitalization, and complications insurgence. Moreover, these studies observed positive results regarding anticancer treatment-related side effects, tumor response, and hospitalization [91,107].

2.4. GLY

Gly, the simplest non-essential AA, is required for protein synthesis as well as being a precursor of fundamental molecules such as purines, heme, creatine, NADPH, and glutathione. In particular, it is involved in the regulation of redox homeostasis, modulating the balance between the two forms of glutathione, the oxidized (GSSG) and the reduced one (GSH) [109]. More specifically, Gly synthesis is stimulated as a mechanism of defense against mitochondrial dysfunction and oxidative stress; indeed, its supplementation is able to enhance NADPH and glutathione content, reducing ROS production and the expression of genes involved in inflammation and muscle macrophage infiltration [109]. Many studies demonstrated that intracellular Gly levels decrease during aging and result lower in association with frailty and in experimental mouse models of muscle wasting [109]. In tumor-bearing mice, Gly administration was able to reduce tumor growth, preventing muscle wasting and preserving muscle strength, suggesting a potential therapeutic use in cancer cachexia [109].

2.5. LEU

Leu is an essential amino acid that belongs to branched-chain amino acids, well known in literature to strongly stimulate skeletal muscle protein synthesis, modulating directly the activity of mTORC1 [110]. Positive effects of Leu supplementation were observed in animals fed with a high fat diet, with attenuation of mitochondrial dysfunction, fat mass, and hyperglycemia [105]. A few studies performed in animal models of cancer cachexia have shown that a diet rich in Leu was able to stimulate, in a dose-dependent manner, protein synthesis in skeletal muscle, resulting in reduced loss of lean body mass and muscle wasting [111]. These data were supported by improvements in muscle strength, physical performance, and inflammatory status [111]. Simultaneously, skeletal muscle mitochondrial biogenesis was ameliorated after Leu supplementation in tumor-bearing rats, together with the increased expression of markers related to oxidative phosphorylation and energy production [111]. Unfortunately, recent evidence suggested an increase of tumor growth rate with a Leu-rich diet, promoting cancer development and for these reasons limiting the clinical potential [111].

2.6. ARG

Arg is a semi-essential AA important for immune function and cell regeneration. 25–30% of the total daily Arg derives from food and the remaining 70–75% can be synthetized endogenously starting from citrulline or from protein turnover [89,106]. During cachexia or other catabolic and inflammatory conditions, Arg levels are decreased even without alterations in the biosynthesis [106]. In cancer patients, Arg supplementation demonstrated immunomodulating properties together with improvement in survival and malnutrition [89,106].

2.7. GLN

Gln is a semi-essential AA necessary for cellular function and immune cell modulation [89,106]. Remembering that Gln is also abundantly used by cancer cells for supporting their metabolism and growth (see above), its use as a supplement may have a dual impact on cancer (stimulating the growth) and on the host (counteracting cachexia). Experimental data seem to discard the first hypothesis since, using the experimental model of Walker-256 tumor-bearing rats, a promising role for Gln in improving energy balance and preventing tumor growth and cancer-induced cachexia was suggested [112,113]. In parallel, clinical trials in cancer patients highlighted that oral Gln supplementation is able to restore glutathione levels with beneficial effects on the antioxidant status and the immune system [89,106].

2.8. Essential AAs

Recent data showed that supplementation with an enriched mixture of branched-chain AAs (BCAAem), a subset of EAAs that comprises Leu, Ile, and Val, integral components of skeletal muscle proteins and powerful stimulators of protein synthesis, increases nitric oxide (NO) production via endothelial NO synthase (eNOS), inducing the expression of PGC-1α, a transcription coactivator and main regulator of mitochondrial biogenesis (reduced in cancer cachexia) and of genes involved in the ROS defense system including superoxide dismutase 1 (SOD1), superoxide dismutase 2 (SOD2), catalase and glutathione peroxidase (GPx1), decreasing oxidative damage and promoting survival [89,105,114]. As a result of PGC-1α increased expression, both glycogen accumulation and fatty acid oxidation improve, preserving mitochondrial metabolism and muscle fiber size, and ameliorating physical endurance and motor coordination in middle-aged mice, suggesting a potential role in the treatment of sarcopenia and cancer cachexia [105,114]. Recent evidence demonstrated that BCAAem was able to preserve skeletal muscle, mitigating muscular dystrophy in an experimental model of Duchenne Muscular Dystrophy (mdx mice), and clinical trials confirmed an improvement of physical performance, muscle mass, and strength in sarcopenic patients [105]. Another relevant study proposed supplementation with BCAA, Tyr, and Cys in order to improve lean muscle mass in cachectic patients with advanced cancer [89,91,101]. Despite some limitations, for example the numerosity, the lack of a control group, and the heterogeneity of patients according to cancer type, ROS reduction and improvements in strength and quality of life were observed [89,91].

Given that AA supplementation could be insufficient to obtain clinically relevant improvements on muscle mass and function, two novel AA formulations containing EAA-BCAA cofactors (citric acid, malic acid, and succinic acid) and precursors of Krebs cycle were explored in experimental models of age-related disorders and in general conditions characterized by mitochondrial dysfunction and altered catabolic state, resulting as more effective than the BCAAem alone [105]. The two mixtures differ in the percentage of each component. The first one (called a5) was able to promote the ROS defense system and mitochondrial biogenesis, preventing cardiac damage induced by doxorubicin; the second one (called PD-E07) was able to improve the expression of PGC-1α and the enzymatic activities of mitochondrial respiratory complexes in the skeletal muscle of mice characterized by age-related muscular alterations [105].

3. Concluding Remarks and Open Challenges

The selected evidence reported in this review highlights multiple aspects of AA biology in either the cancer itself or in the cancer host, meaning that any conclusion based on the study of only one of these two components is of limited value in its translation into a cure for the cancer disease in humans. Beyond this critical point, the narrative of AA relevance in cancer diagnosis and treatment provided here is definitively non-exhaustive. Several potential fields where deeper AA investigation may provide useful knowledge and tools against cancer, translating into innovative clinical applications, are described below.

Biomarkers. AA plasma levels may serve as disease biomarkers, guiding diagnosis and the choice of a potentially more effective treatment. As recently shown [115], the metabolomics era will soon produce breakthrough discoveries, unpredictable using the previous generation of targeted analyses. In this context, experts in cancer and host metabolism must interact to correctly interpret the significance of circulating AA levels resulting from both cancer and host metabolic activities.

Supplementation vs. *diet*. Although whole foods look more effective than oral nutritional supplements, at least in head and neck cancer patients undergoing cachexia [116], AA supplementation provides a precise dosage, allowing adjustments according to response (either by biochemical assessments or by disease follow-up). More comparative clinical trials are needed to define the best strategy.

AA supplementation during chemotherapy. Similarly to the dualism described in this review, AA may improve the host's ability to tolerate chemotherapy and to support or even stimulate tumor immunity as a combined treatment with immunotherapy in the emerging field of immunonutrition [117].

AA and microbiota in cancer patients. Microbiota dysbiosis has been reported in both pre-clinical animal models and in cancer patients, resulting in altered AA metabolism [118,119]. AA supplements may impact on the microbiota, helping controlling tumor growth and cachexia.

In conclusion, personalized (P4) medicine is the only reasonable way of introducing AA-based supportive oncology strategies which, by treating the cancer patient as a whole (i.e., by fighting the cancer and supporting the host), will likely improve the outcome of several incurable cancers. However, fasting the tumor to impair cellular proliferation remains a goal to pursue. Consistently, Fasting Mimicking Diets (FMD) were proven effective in maximizing the chemotherapy response [120]. In this context, AA supplementation may accelerate the recovery after FMD-induced weight loss by shortening the interval between the therapy cycles, given that the best refeeding strategy after FMD is still unknown and deserves further research. Similarly, a recent report shows an attractive alternative strategy for starving cancer cells by means of cold exposure [121], suggesting that nutrient deprivation may be obtained with alternative approaches, avoiding feeding restrictions.

Author Contributions: Conceptualization: E.N. and F.P.; investigation: M.R., C.F., E.N. and F.P.; writing—original draft: M.R., C.F., E.N. and F.P.; writing—review and editing: F.P. All authors have read and agreed to the published version of the manuscript.

Funding: The research leading to these results received funding from Fondazione AIRC under IG 2018—ID. 21963 project (Principal Investigator Fabio Penna). Enzo Nisoli is grateful to Professional Dietetics, Milan (Italy) for the liberal support.

Conflicts of Interest: The authors have no relevant conflicts of interest to disclose.

References

1. Martínez-Reyes, I.; Chandel, N.S. Cancer metabolism: Looking forward. *Nat. Rev. Cancer* **2021**, *21*, 669–680. [CrossRef] [PubMed]
2. Hanahan, D. Hallmarks of Cancer: New Dimensions. *Cancer Discov.* **2022**, *12*, 31–46. [CrossRef] [PubMed]
3. Warburg, O. The metabolism of carcinoma cells 1. *J. Cancer Res.* **1925**, *9*, 148–163. [CrossRef]
4. Altman, B.J.; Stine, Z.E.; Dang, C.V. From Krebs to clinic: Glutamine metabolism to cancer therapy. *Nat. Rev. Cancer* **2016**, *16*, 619–634. [CrossRef] [PubMed]
5. Lunt, S.Y.; Vander Heiden, M.G. Aerobic glycolysis: Meeting the metabolic requirements of cell proliferation. *Annu. Rev. Cell Dev. Biol.* **2011**, *27*, 441–464. [CrossRef]
6. Heiden, M.G.V.; Cantley, L.C.; Thompson, C.B. Understanding the Warburg effect: The metabolic requirements of cell proliferation. *Science* **2009**, *324*, 1029–1033. [CrossRef]
7. Hosios, A.M.; Hecht, V.C.; Danai, L.V.; Johnson, M.O.; Rathmell, J.C.; Steinhauser, M.L.; Manalis, S.R.; Vander Heiden, M.G. Amino Acids Rather than Glucose Account for the Majority of Cell Mass in Proliferating Mammalian Cells. *Dev. Cell* **2016**, *36*, 540–549. [CrossRef]
8. Condon, K.J.; Sabatini, D.M. Nutrient regulation of mTORC1 at a glance. *J. Cell Sci.* **2019**, *132*, cs222570. [CrossRef]
9. Kim, E. Mechanisms of amino acid sensing in mTOR signaling pathway. *Nutr. Res. Pract.* **2009**, *3*, 64. [CrossRef]
10. Shen, J.Z.; Wu, G.; Guo, S. Amino Acids in Autophagy: Regulation and Function. *Adv. Exp. Med. Biol.* **2021**, *1332*, 51–66. [CrossRef]
11. Eagle, B.H. The Minimum Vitamin Requirements of the L and I~A Cells in Tissue Culture, The Production of Specific Vitamin Deficiencies, and Their Cure (From the Section on Experimental Therapeutics, Laboratory of Infergious Diseases, National Microbiological Institute, National Institutes of Health, * Bethesda). *J. Exp. Med.* **1955**, *102*, 595–600. [CrossRef] [PubMed]
12. Reitzer, L.J.; Wice, B.M.; Kennell, D. Evidence that glutamine, not sugar, is the major energy source for cultured HeLa cells. *J. Biol. Chem.* **1979**, *254*, 2669–2676. [CrossRef]
13. DeBerardinis, R.J.; Mancuso, A.; Daikhin, E.; Nissim, I.; Yudkoff, M.; Wehrli, S.; Thompson, C.B. Beyond aerobic glycolysis: Transformed cells can engage in glutamine metabolism that exceeds the requirement for protein and nucleotide synthesis. *Proc. Natl. Acad. Sci. USA* **2007**, *104*, 19345–19350. [CrossRef] [PubMed]
14. Yang, L.; Moss, T.; Mangala, L.S.; Marini, J.; Zhao, H.; Wahlig, S.; Armaiz-Pena, G.; Jiang, D.; Achreja, A.; Win, J.; et al. Metabolic shifts toward glutamine regulate tumor growth, invasion and bioenergetics in ovarian cancer. *Mol. Syst. Biol.* **2014**, *10*, 728. [CrossRef]
15. Cardoso, H.J.; Figueira, M.I.; Vaz, C.V.; Carvalho, T.M.A.; Brás, L.A.; Madureira, P.A.; Oliveira, P.J.; Sardão, V.A.; Socorro, S. Glutaminolysis is a metabolic route essential for survival and growth of prostate cancer cells and a target of 5α-dihydrotestosterone regulation. *Cell Oncol.* **2021**, *44*, 385–403. [CrossRef]
16. Van Geldermalsen, M.; Wang, Q.; Nagarajah, R.; Marshall, A.D.; Thoeng, A.; Gao, D.; Ritchie, W.; Feng, Y.; Bailey, C.G.; Deng, N.; et al. ASCT2/SLC1A5 controls glutamine uptake and tumour growth in triple-negative basal-like breast cancer. *Oncogene* **2016**, *35*, 3201–3208. [CrossRef]
17. Owen, O.E.; Kalhan, S.C.; Hanson, R.W. The key role of anaplerosis and cataplerosis for citric acid cycle function. *J. Biol. Chem.* **2002**, *277*, 30409–30412. [CrossRef]
18. Sullivan, L.B.; Gui, D.Y.; Hosios, A.M.; Bush, L.N.; Freinkman, E.H.M. Vander Differential Glutamate Metabolism in Proliferating and Quiescent Mammary Epithelial Cells. *Cell Metab.* **2016**, *23*, 867–880. [CrossRef]
19. Chendong, Y.; Sudderth, J.; Tuyen, D.; Bachoo, R.G.; McDonald, J.G.; DeBerardinis, R.J. Glioblastoma cells require glutamate dehydrogenase to survive impairments of glucose metabolism or Akt signaling. *Cancer Res.* **2009**, *69*, 7986–7993. [CrossRef]
20. Choo, A.Y.; Kim, S.G.; Vander Heiden, M.G.; Mahoney, S.J.; Vu, H.; Yoon, S.O.; Cantley, L.C.; Blenis, J. Glucose addiction of TSC null cells is caused by failed mTORC1-dependent balancing of metabolic demand with supply. *Mol. Cell* **2010**, *38*, 487–499. [CrossRef]
21. Eng, C.H.; Yu, K.; Lucas, J.; White, E.; Abraham, R.T. Ammonia derived from glutaminolysis is a diffusible regulator of autophagy. *Sci. Signal.* **2010**, *3*, ra31. [CrossRef] [PubMed]
22. Spinelli, J.B.; Yoon, H.; Ringel, A.E.; Jeanfavre, S.; Clish, C.B.; Haigis, M.C. Metabolic recycling of ammonia via glutamate dehydrogenase supports breast cancer biomass. *Science* **2017**, *358*, 941. [CrossRef] [PubMed]

23. Cheng, C.; Geng, F.; Li, Z.; Zhong, Y.; Wang, H.; Cheng, X.; Zhao, Y.; Mo, X.; Horbinski, C.; Duan, W.; et al. Ammonia stimulates SCAP/Insig dissociation and SREBP-1 activation to promote lipogenesis and tumour growth. *Nat. Metab.* **2022**, *4*, 575–588. [CrossRef] [PubMed]
24. Jiang, L.; Shestov, A.A.; Swain, P.; Yang, C.; Parker, S.J.; Wang, Q.A.; Terada, L.S.; Adams, N.D.; McCabe, M.T.; Pietrak, B.; et al. Reductive carboxylation supports redox homeostasis during anchorage-independent growth. *Nature* **2016**, *73*, 389–400. [CrossRef]
25. Metallo, C.M.; Gameiro, P.A.; Bell, E.L.; Mattaini, K.R.; Yang, J.; Hiller, K.; Jewell, C.M.; Johnson, Z.R.; Irvine, D.J.; Guarente, L.; et al. Reductive glutamine metabolism by IDH1 mediates lipogenesis under hypoxia. *Nature* **2011**, *481*, 380–384. [CrossRef] [PubMed]
26. Wise, D.R.; Ward, P.S.; Shay, J.E.S.; Cross, J.R.; Gruber, J.J.; Sachdeva, U.M.; Platt, J.M.; DeMatteo, R.G.; Simon, M.C.; Thompson, C.B. Hypoxia promotes isocitrate dehydrogenasedependent carboxylation of α-ketoglutarate to citrate to support cell growth and viability. *Proc. Natl. Acad. Sci. USA* **2011**, *108*, 19611–19616. [CrossRef] [PubMed]
27. Cheng, T.; Yang, Y.; Linehan, W.M.; Chandel, N.S.; Mullen, A.R.; Wheaton, W.W.; Jin, E.S.; Chen, P.H.; Sullivan, L.B.; Cheng, T.; et al. Reductive carboxylation supports growth in tumour cells with defective mitochondria. *Nature* **2012**, *481*, 385–388. [CrossRef]
28. Gameiro, P.A.; Yang, J.; Metelo, A.M.; Pérez-Carro, R.; Baker, R.; Wang, Z.; Arreola, A.; Rathmell, W.K.; Olumi, A.; López-Larrubia, P.; et al. In vivo HIF-mediated reductive carboxylation is regulated by citrate levels and sensitizes VHL-deficient cells to glutamine deprivation. *Cell Metab.* **2013**, *17*, 372–385. [CrossRef]
29. Dasgupta, S.; Putluri, N.; Long, W.; Zhang, B.; Wang, J.; Kaushik, A.K.; Arnold, J.M.; Bhowmik, S.K.; Stashi, E.; Brennan, C.A.; et al. Coactivator SRC-2'dependent metabolic reprogramming mediates prostate cancer survival and metastasis. *J. Clin. Invest.* **2015**, *125*, 1174–1188. [CrossRef]
30. Birsoy, K.; Wang, T.; Chen, W.W.; Freinkman, E.; Abu-Remaileh, M.; Sabatini, D.M. An Essential Role of the Mitochondrial Electron Transport Chain in Cell Proliferation Is to Enable Aspartate Synthesis. *Cell* **2015**, *162*, 540–551. [CrossRef]
31. Sullivan, L.B.; Gui, D.Y.; Hosios, A.M.; Bush, L.N.; Freinkman, E.; Vander Heiden, M.G. Supporting Aspartate Biosynthesis Is an Essential Function of Respiration in Proliferating Cells. *Cell* **2015**, *162*, 552–563. [CrossRef] [PubMed]
32. Molina, J.R.; Sun, Y.; Protopopova, M.; Gera, S.; Bandi, M.; Bristow, C.; McAfoos, T.; Morlacchi, P.; Ackroyd, J.; Agip, A.N.A.; et al. An inhibitor of oxidative phosphorylation exploits cancer vulnerability. *Nat. Med.* **2018**, *24*, 1036–1046. [CrossRef] [PubMed]
33. Pachnis, P.; Wu, Z.; Faubert, B.; Tasdogan, A.; Gu, W.; Shelton, S.; Solmonson, A.; Rao, A.D.; Kaushik, A.K.; Rogers, T.J.; et al. In vivo isotope tracing reveals a requirement for the electron transport chain in glucose and glutamine metabolism by tumors. *Sci. Adv.* **2022**, *8*, 1–14. [CrossRef] [PubMed]
34. Gui, D.Y.; Sullivan, L.B.; Luengo, A.; Hosios, A.M.; Bush, L.N.; Gitego, N.; Davidson, S.M.; Freinkman, E.; Thomas, C.J.; Heiden, M.G.V.; et al. Environment Dictates Dependence on Mitochondrial Complex I for NAD+ and Aspartate Production and Determines Cancer Cell Sensitivity to Metformin. *Cell Metab.* **2016**, *24*, 716–727. [CrossRef]
35. Cardaci, S.; Zheng, L.; Mackay, G.; Van Den Broek, N.J.F.; Mackenzie, E.D.; Nixon, C.; Stevenson, D.; Tumanov, S.; Bulusu, V.; Kamphorst, J.J.; et al. Pyruvate carboxylation enables growth of SDH-deficient cells by supporting aspartate biosynthesis. *Nat. Cell Biol.* **2015**, *17*, 1317–1326. [CrossRef]
36. Altea-Manzano, P.; Vandekeere, A.; Edwards-Hicks, J.; Roldan, M.; Abraham, E.; Lleshi, X.; Guerrieri, A.N.; Berardi, D.; Wills, J.; Junior, J.M.; et al. Reversal of mitochondrial malate dehydrogenase 2 enables anaplerosis via redox rescue in respiration-deficient cells. *Mol. Cell* **2022**. Online ahead of print. [CrossRef]
37. Diehl, F.F.; Lewis, C.A.; Fiske, B.P.; Vander Heiden, M.G. Cellular redox state constrains serine synthesis and nucleotide production to impact cell proliferation. *Nat. Metab.* **2019**, *1*, 861–867. [CrossRef]
38. Kilberg, M.S.; Balasubramanian, M.; Fu, L.; Shan, J. The transcription factor network associated with the amino acid response in mammalian cells. *Adv. Nutr.* **2012**, *3*, 295–306. [CrossRef]
39. Bao, X.R.; Ong, S.E.; Goldberger, O.; Peng, J.; Sharma, R.; Thompson, D.A.; Vafai, S.B.; Cox, A.G.; Marutani, E.; Ichinose, F.; et al. Mitochondrial dysfunction remodels one-carbon metabolism in human cells. *Elife* **2016**, *5*, e10575. [CrossRef]
40. Locasale, J.W. Serine, glycine and one-carbon units: Cancer metabolism in full circle. *Nat. Rev. Cancer* **2013**, *13*, 572–583. [CrossRef]
41. Pollari, S.; Käkönen, S.M.; Edgren, H.; Wolf, M.; Kohonen, P.; Sara, H.; Guise, T.; Nees, M.; Kallioniemi, O. Enhanced serine production by bone metastatic breast cancer cells stimulates osteoclastogenesis. *Breast Cancer Res. Treat.* **2011**, *125*, 421–430. [CrossRef] [PubMed]
42. Possemato, R.; Marks, K.M.; Shaul, Y.D.; Pacold, M.E.; Kim, D.; Birsoy, K.; Sethumadhavan, S.; Woo, H.K.; Jang, H.G.; Jha, A.K.; et al. Functional genomics reveal that the serine synthesis pathway is essential in breast cancer. *Nature* **2011**, *476*, 346–350. [CrossRef] [PubMed]
43. Snell, K. Enzymes of serine metabolism in normal, developing and neoplastic rat tissues. *Adv. Enzyme Regul.* **1984**, *22*, 325–400. [CrossRef]
44. Locasale, J.W.; Grassian, A.R.; Melman, T.; Lyssiotis, C.A.; Mattaini, K.R.; Bass, A.J.; Heffron, G.; Metallo, C.M.; Muranen, T.; Sharfi, H.; et al. Phosphoglycerate dehydrogenase diverts glycolytic flux and contributes to oncogenesis. *Nat. Genet.* **2011**, *43*, 869–874. [CrossRef] [PubMed]
45. Zahra, K.; Dey, T.; Ashish; Mishra, S.P.; Pandey, U. Pyruvate Kinase M2 and Cancer: The Role of PKM2 in Promoting Tumorigenesis. *Front. Oncol.* **2020**, *10*, 159. [CrossRef] [PubMed]

46. Chaneton, B.; Hillmann, P.; Zheng, L.; Martin, A.C.L.; Maddocks, O.D.K.; Chokkathukalam, A.; Coyle, J.E.; Jankevics, A.; Holding, F.P.; Vousden, K.H.; et al. Serine is a natural ligand and allosteric activator of pyruvate kinase M2. *Nature* **2012**, *491*, 458–462. [CrossRef]
47. Lee, G.Y.; Haverty, P.M.; Li, L.; Kljavin, N.M.; Bourgon, R.; Lee, J.; Stern, H.; Modrusan, Z.; Seshagiri, S.; Zhang, Z.; et al. Comparative oncogenomics identifies psmb4 and shmt2 as potential cancer driver genes. *Cancer Res.* **2014**, *74*, 3114–3126. [CrossRef]
48. Minton, D.R.; Nam, M.; McLaughlin, D.J.; Shin, J.; Bayraktar, E.C.; Alvarez, S.W.; Sviderskiy, V.O.; Papagiannakopoulos, T.; Sabatini, D.M.; Birsoy, K.; et al. Serine Catabolism by SHMT2 Is Required for Proper Mitochondrial Translation Initiation and Maintenance of Formylmethionyl-tRNAs. *Mol. Cell* **2018**, *69*, 610–621.e5. [CrossRef]
49. Morscher, R.J.; Ducker, G.S.; Li, S.H.J.; Mayer, J.A.; Gitai, Z.; Sperl, W.; Rabinowitz, J.D. Mitochondrial translation requires folate-dependent tRNA methylation. *Nature* **2018**, *554*, 128–132. [CrossRef]
50. Lucas, S.; Chen, G.; Aras, S.; Wang, J. Serine catabolism is essential to maintain mitochondrial respiration in mammalian cells. *Life Sci. Alliance* **2018**, *1*, e201800036. [CrossRef] [PubMed]
51. Tani, H.; Ohnishi, S.; Shitara, H.; Mito, T.; Yamaguchi, M.; Yonekawa, H.; Hashizume, O.; Ishikawa, K.; Nakada, K.; Hayashi, J.I. Mice deficient in the Shmt2 gene have mitochondrial respiration defects and are embryonic lethal. *Sci. Rep.* **2018**, *8*, 8–15. [CrossRef] [PubMed]
52. Butler, M.; van der Meer, L.T.; van Leeuwen, F.N. Amino Acid Depletion Therapies: Starving Cancer Cells to Death. *Trends Endocrinol. Metab.* **2021**, *32*, 367–381. [CrossRef] [PubMed]
53. Wang, Z.; Liu, F.; Fan, N.; Zhou, C.; Li, D.; Macvicar, T.; Dong, Q.; Bruns, C.J.; Zhao, Y. Targeting Glutaminolysis: New Perspectives to Understand Cancer Development and Novel Strategies for Potential Target Therapies. *Front. Oncol.* **2020**, *10*, 589508. [CrossRef] [PubMed]
54. Sallan, S.E.; Hitchcock-Bryan, S.; Gelber, R.; Cassady, J.R.; Frei, E.; Nathan, D.G. Influence of Intensive Asparaginase in the Treatment of Childhood Non-T-Cell Acute Lymphoblastic Leukemia. *Cancer Res.* **1983**, *43*, 5601–5607. [PubMed]
55. Nachman, J.B.; Harland, N.S.; Sensel, M.G.; Trigg, M.E.; Cherlow, J.M.; Lunkens, J.N.; Wolfl, L.; Uckun, F.M.; Gaynon, P.S. Augmented Post-Induction Therapy for Children With High-Risk To Initial Therapy. *N. Engl. J. Med.* **1998**, *338*, 1663–1671. [CrossRef]
56. Cools, J. Improvements in the survival of children and adolescents with acute lymphoblastic leukemia. *Haematologica* **2012**, *97*, 635. [CrossRef]
57. Curran, E.; Stock, W. How I treat acute lymphoblastic leukemia in older adolescents and young adults. *Blood* **2015**, *125*, 3702–3710.
58. Bach, S.J.; Simon-Reuss, I. Arginase, an antimitotic agent in tissue culture. *Biochim. Biophys. Acta* **1953**, *11*, 396–402. [CrossRef]
59. Feun, L.G.; Marini, A.; Walker, G.; Elgart, G.; Moffat, F.; Rodgers, S.E.; Wu, C.J.; You, M.; Wangpaichitr, M.; Kuo, M.T.; et al. Negative argininosuccinate synthetase expression in melanoma tumours may predict clinical benefit from arginine-depleting therapy with pegylated arginine deiminase. *Br. J. Cancer* **2012**, *106*, 1481–1485. [CrossRef]
60. Dillon, B.J.; Prieto, V.G.; Curley, S.A.; Ensor, C.M.; Holtsberg, F.W.; Bomalaski, J.S.; Clark, M.A. Incidence and Distribution of Argininosuccinate Synthetase Deficiency in Human Cancers: A Method for Identifying Cancers Sensitive to Arginine Deprivation. *Cancer* **2004**, *100*, 826–833. [CrossRef]
61. Szlosarek, P.W.; Klabatsa, A.; Pallaska, A.; Sheaff, M.; Smith, P.; Crook, T.; Grimshaw, M.J.; Steele, J.P.; Rudd, R.M.; Balkwill, F.R.; et al. In vivo loss of expression of argininosuccinate synthetase in malignant pleural mesothelioma is a biomarker for susceptibility to arginine depletion. *Clin. Cancer Res.* **2006**, *12*, 7126–7131. [CrossRef] [PubMed]
62. Yoon, C.Y.; Shim, Y.J.; Kim, E.H.; Lee, J.H.; Won, N.H.; Kim, J.H.; Park, I.S.; Yoon, D.K.; Min, B.H. Renal cell carcinoma does not express argininosuccinate synthetase and is highly sensitive to arginine deprivation via arginine deiminase. *Int. J. Cancer* **2007**, *120*, 897–905. [CrossRef] [PubMed]
63. Scott, L.; Lamb, J.; Smith, S.; Wheatley, D.N. Single amino acid (arginine) deprivation: Rapid and selective death of cultured transformed and malignant cells. *Br. J. Cancer* **2000**, *83*, 800–810. [CrossRef] [PubMed]
64. Kawatra, A.; Dhankhar, R.; Gulati, P. Microbial arginine deiminase: A multifaceted green catalyst in biomedical sciences. *Int. J. Biol. Macromol.* **2022**, *196*, 151–162. [CrossRef]
65. Farber, S.; Diamond, L.K.; Mercer, R.D.; Sylvester, R.F.; Wolff, J.A. Temporary remissions in acute leukemia in children produced by folic acid antagonist, 4-aminopteroyl-glutamic acid. *N. Engl. J. Med.* **1948**, *238*, 787–793. [CrossRef] [PubMed]
66. Howard, S.C.; McCormick, J.; Pui, C.-H.; Buddington, R.K.; Harvey, R.D. Preventing and Managing Toxicities of High-Dose Methotrexate. *Oncologist* **2016**, *21*, 1471–1482. [CrossRef]
67. Dekhne, A.S.; Hou, Z.; Gangjee, A.; Matherly, L.H. Therapeutic targeting of mitochondrial one-carbon metabolism in cancer. *Mol. Cancer Ther.* **2020**, *19*, 2245–2255. [CrossRef]
68. Marani, M.; Paone, A.; Fiascarelli, A.; Macone, A.; Gargano, M.; Rinaldo, S.; Giardina, G.; Pontecorvi, V.; Koes, D.; McDermott, L.; et al. A pyrazolopyran derivative preferentially inhibits the activity of human cytosolic serine hydroxymethyltransferase and induces cell death in lung cancer cells. *Oncotarget* **2016**, *7*, 4570–4583. [CrossRef]
69. Tajan, M.; Hennequart, M.; Cheung, E.C.; Zani, F.; Hock, A.K.; Legrave, N.; Maddocks, O.D.K.; Ridgway, R.A.; Athineos, D.; Suárez-Bonnet, A.; et al. Serine synthesis pathway inhibition cooperates with dietary serine and glycine limitation for cancer therapy. *Nat. Commun.* **2021**, *12*, 1–16. [CrossRef]

70. Vilstrup, H.; Amodio, P.; Bajaj, J.; Cordoba, J.; Ferenci, P.; Mullen, K.D.; Weissenborn, K.; Wong, P. Hepatic encephalopathy in chronic liver disease: 2014 Practice Guideline by the American Association for the Study Of Liver Diseases and the European Association for the Study of the Liver. *Hepatology* **2014**, *60*, 715–735. [CrossRef]
71. Maddocks, O.D.K.; Athineos, D.; Cheung, E.C.; Lee, P.; Zhang, T.; Van Den Broek, N.J.F.; Mackay, G.M.; Labuschagne, C.F.; Gay, D.; Kruiswijk, F.; et al. Modulating the therapeutic response of tumours to dietary serine and glycine starvation. *Nature* **2017**, *544*, 372–376. [CrossRef] [PubMed]
72. Kuo, M.T.; Chen, H.H.W.; Feun, L.G.; Savaraj, N. Targeting the proline–glutamine–asparagine–arginine metabolic axis in amino acid starvation cancer therapy. *Pharmaceuticals* **2021**, *14*, 72. [CrossRef] [PubMed]
73. Hayaishi, S.; Chung, H.; Kudo, M.; Ishikawa, E.; Takita, M.; Ueda, T.; Kitai, S.; Inoue, T.; Yada, N.; Hagiwara, S.; et al. Oral branched-chain amino acid granules reduce the incidence of hepatocellular carcinoma and improve event-free survival in patients with liver cirrhosis. *Dig. Dis.* **2011**, *29*, 326–332. [CrossRef] [PubMed]
74. Poon, R.T.P.; Yu, W.C.; Fan, S.T.; Wong, J. Long-term oral branched chain amino acids in patients undergoing chemoembolization for hepatocellular carcinoma: A randomized trial. *Aliment. Pharmacol. Ther.* **2004**, *19*, 779–788. [CrossRef]
75. Park, J.G.; Tak, W.Y.; Park, S.Y.; Kweon, Y.O.; Chung, W.J.; Jang, B.K.; Bae, S.H.; Lee, H.J.; Jang, J.Y.; Suk, K.T.; et al. Effects of Branched-Chain Amino Acid (BCAA) Supplementation on the Progression of Advanced Liver Disease: A Korean Nationwide, Multicenter, Prospective, Observational, Cohort Study. *Nutrients* **2020**, *12*, 1429. [CrossRef] [PubMed]
76. Marchesini, G.; Bianchi, G.; Merli, M.; Amodio, P.; Panella, C.; Loguercio, C.; Fanelli, F.R.; Abbiati, R. Nutritional supplementation with branched-chain amino acids in advanced cirrhosis: A double-blind, randomized trial. *Gastroenterology* **2003**, *124*, 1792–1801. [CrossRef]
77. Ishak Gabra, M.B.; Yang, Y.; Li, H.; Senapati, P.; Hanse, E.A.; Lowman, X.H.; Tran, T.Q.; Zhang, L.; Doan, L.T.; Xu, X.; et al. Dietary glutamine supplementation suppresses epigenetically-activated oncogenic pathways to inhibit melanoma tumour growth. *Nat. Commun.* **2020**, *11*, 1–15. [CrossRef]
78. Kanarek, N.; Keys, H.R.; Cantor, J.R.; Lewis, C.A.; Chan, S.H.; Kunchok, T.; Abu-Remaileh, M.; Freinkman, E.; Schweitzer, L.D.; Sabatini, D.M.; et al. Histidine catabolism is a major determinant of methotrexate sensitivity. *Nature* **2018**, *559*, 632–636. [CrossRef]
79. Ragni, M.; Ruocco, C.; Tedesco, L.; Carruba, M.O.; Valerio, A.; Nisoli, E. An amino acid-defined diet impairs tumour growth in mice by promoting endoplasmic reticulum stress and mTOR inhibition. *Mol. Metab.* **2022**, *60*, 101478. [CrossRef]
80. Hamill, M.J.; Afeyan, R.; Chakravarthy, M.V.; Tramontin, T. Endogenous Metabolic Modulators: Emerging Therapeutic Potential of Amino Acids. *iScience* **2020**, *23*, 101628. [CrossRef]
81. Saha, S.K.; Riazul Islam, S.M.; Abdullah-Al-Wadud, M.; Islam, S.; Ali, F.; Park, K.S. Multiomics analysis reveals that GLS and GLS2 differentially modulate the clinical outcomes of cancer. *J. Clin. Med.* **2019**, *8*, 355. [CrossRef] [PubMed]
82. Hagiwara, A.; Nishiyama, M.; Ishizaki, S. Branched-chain amino acids prevent insulin-induced hepatic tumor cell proliferation by inducing apoptosis through mTORC1 and mTORC2-dependent mechanisms. *J. Cell Physiol.* **2012**, *227*, 2097–2105. [CrossRef] [PubMed]
83. Harrison, S.A.; Baum, S.J.; Gunn, N.T.; Younes, Z.H.; Kohli, A.; Patil, R.; Koziel, M.J.; Chera, H.; Zhao, J.; Chakravarthy, M.V. Safety, Tolerability, and Biologic Activity of AXA1125 and AXA1957 in Subjects with Nonalcoholic Fatty Liver Disease. *Am. J. Gastroenterol.* **2021**, *116*, 2399–2409. [CrossRef] [PubMed]
84. Argilés, J.M.; Busquets, S.; Stemmler, B.; López-Soriano, F.J. Cancer cachexia: Understanding the molecular basis. *Nat. Rev. Cancer* **2014**, *14*, 754–762. [CrossRef]
85. Penna, F.; Ballarò, R.; Beltrà, M.; De Lucia, S.; Castillo, L.G.; Costelli, P. The Skeletal Muscle as an Active Player Against Cancer Cachexia. *Front. Physiol.* **2019**, *10*, 41. [CrossRef] [PubMed]
86. Robinder, J.S.; Dhillon, M.D.M.; Sarfaraz, H.M. Pathogenesis and management of sarcopenia. *Clin. Geriatr. Med.* **2017**, *33*, 17–36. [CrossRef]
87. Bruggeman, A.R.; Kamal, A.H.; LeBlanc, T.W.; Ma, J.D.; Baracos, V.E.; Roeland, E.J. Cancer cachexia: Beyond weight loss. *J. Oncol. Pract.* **2016**, *12*, 1163–1171. [CrossRef]
88. Fearon, K.; Arends, J.; Baracos, V. Understanding the mechanisms and treatment options in cancer cachexia. *Nat. Rev. Clin. Oncol.* **2013**, *10*, 90–99. [CrossRef]
89. van der Meij, B.S.; Teleni, L.; Engelen, M.P.K.J.; Deutz, N.E.P. Amino acid kinetics and the response to nutrition in patients with cancer. *Int. J. Radiat. Biol.* **2019**, *95*, 480–492. [CrossRef]
90. Cruz-Jentoft, A.J.; Bahat, G.; Bauer, J.; Boirie, Y.; Bruyère, O.; Cederholm, T.; Cooper, C.; Landi, F.; Rolland, Y.; Sayer, A.A.; et al. Sarcopenia: Revised European consensus on definition and diagnosis. *Age Ageing* **2019**, *48*, 601. [CrossRef]
91. Zanetti, M.; Cappellari, G.G.; Barazzoni, R.; Sanson, G. The impact of protein supplementation targeted at improving muscle mass on strength in cancer patients: A scoping review. *Nutrients* **2020**, *12*, 2099. [CrossRef]
92. Marzetti, E.; Calvani, R.; Cesari, M.; Buford, T.W.; Lorenzi, M.; Behnke, B.J.; Leeuwenburgh, C. Mitochondrial dysfunction and sarcopenia of aging: From signaling pathways to clinical trials. *Int. J. Biochem. Cell Biol.* **2013**, *45*, 2288–2301. [CrossRef]
93. Dao, T.; Green, A.E.; Kim, Y.A.; Bae, S.J.; Ha, K.T.; Gariani, K.; Lee, M.R.; Menzies, K.J.; Ryu, D. Sarcopenia and muscle aging: A brief overview. *Endocrinol. Metab.* **2020**, *35*, 716–732. [CrossRef]
94. Beltrà, M.; Pin, F.; Ballarò, R.; Costelli, P.; Penna, F. Mitochondrial Dysfunction in Cancer Cachexia: Impact on Muscle Health and Regeneration. *Cells* **2021**, *10*, 3150. [CrossRef] [PubMed]
95. Sandri, M. Protein breakdown in cancer cachexia. *Semin. Cell Dev. Biol.* **2016**, *54*, 11–19. [CrossRef] [PubMed]

96. Penna, F.; Baccino, F.M.; Costelli, P. Coming back: Autophagy in cachexia. *Curr. Opin. Clin. Nutr. Metab. Care* **2014**, *17*, 241–246. [CrossRef]
97. Argilés, J.M.; López-Soriano, F.J.; Busquets, S. Muscle wasting in cancer: The role of mitochondria. *Curr. Opin. Clin. Nutr. Metab. Care* **2015**, *18*, 221–225. [CrossRef] [PubMed]
98. Penna, F.; Costamagna, D.; Pin, F.; Camperi, A.; Fanzani, A.; Chiarpotto, E.M.E.M.; Cavallini, G.; Bonelli, G.; Baccino, F.M.F.M.; Costelli, P. Autophagic degradation contributes to muscle wasting in cancer cachexia. *Am. J. Pathol.* **2013**, *182*, 1367–1378. [CrossRef]
99. Ballarò, R.; Beltrà, M.; De Lucia, S.; Pin, F.; Ranjbar, K.; Hulmi, J.J.; Costelli, P.; Penna, F. Moderate exercise in mice improves cancer plus chemotherapy-induced muscle wasting and mitochondrial alterations. *FASEB J.* **2019**, *33*, 5482–5494. [CrossRef]
100. Sadeghi, M.; Keshavarz-Fathi, M.; Baracos, V.; Arends, J.; Mahmoudi, M.; Rezaei, N. Cancer cachexia: Diagnosis, assessment, and treatment. *Crit. Rev. Oncol. Hematol.* **2018**, *127*, 91–104. [CrossRef]
101. Madeddu, C.; Maccio, A.; Mantovani, G. Multitargeted treatment of cancer cachexia. *Crit. Rev. Oncog.* **2012**, *17*, 305–314. [CrossRef] [PubMed]
102. Penna, F.; Ballarò, R.; Beltrá, M.; De Lucia, S.; Costelli, P. Modulating Metabolism to Improve Cancer-Induced Muscle Wasting. *Oxid. Med. Cell Longev.* **2018**, *2018*, 1–11. [CrossRef] [PubMed]
103. Muscaritoli, M.; Arends, J.; Bachmann, P.; Baracos, V.; Barthelemy, N.; Bertz, H.; Bozzetti, F.; Hütterer, E.; Isenring, E.; Kaasa, S.; et al. ESPEN practical guideline: Clinical Nutrition in cancer. *Clin. Nutr.* **2021**, *40*, 2898–2913. [CrossRef] [PubMed]
104. McCurdy, B.; Nejatinamini, S.; Debenham, B.J.; Álvarez-Camacho, M.; Kubrak, C.; Wismer, W.V.; Mazurak, V.C. Meeting Minimum ESPEN Energy Recommendations Is Not Enough to Maintain Muscle Mass in Head and Neck Cancer Patients. *Nutrients* **2019**, *11*, 2743. [CrossRef] [PubMed]
105. Ruocco, C.; Segala, A.; Valerio, A.; Nisoli, E. Essential amino acid formulations to prevent mitochondrial dysfunction and oxidative stress. *Curr. Opin. Clin. Nutr. Metab. Care* **2021**, *24*, 88–95. [CrossRef]
106. Soares, J.D.P.; Howell, S.L.; Teixeira, F.J.; Pimentel, G.D. Dietary Amino Acids and Immunonutrition Supplementation in Cancer-Induced Skeletal Muscle Mass Depletion: A Mini-Review. *Curr. Pharm. Des.* **2020**, *26*, 970–978. [CrossRef]
107. Prado, C.M.; Orsso, C.E.; Pereira, S.L.; Atherton, P.J.; Deutz, N.E.P. Effects of β-hydroxy β-methylbutyrate (HMB) supplementation on muscle mass, function, and other outcomes in patients with cancer: A systematic review. *J. Cachexia. Sarcopenia Muscle* **2022**, *13*, 1623–1641. [CrossRef]
108. Molfino, A.; Gioia, G.; Rossi Fanelli, F.; Muscaritoli, M. Beta-hydroxy-beta-methylbutyrate supplementation in health and disease: A systematic review of randomized trials. *Amino Acids* **2013**, *45*, 1273–1292. [CrossRef]
109. Koopman, R.; Caldow, M.K.; Ham, D.J.; Lynch, G.S. Glycine metabolism in skeletal muscle: Implications for metabolic homeostasis. *Curr. Opin. Clin. Nutr. Metab. Care* **2017**, *20*, 237–242. [CrossRef]
110. de Bandt, J.P. Leucine and Mammalian Target of Rapamycin-Dependent Activation of Muscle Protein Synthesis in Aging. *J. Nutr.* **2016**, *146*, 2616S–2624S. [CrossRef]
111. Beaudry, A.G.; Law, M.L. Leucine Supplementation in Cancer Cachexia: Mechanisms and a Review of the Pre-Clinical Literature. *Nutrients* **2022**, *14*, 2824. [CrossRef] [PubMed]
112. Martins, H.A.; Bazotte, R.B.; Vicentini, G.E.; Lima, M.M.; Guarnier, F.A.; Hermes-Uliana, C.; Frez, F.C.V.; Bossolani, G.D.P.; Fracaro, L.; Fávaro, L.D.S.; et al. l-Glutamine supplementation promotes an improved energetic balance in Walker-256 tumor–bearing rats. *Tumor Biol.* **2017**, *39*, 1010428317695960. [CrossRef]
113. Martins, H.A.; Sehaber, C.C.; Hermes-Uliana, C.; Mariani, F.A.; Guarnier, F.A.; Vicentini, G.E.; Bossolani, G.D.P.; Jussani, L.A.; Lima, M.M.; Bazotte, R.B.; et al. Supplementation with l-glutamine prevents tumor growth and cancer-induced cachexia as well as restores cell proliferation of intestinal mucosa of Walker-256 tumor-bearing rats. *Amino Acids* **2016**, *48*, 2773–2784. [CrossRef] [PubMed]
114. D'Antona, G.; Ragni, M.; Cardile, A.; Tedesco, L.; Dossena, M.; Bruttini, F.; Caliaro, F.; Corsetti, G.; Bottinelli, R.; Carruba, M.O.; et al. Branched-chain amino acid supplementation promotes survival and supports cardiac and skeletal muscle mitochondrial biogenesis in middle-aged mice. *Cell Metab.* **2010**, *12*, 362–372. [CrossRef] [PubMed]
115. Larkin, J.R.; Anthony, S.; Johanssen, V.A.; Yeo, T.; Sealey, M.; Yates, A.G.; Smith, C.F.; Claridge, T.D.W.; Nicholson, B.D.; Moreland, J.A.; et al. Metabolomic Biomarkers in Blood Samples Identify Cancers in a Mixed Population of Patients with Nonspecific Symptoms. *Clin. Cancer Res.* **2022**, *28*, 1651–1661. [CrossRef] [PubMed]
116. Leoncini, E.; Ricciardi, W.; Cadoni, G.; Arzani, D.; Petrelli, L.; Paludetti, G.; Brennan, P.; Luce, D.; Stucker, I.; Matsuo, K.; et al. Recommended European Society of Parenteral and Enteral Nutrition protein and energy intakes and weight loss in patients with head and neck cancer. *Head Neck* **2014**, *36*, 1391. [CrossRef]
117. Ala, M. Tryptophan metabolites modulate inflammatory bowel disease and colorectal cancer by affecting immune system. *Int. Rev. Immunol.* **2022**, *41*, 326–345. [CrossRef]
118. Ni, Y.; Lohinai, Z.; Heshiki, Y.; Dome, B.; Moldvay, J.; Dulka, E.; Galffy, G.; Berta, J.; Weiss, G.J.; Sommer, M.O.A.; et al. Distinct composition and metabolic functions of human gut microbiota are associated with cachexia in lung cancer patients. *ISME J.* **2021**, *15*, 3207–3220. [CrossRef]
119. Genton, L.; Mareschal, J.; Charretier, Y.; Lazarevic, V.; Bindels, L.B.; Schrenzel, J. Targeting the Gut Microbiota to Treat Cachexia. *Front. Cell Infect. Microbiol.* **2019**, *9*, 305. [CrossRef]

120. Vernieri, C.; Fucà, G.; Ligorio, F.; Huber, V.; Vingiani, A.; Iannelli, F.; Raimondi, A.; Rinchai, D.; Frigè, G.; Belfiore, A.; et al. Fasting-Mimicking Diet Is Safe and Reshapes Metabolism and Antitumor Immunity in Patients with Cancer. *Cancer Discov.* **2022**, *12*, 90–107. [CrossRef]
121. Seki, T.; Yang, Y.; Sun, X.; Lim, S.; Xie, S.; Guo, Z.; Xiong, W.; Kuroda, M.; Sakaue, H.; Hosaka, K.; et al. Brown-fat-mediated tumour suppression by cold-altered global metabolism. *Nature* **2022**, *608*, 421–428. [CrossRef] [PubMed]

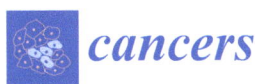

Review

The Mechanism of Action of Biguanides: New Answers to a Complex Question

Laura Di Magno [1], Fiorella Di Pastena [1], Rosa Bordone [1], Sonia Coni [1] and Gianluca Canettieri [1,2,*]

[1] Department of Molecular Medicine, Sapienza University of Rome, 00189 Rome, Italy; laura.dimagno@uniroma1.it (L.D.M.); fiorella.dipastena@uniroma1.it (F.D.P.); rosa.bordone@uniroma1.it (R.B.); sonia.coni@uniroma1.it (S.C.)
[2] Istituto Pasteur—Fondazione Cenci—Bolognetti, 00161 Rome, Italy
* Correspondence: gianluca.canettieri@uniroma1.it

Simple Summary: In the last two decades, the antidiabetic drugs, biguanides, have received considerable interest owing to their presumed antitumor properties. A critical issue that has been at the center of many studies is how they act at the molecular level. Most works propose that biguanides inhibit mitochondrial complex I, which causes ATP depletion and activation of compensatory responses, responsible for the therapeutic properties. However, complex I can only be inhibited with concentrations of biguanides that cannot be tolerated by animals and patients, suggesting that alternative targets and intracellular perturbations are involved. Here, we will discuss the current knowledge of the mechanisms of action of biguanides, when used under clinically relevant conditions. The ongoing clinical trials in cancer and the proper conditions of usage will also be addressed. Understanding the mode of action of these drugs represents critical information for further investigation and usage in cancer models.

Abstract: Biguanides are a family of antidiabetic drugs with documented anticancer properties in preclinical and clinical settings. Despite intensive investigation, how they exert their therapeutic effects is still debated. Many studies support the hypothesis that biguanides inhibit mitochondrial complex I, inducing energy stress and activating compensatory responses mediated by energy sensors. However, a major concern related to this "complex" model is that the therapeutic concentrations of biguanides found in the blood and tissues are much lower than the doses required to inhibit complex I, suggesting the involvement of additional mechanisms. This comprehensive review illustrates the current knowledge of pharmacokinetics, receptors, sensors, intracellular alterations, and the mechanism of action of biguanides in diabetes and cancer. The conditions of usage and variables affecting the response to these drugs, the effect on the immune system and microbiota, as well as the results from the most relevant clinical trials in cancer are also discussed.

Keywords: biguanides; complex I; metabolism; redox; metformin; cancer

Citation: Di Magno, L.; Di Pastena, F.; Bordone, R.; Coni, S.; Canettieri, G. The Mechanism of Action of Biguanides: New Answers to a Complex Question. *Cancers* **2022**, *14*, 3220. https://doi.org/10.3390/cancers14133220

Academic Editor: Paola Tucci

Received: 25 May 2022
Accepted: 23 June 2022
Published: 30 June 2022

Publisher's Note: MDPI stays neutral with regard to jurisdictional claims in published maps and institutional affiliations.

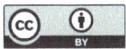

Copyright: © 2022 by the authors. Licensee MDPI, Basel, Switzerland. This article is an open access article distributed under the terms and conditions of the Creative Commons Attribution (CC BY) license (https://creativecommons.org/licenses/by/4.0/).

1. Introduction

The history of biguanides began in the 19th century when it was found that the blood-glucose-lowering properties of the herb *Galega officinalis* (French lilac), used since the medieval age to treat polyuria and other diseases, were due to galegine, a derivative of guanidine contained in the plant seeds and flowers. The identification of galegine led to the synthesis of various biguanides (synthelin A and B, biguanide, metformin, phenformin, and buformin) in the early 20th century that were tested as antidiabetic agents but shortly discontinued due to toxicity issues or presumed low potency.

Starting from the 1980s, further studies led to the re-evaluation of the use of metformin in type 2 diabetes mellitus (T2DM), providing strong evidence for its effectiveness and safety [1] and leading to FDA approval in 1994. Since then, metformin has progressively gained ground, to become the most widely prescribed oral antidiabetic drug and first-line therapy for the treatment of T2D in the last two decades.

The broad utilization of metformin has also allowed epidemiological observations reporting a significant reduction of the risk of cancer in diabetic patients treated with this drug [2–4], which has prompted a significant effort aimed at establishing the therapeutic efficacy of metformin against cancer in cells culture, animal models, and patients.

Phenformin and buformin were prescribed for the treatment of T2D starting from the 1950s but were withdrawn from the market in the 1970s because of the higher risk of cardiac mortality and lactic acidosis [5,6]. Following the increased interest in the anticancer properties of metformin, these drugs (particularly phenformin) have been re-considered for cancer treatment, showing significant antitumor effects, often stronger than metformin, in numerous preclinical studies, likely related to their higher cell permeability.

A substantial amount of effort has been devoted to understanding how biguanides act at the molecular level, an issue that has not yielded unique conclusions but rather has been quite controversial.

According to a widely accepted interpretation, the primary target of biguanides underlying both their antidiabetic and anticancer effects, is mitochondrial complex I of the respiratory transport chain. All biguanides display an inhibitory effect on complex I and inhibit the rate of oxygen consumption, thereby causing energy stress, increase in AMP/ATP ratio, and activation of AMP Kinase (AMPK), which is believed to be a master mediator of the therapeutic effects of these drugs, through phosphorylation-mediated regulation of key targets such as hepatic CRTCs in diabetes and mTOR in tumors.

However, while this model is generally accepted and used to support many experimental findings, it has also raised concerns that have led to alternative interpretations.

A primary reason for this lack of consensus is the inconsistencies in the drug concentrations and conditions used in the experimental settings.

Indeed, most of the reported mechanisms of action of biguanides have been demonstrated in cell culture using doses of the drugs and culturing conditions that are different from those found in patients or animal tissues. Even if many studies have shown that these parameters have a profound influence on the drug response, these pieces of information have been often poorly considered when addressing the mechanism of action of these drugs.

In the first part of this article, we review the available information about the pharmacological properties of biguanides, describing the structure, the dosage administered in patients and animal models, the concentrations reached in the circulation and tissues over time, the cellular transporters, and how these drugs travel across the cells. In the second section, we illustrate what is known about the mechanism of action of these drugs as glucose-lowering agents, in terms of target tissues and target molecules. In the third part of this work, we describe the current knowledge on the mechanism of action of biguanides in cancer, the variables affecting the cellular responses, and the available data arising from clinical trials.

2. Pharmacological Properties

Biguanides are a class of compounds in which two guanidine groups are bound by a common nitrogen atom. They all share the feature of being both polar and hydrophilic molecules, highly soluble in aqueous media because of two imino and three amino groups in tautomerism. However, they also differ in some chemical peculiarities, responsible for the pharmacokinetic and pharmacodynamic properties in each of them.

2.1. Metformin: Uptake, Therapeutic Concentration, Excretion

Metformin (3-(diaminomethylidene)-1,1-dimethylguanidine) carries two methyl substituents in position 1 and is synthesized from 2-cyanoguanidine and dimethylammonium chloride [7]. The first evidence of the hypoglycemic activity of metformin in animal models was from Slotta and Tschesche in 1929 [8], and its clinical use was first reported by Sterne in 1957 [9]. In type 2 diabetic patients, metformin is administered orally as immediate or extended-release tablets. The immediate release is generally taken 2–3 times a day, while the extended release is administered once daily.

The daily dose ranges from 500 to 2550 mg. Metformin is rapidly dissolved in the gastrointestinal tract [10] but, due to its hydrophilic nature, the absorption cannot occur passively through the plasma membrane but requires active transport. Multiple organic cation transporters are involved in the uptake of metformin, and many of them are important in its pharmacological action, as mediators of metformin entry into target tissues. Metformin is a substrate of various organic cation transporters (OCT), including OCT1 (SLC22A1), OCT2 (SLC22A2), OCT3 (SLC22A3), MATE1 (SLC47A1), MATE2 (SLC47A2), PMAT (SLC29A4), and OCTN1 (SLC22A4) [11–16]. Several transporters have been implicated in metformin intestinal absorption. PMAT is primarily located on the apical membrane of polarized epithelial cells [17], while transporters in the SLC22 family are expressed in the small intestine and play a role in metformin absorption.

Metformin can also cross the enterocytes through the organic cation transporters 1 and 3 (OCT1 and OCT3) [18,19]. OCT3 is localized in the apical membrane and carries metformin into enterocytes, while OCT1 is localized in basolateral membranes and transports metformin into the interstitial fluid [20]. OCT1 and 3 are also expressed on the basolateral membrane of hepatocytes and mediate metformin liver uptake [21]. High expression of OCTs is responsible for the elevated metformin accumulation in mouse liver (~40 µM) when compared to serum (~5 µM) [22]. In agreement with this value, Ma and colleagues recently showed that in mouse primary hepatocytes treated with 5 µM metformin for up to 48 h, the intracellular concentration was 25–40 µM, suggesting the ability to accumulate 5–8-fold in these cells [23]. Similarly, Moonira et al. measured an intracellular/extracellular metformin concentration ratio of about 5-fold after 3 h incubation of mouse hepatocytes with 100–200 µM of the biguanide [24].

OCT transporters could also move metformin from the liver to the blood thus causing its rapid distribution into peripheral body tissues and fluids. Both OCT1 and 3 are also expressed in skeletal muscles where they mediate metformin uptake.

Metformin does not bind to plasma proteins, and this causes its rapid distribution throughout the body [25] (Table 1). The plasma concentration measured in subjects taking 1.5–2.5 g of metformin orally per day (~30 mg/kg/day) ranges between 4 and 15 µM [10]. In particular, 3 h after receiving a single dose of 0.5 g metformin orally, the peak plasma concentration ranges between 7.74–12.39 µM; 3 h after a single dose of 1.5 g metformin, the peak plasma concentration is 23.23 µM. Assumption of 1 g metformin twice a day determines a plasma mean concentration of 3.1–10.07 µM. The mean concentration over a dosage interval is 6.66 µM. Lalau et al., in 2003, measured metformin plasma concentration in subjects with type 2 diabetes mellitus under metformin therapy within the recommended dosage range (1700–2550 mg/day) and reported a mean metformin concentration of 3.8 µM [26].

Madiraju et al. in 2018 detected metformin plasma concentration in human subjects 3 h after 1 g of metformin by oral administration, and values ranged from 14 µM to 22 µM [27]. In contrast to the rapid decrease of plasma concentrations, Bailey et al. detected metformin accumulation in the gut after administering 850 mg daily for 2–3 weeks and then twice daily for other 3–5 weeks to T2 diabetes patients [28]. Metformin levels detected 12–16 h after the last 850 mg dose (pre-dose jejunal sample) corresponded to 33 ± 26 ng/mg wet weight of tissue (approximately 250 µmol/kg), while the concentration reached 3 h after the last 850 mg morning dose (post-dose sample) was 504 ± 232 ng/mg wet weight of tissue (approximately 4 mmol/kg). These values were 30–300 times higher than metformin plasma concentration (8–24 µM).

Pentikainen and colleagues [29] measured metformin plasma concentration in three patients, following i.v. injection of 500 mg [29] After 1 h, they observed a peak of 5 µg/mL (=38.68 µM), which rapidly decreased at 1.5 µg/mL (=11.6 µM) 2h after administration. Renal clearance after intravenous administration calculated in this study (454 ± 47 mL/min) was comparable to that calculated after oral administration (507 ± 129 mL/min) by Graham et al. in 2011 [10].

Data on liver concentrations of metformin in humans are not available and it is, therefore, difficult to establish the exact therapeutic values. However, based on a presumed three-fold higher liver concentration compared to plasma content (where the calculated range is 20–30 µM), the estimated hepatic exposure is believed to be 60–90 µM, corresponding to 2 g/day in patients or to oral dosing in rodents of 50–100 mg/kg [30].

As for dosing in rodents, other authors indicate that the oral dose of 250 mg/kg/day in mice corresponds to 30 mg/kg/day in humans (2–2.5g/day), considering the interspecies scaling in pharmacokinetics [22].

Metformin concentration reached in plasma and tumor tissue ranges from 3.2 to 12.4 µM [22]. These data are consistent with work from Madiraju and colleagues where after ad libitum administration of 200–300 mg/kg/day of metformin, plasma concentration was 15 µM and liver concentration was 40 µM [27].

Madiraju et al. also reported that 30 minutes after intravenous injection of 50 mg/kg metformin in rats, plasma concentration was 74 µM, while in the liver it was 100 µM.

Chandel and collaborators [22] observed that administration of 350 mg/kg metformin by oral gavage for 3 weeks caused a peak of 1500 µM in the liver and 200 µM in the tumor, in a mouse model of lung adenocarcinoma. However, these concentrations were considered supra-pharmacological by others [30]. Time-averaged plasma concentration was 47 µM. The authors also injected metformin 350 mg/kg intraperitoneally (i.p.) for 2 weeks and detected a concentration peak of 100 µM in the liver and tumor after 25 h from the last administration, while the time-averaged plasma concentration was 7.5 µM [22]. Acute IP administration is reported also by Dowling and colleagues [31] after 30 minutes from an injection of 125 mg/kg metformin, mean plasma concentration was 184 µM and it decreased to 42 µM after 1 h.

Wilcock and Bailey, in 1993, analyzed metformin concentration reached in tissues such as the liver and gut after acute administration (50 mg/kg) via oral gavage or intravenous route [32]. Oral gavage seems to be more efficient in achieving higher concentrations: 51.7 µM measured in hepatic portal vein after 30 minutes vs 21.9 µM in inferior vena cava detected after the intravenous injection. Moreover, liver tissue concentration was 37 µM after oral gavage and 22 µM after i.v. As for the gut, they measured different grades of accumulation along the tract with a maximum of 1206 µM and a minimum of 147 µM after oral gavage; the highest concentration reached in the gut after i.v. injection was 55 µM and the lowest 38 µM.

Metformin is not metabolized and is secreted unmodified by the kidney [33], after being transported through OCT2 [34] located on the basolateral side of renal tubular cells. The multidrug and toxin extrusion (MATE) transporters, such as MATE1 and MATE2K contribute to the transport of metformin into urine [35]. The mean renal clearance rate is around 552–642 mL/min. Its mean plasma elimination half-life is 1.5–4.7 h [25,36].

Metformin renal clearance decreases along with the impairment of kidney function and depends on the genetic pool of transporters expressed in kidney cells: OCT2 is the principal carrier involved in the uptake from tubular cells, and OCT1 mediates its secretion but it could also participate in the entry process. OCT3 is also expressed in the kidney. MATE1 is thought to carry metformin out of tubular cells and into the urine, while MATE2K could be the principal extrusion transporter [35,37]. Metformin is excreted in the urine unchanged, and no metabolites have been reported.

2.2. Phenformin: Uptake, Therapeutic Concentration, Excretion

Phenformin (1-(diaminomethylidene)-2-(2-phenylethyl)guanidine) is a phenethyl biguanide derivative of metformin that is characterized by the substitution of one of the terminal nitrogen atoms with a 2-phenylethyl group. Phenformin is obtained by heating phenethylamine and cyanoguanidine (37% yield) [38]. It was used as an antidiabetic agent but was later withdrawn from many countries because it was associated with a greater incidence of lactic acidosis [1,39].

Phenformin is more lipophilic than metformin and therefore it is generally thought to passively cross the cell membrane and display a higher potency. This makes phenformin less dependent on active transport, while metformin requires transporters to enter cells [40]. Supporting this idea, Hawley et al., [41] showed that while OCT1 is required to transport metformin in rat hepatoma cells, it is not necessary for phenformin uptake. Other studies revealed that an active phenformin transport is required to cross the mitochondrial membrane: Shitara et al., in 2013, described the role of organic cation/carnitine transporter 1 (OCTN1) in mitochondrial accumulation of phenformin [42]. Bridges et al. (2016) confirmed these data (selective transport) by comparing the ability of biguanides with the same lipophilicity in mitochondria entry [43]. Moreover, work by Sogame et al., (2013) revealed that phenformin has an affinity for hOCT2, which is majorly involved in biguanides uptake from blood to kidney cells, stronger than metformin [44].

Phenformin is rapidly absorbed after oral administration and is not significantly bound to plasma proteins [45] (Table 1). It undergoes hydroxylation in the liver to 4-hydroxyphenformin [46]. The half-life of circulating phenformin is about 11 h [47]. Both phenformin and its hydroxylated metabolite are predominantly eliminated in the urine [46].

Beckmann and colleagues measured a phenformin plasma concentration of 0.97 µM 2 h after a single oral dose of 100 mg in patients, with a half-life of 3.2 h [45]. Matin et al. also measured phenformin concentration after administration of 100 mg to a diabetic patient. Maximum plasma concentration, measured with mass spectrometry, was reached after 3 h and was 147 ng/mL, corresponding to 0.72 µM [48]. Nattrass et al. in 1980 [49] measured a sustained release formulation of 50 mg of phenformin administered to six healthy volunteers. The values obtained from their analysis (0.19 µM 3.5 h after ingestion) were lower than those obtained by Beckmann and collaborators, although the authors pointed out that the time course could have been altered using a sustained-release capsule. Similar steady-state concentrations were reported by Marchetti and Navalesi [50] and were between 0.13 and 0.56 µM.

More data about phenformin circulating levels in patients were reported by Karam et al. [51]. They commented on the results obtained from the University Group Diabetes Program (UGDP) in which patients with hyperglycemic reactions to oral glucose assumption were treated with different anti-diabetic drugs. Circulating phenformin concentrations measured in these patients using gas chromatography were comprised between 102–241 ng/mL (0.5–1.17 µM).

As for animal models, in a recent work, HPLC analysis was used to measure plasma phenformin in C57BL/6J mice. After 10 days of treatment with phenformin (300 mg/Kg/day) in the drinking water, a 1.4 µM phenformin concentration was detected in the blood [52]. The same dose of 300 mg/Kg/day in the drinking water was used also by Huang et al. [53] and Appleyard et al. [39] for xenografts experiments.

After i.v. administration in the tail vein of 12.5 mg/kg phenformin, the maximum concentration (3.4 µM) was achieved 30 minutes after injection (maximum tolerated dose), while higher doses were not tolerated [52].

Phenformin blood concentrations in mice treated for 5- and 7-days ad libitum per os are described also in Shackelford et al. [54] and are in a range between 1–1.5 µM. Similar data were obtained by Bando et al. in 2010 [55] using oral gavage to administer different phenformin doses. Here, 28 days after daily ingestion of 200 mg/kg phenformin, the mean plasma concentration was 1.49 µM.

Various studies have been carried out in animal models highlighting the higher accumulation of the drug in the liver and gut. Wick et al. in 1960 [56] administered 100 mg/kg of phenformin orally or intraperitoneally. In the first case, they detected the maximum liver concentration (2 mM tissue water) after 1h and the maximum GI concentration (3.1 mM tissue water) after 2 h. The intraperitoneal route determined a liver Cmax of 2.6mM tissue water after 2 h and a GI tract Cmax of 0.9 mM after 1 h.

Sogame et al. in 2011 measured phenformin levels in rats after oral gavage administration of 50 mg/kg. The portal vein and liver concentrations after 30′ from ingestion were 2.5 µM and 147.1 µM respectively, while the highest plasma concentration (3.49 µM) was reached 4 h later [57].

Another study by Conlay (1977) measured phenformin serum concentration in patients manifesting lactic acidosis [58]. They received 50 mg of phenformin three times a day. Five of seven patients presented phenformin concentration under 241 ng/mL (1.17 µM) confirming the previous data.

Phenformin is partially metabolized in the liver in N1-p-hydroxy-β-phenethyl biguanide by CYP2D6, and about one-third is excreted in this form, whereas the other two-thirds are eliminated unmodified. It is reported in Beckmann [45] that the maximal excretion rate is 4.1 mg/h. The average half-life of excretion is 3.2 h, which is equivalent to an average rate constant of 0.22 mg/h.

Although the use of phenformin has been discontinued due to the high incidence of lactic acidosis, many studies demonstrated that the increased frequency may be principally related to the subjects receiving this drug. First, kidney dysfunction, which is often associated with diabetes, may reduce the clearance of the drug. Second, some genetic features, such as the expression level of transporters involved in phenformin excretion (OCT2 or MATE), may also affect its plasma levels. Third, alterations of the enzymes that metabolize phenformin (CYP2D6 and P-glycoprotein) can modulate phenformin circulating levels and consequentially the risk of lactic acidosis. Indeed, it has been demonstrated that patients that are poor CYP2D6 metabolizers show higher levels of phenformin plasma concentrations that lead to higher toxicity [59]. The risk of lactic acidosis is also increased by CYP2D6 gene mutations that lead to high levels of unmetabolized phenformin [1,59].

2.3. Buformin: Uptake, Therapeutic Concentration, Excretion

Buformin (2-butyl-1-(diaminomethylidene)guanidine) was synthesized and tested as a hypoglycemic agent in the 1950s [60]. Like phenformin, this drug is more lipophilic and effective than metformin, but the major limitation to its usage is the associated high risk of lactic acidosis [61]. For this reason, buformin was withdrawn from clinical use in the 1970s in most countries (except for Romania where it is still commercially available and administered in doses ranging from 50 mg to 300 mg daily).

Buformin is not metabolized [62–64] and only 10% has been found to interact with serum proteins [64,65] (Table 1). Data regarding buformin concentration and pharmacokinetics are reported by Lintz et al. [66]. Four diabetic patients were treated with 50 mg of ^{14}C-butylbiguanide intravenously. 1 h and 5 h after administration, buformin plasma concentrations were 1.8–2.13 µM and 0.45–0.64 µM, respectively. The biological half-life of butylbiguanide calculated after intravenous administration was 3.7–6.0 h with a mean of 4.6 h. In this study, the authors also measured the total clearance, which ranged from 439 to 618 mL/min, and averaged 536 mL/min. A mean value of 72.4% (61.2–90.2%) of the administered drug was excreted in the urine. Mean renal clearance was 393 mL/min (282–518 mL/min). The value given here for the total clearance (536 + 78 mL/min) corresponds to previously described values. Buformin renal clearance was significantly higher than insulin clearance, and this suggested that the drug was excreted both via glomerular filtration and active tubular secretion. It was observed that only 72.4% of the drug was detectable in the urine without any of its metabolites [45,62,63], and this suggested that additional mechanisms were required for its excretion. Animal experiments described in Beckmann et al. [64] and Yoh et al. [67] highlighted the presence of buformin in the bile and the transport of this biguanide from the blood to the intestinal lumen. Lintz et al. confirmed this data in patients by detecting radioactive signals in the intestinal fluid after intravenous administration of butylbiguanide [66]. However, it was not clear if the drug could reach the intestinal lumen via the bile or via the intestinal mucosa.

In additional studies, five fasted diabetic patients received 100 mg micronized ^{14}C-butylbiguanide (50 IxCi) in hard-shell capsules orally. Mean plasma concentration after

1 h from administration extrapolated from their report was 4.33 µM [66]. An average of 74.4% of the amount of drug administered was excreted by the kidneys of the 4 test subjects, whereas a higher value had been found in previous investigations [45,62,64,68].

After oral administration of butylbiguanide, high concentrations of the drug were detected in intestinal fluid, with a maximum value of 700 µg/mL. The concentration of butylbiguanide in the intestinal fluid of the jejunum 4–5 h after oral administration was still significantly higher than the amount detected after intravenous administration, and remained almost constant for a long period, indicating that there was a significant accumulation of butylbiguanide in the intestinal mucosa, which was more significant after oral administration rather than intravenous administration. After intravenous injection, the concentration of butylbiguanide in the intestinal epithelium was 6–11 times higher than in plasma, and after oral administration, it was 10–35 times higher than in plasma, with only one exception. Accumulation of butylbiguanide in the intestinal mucosa in humans corresponds to that found in animal studies [66,67,69,70]. For example, 3 h after oral administration of 10 mg/kg butylbiguanide, a concentration of 13 µg/g was found in the intestinal wall of rats, while in plasma concentration was 5.72 µM [69]. After intravenous administration of 50 mg butylbiguanide, its concentration in the liver was 12.72–25.44 µM [66]. The accumulation was even greater after oral administration: in two patients, 2–3 h after oral administration, the detected liver concentrations were 63.61–127.21 µM [66].

Table 1. Therapeutic concentrations of biguanides.

No.	Drug	Dosage	Mean of Administration	Concentration	Treatment Duration	Model	References
1	Metformin	1.5–2.5 g/day	Oral	4–15 µM	1.5–3 h	Human	[10]
2	Metformin	1.7/2.55 g/day	Oral	3.8 µM	0.3–2.5 h	Human	[26]
3	Metformin	1 g	Oral	14–22 µM	3 h	Human	[27]
4	Metformin	0.85–1.70 g/day	Oral	250 µmol/Kg –4 mmol/Kg	2–3/3V5 weeks	Human	[28]
5	Metformin	0.5 g	Intravenous	11.6–38.68 µM	1–2 h	Human	[29]
6	Metformin	0.35 g/Kg	Oral	200–1500 µM	3 weeks	Mouse	[22]
7	Metformin	0.35 g/Kg	Intraperitoneal	7.5–100 µM	2 weeks	Mouse	[22]
8	Metformin	0.125 g/Kg	Intraperitoneal	42–184 µM	0.5 h	Mouse	[31]
9	Metformin	0.05 g/Kg	Oral	147–1206 µM	0.5 h	Mouse	[32]
10	Metformin	0.05 g/Kg	Intravenous	38–55 µM	0.5 h	Mouse	[32]
11	Phenformin	0.1 g	Oral	0.97 µM	2 h	Human	[45]
12	Phenformin	0.1 g	Oral	0.72 µM	3 h	Human	[48]
13	Phenformin	0.05 g	Intravenous	0.19 µM	3.5 h	Human	[49]
14	Phenformin	66 ± 20 mg/day	Oral	0.14–0.56 µM	5 ± 3 years	Human	[50]
15	Phenformin	0.15 g/day	Oral	0.5–1.17 µM	N/A	Human	[51]
16	Phenformin	0.3 g/Kg/day	Oral	1.4 µM	10 days	Mouse	[52]
17	Phenformin	0.0125 g/Kg	Intravenous	3.4 µM	0.5 h	Mouse	[52]
18	Phenformin	1.8 mg/mL	Oral	1–1.5 µM	5–7 days	Mouse	[54]
19	Phenformin	0.2 g/Kg	Oral	1.49 µM	28 days	Mouse	[55]
20	Phenformin	0.1 g/Kg	Oral	2–3.1 mM	1–2 h	Mouse	[56]

Table 1. Cont.

No.	Drug	Dosage	Mean of Administration	Concentration	Treatment Duration	Model	References
21	Phenformin	0.1 g/Kg	Intraperitoneal	0.9–2.6 mM	1–2 h	Mouse	[56]
22	Phenformin	0.05 g/Kg	Oral	2.5 µM–3.49 µM	0.5–4 h	Rat	[57]
23	Phenformin	1.5 g	Oral	1.17 µM	N/A	Human	[58]
24	Buformin	0.05 g	Intravenous	0.45–2.13 µM	1–5 h	Human	[66]
25	Buformin	0.1 g	Oral	4.33 µM	1 h	Human	[66]
26	Buformin	0.01 g/Kg	Oral	5.72 µM	3 h	Rat	[69]
27	Buformin	0.05g	Intravenous	12.72–25.44 µM	2–3 h	Human	[66]
28	Buformin	0.1g	Oral	63.61–127.21 µM	2–3 h	Human	[66]

3. The Mechanism of Action of Biguanides: Lessons from Type 2 Diabetes Mellitus (T2DM)

Type 2 diabetes mellitus (T2DM) is the most common type of diabetes observed in the population and a leading cause of death [71]. T2DM is characterized by insulin resistance, βcell dysfunction, and elevated hepatic glucose output mainly attributed to an increase in gluconeogenesis [72,73].

Biguanides have been used for the treatment of type 2 diabetes mellitus (T2DM) for more than 70 years and metformin is the most prescribed oral anti-diabetic agent worldwide, taken by over 150 million people annually [74]. Metformin prevents body weight gain and does not cause hypoglycemia, which is frequently associated with the use of other antidiabetic drugs [75]. Moreover, metformin may have therapeutic potential in the treatment of conditions such as nephropathy [76], polycystic ovary syndrome [77], and cardiovascular diseases [78,79], often associated with diabetes or insulin resistance.

The pleiotropic properties of metformin suggest that the drug acts on multiple tissues, but the underlying mechanism of action remains debated.

Most of the studies on the mechanism of action of biguanides, especially metformin, have been conducted in T2DM models, trying to identify the primary target and the consequences of its alteration. These studies have then ignited investigation in tumor models, to determine if the effectors and mechanisms operating in diabetes could also be responsible for the antitumor properties of these drugs.

The main and best studied site of the antidiabetic action of biguanides is the liver, where these drugs reduce hepatic gluconeogenesis, through various mechanisms discussed below. However, other studies have also proposed the gut and skeletal muscle as additional sites responsible for the blood-glucose-lowering properties of biguanides.

3.1. Liver as a Target Tissue

A clinical study using ^{13}C nuclear magnetic resonance spectroscopy showed that metformin reduces fasting plasma glucose concentrations in diabetic patients by decreasing hepatic glucose production (HGP) by about 25% and gluconeogenesis (two to three times higher in diabetics than in control patients) by about 35%, without affecting glycogenolysis [80].

Several mechanisms have been identified for the action of biguanides in hepatic gluconeogenesis and glucose production, which are generally thought to be mediated by the interaction of the drugs with two main cell compartments: mitochondria (energy or redox alterations) or lysosomes.

3.1.1. Energy-Dependent Mechanisms: The Controversial Role of the Complex I—AMPK Axis

In 2000, two independent groups reported for the first time that metformin inhibits the mitochondrial respiratory chain complex I thus decreasing NADH oxidation, proton pumping across the inner mitochondrial membrane, and oxygen consumption rate [81,82].

The mammalian mitochondrial respiratory complex I, also known as NADH-ubiquinone oxidoreductase, is a large L-shaped membrane-bound enzyme consisting of many core and accessory subunits, that oxidizes NADH to NAD$^+$ and transfers four protons from the mitochondrial matrix to the transmembrane space and electrons to the ubiquinone pool [83].

The molecular interaction mechanism between biguanides and the mitochondrial respiratory chain complex I has not been completely understood (Figure 1). A proposed mechanism suggests that metformin binds the Cys-39 in the amphipathic region at the interface of the hydrophilic and membrane domains, trapping the enzyme in a deactive-like open-loop conformation [84]. Complex I inhibition causes a decline in intracellular ATP levels concomitantly with an increase in intracellular ADP and AMP. This altered cellular energy charge activates the energy sensor AMPK [85], already reported to be activated by metformin in 2001 [86]. These two seminal discoveries, the decrease of energy metabolism and activation of AMPK, were at the center of the proposed mechanism of action of biguanides for the following years. In 2005, Shaw and colleagues showed that metformin requires LKB1, a kinase that phosphorylates and activates AMPK, to lower blood glucose levels in the liver of adult mice. Loss of LKB1 increased gluconeogenesis and abolished metformin glucose-lowering activity [87]. Once activated by LKB1, AMPK phosphorylates TORC2/CRTC2, the CREB (cAMP response element-binding protein) transcriptional coactivator, and sequesters this factor into the cytoplasm, preventing PPARγ coactivator 1α (PGC1α) transcription and subsequent increase of gluconeogenic phosphoenolpyruvate carboxylase (PEPCK) and glucose-6-phosphatase (G6Pase) target gene expression [87]. A few years later, this mechanism of action was challenged by the evidence that, in response to metformin administration, blood glucose levels, hepatocytes glucose production, and gluconeogenic gene expression were not changed in mice lacking AMPK in the liver, compared to wild-type littermates. Moreover, the metformin glucose-lowering effect was maintained even under forced expression of gluconeogenic genes through PGC-1α overexpression [88]. Thus, metformin inhibited gluconeogenesis independently of LKB1/AMPK.

The gluconeogenic pathway is a high-energy-consuming process that requires six ATP equivalents for each molecule of glucose produced. Since AMP is a potent allosteric inhibitor of fructose 1,6-bisphosphatase (FBP1), a key enzyme in gluconeogenesis, it was proposed that by raising AMP levels metformin inhibits gluconeogenesis through FBP1 inhibition. Supporting this hypothesis, a point mutation in FBP1 that renders the enzyme insensitive to AMP was found to abrogate the response to metformin in vivo [89]. A further breakthrough study in 2013 showed a novel mechanism of action for biguanides-driven hypoglycemic function independent of AMPK [90] whereby biguanides were suggested to antagonize the action of glucagon by inhibiting the activity of the cAMP-activated protein kinase A (PKA). Through their effect on complex I and consequent accumulation of cellular AMP, biguanides inhibit adenylate cyclase and reduce the levels of cyclic AMP, abrogating the phosphorylation of critical PKA substrates, including the 6-phosphofructo-2-kinase isoform 1 (PFKFB1). Phosphorylation of PFKFB1 inhibits the formation of fructose-2,6-bisphosphate, an intracellular mediator that acutely activates the glycolytic enzyme 6-phosphofructo-1-kinase and inhibits the gluconeogenic enzyme fructose-1,6-bisphosphatase. Lowering of cAMP would therefore inhibit the switch from glycolysis to gluconeogenesis triggered by glucagon [91]. Hence, according to these studies, the metformin-driven complex I inhibition, and consequent decrease of ATP/AMP ratio, could block the gluconeogenic flux independently of AMPK. Other studies added further evidence arguing against the involvement of AMPK in hepatic glucose production. Using liver-specific AMPK knock-out mice, Hasenour and colleagues showed that AMPK is not required for suppression of hepatic glucose production induced by AICAR, an inducer of metabolic stress [92]. More recently, Cokorinos et al. showed that a non-selective AMPK agonist lowered blood glucose levels by inducing an AMPK-mediated increase of glucose disposal in skeletal muscle, without inhibiting hepatic glucose production [93].

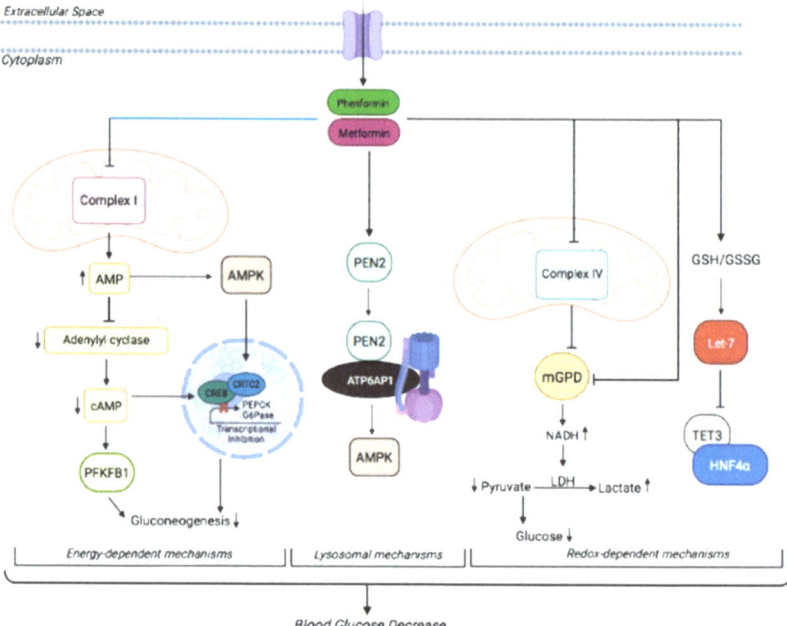

Figure 1. Proposed mechanisms for the glucose-lowering properties of biguanides. (Left) Energy-dependent mechanisms. Supra-pharmacological concentrations of biguanides suppress glucose production through the inhibition of complex I, which leads to the activation of AMPK and inhibition of the cAMP-PKA pathway. (Middle) Lysosomal mechanisms. Pharmacological concentrations activate PEN2, which inhibits lysosomal v-ATPase and activates AMPK in the intestine, decreasing blood glucose levels. (Right) Redox-dependent mechanisms. Biguanides inhibit mitochondrial complex IV, which results in inhibition of mitochondrial glycerol 3-phosphate dehydrogenase (mGPD) activity and gluconeogenic program. Alternatively, pharmacologic biguanides concentrations directly inhibit mGPD, leading to an increase in cytosolic NADH levels, which prevents lactate utilization and decreases hepatic glucose output. On the other hand, clinically relevant concentrations of biguanides up-regulate microRNA let-7, leading to the downregulation of TET3 and changes in the ratio of HNF4α isoforms, with consequent gluconeogenesis inhibition.

In addition to the growing skepticism about the involvement of AMPK in the inhibition of gluconeogenesis in response to metformin, in more recent years, some researchers started also being concerned that only supra-physiological concentrations of biguanides could directly inhibit mitochondrial complex I activity [74]. In isolated mitochondria or in sub-mitochondrial particles, concentrations of metformin between 20 and 100 mM are required for complex I inhibition [94], and the half-maximal inhibitory concentration (IC50) for complex I inhibition is reported to fall within the micromolar range (~500 μM) for phenformin [84]. Furthermore, it has been reported that the concentration of metformin required to inhibit complex I is lower in intact cells than in isolated mitochondria. An explanation that was proposed to solve this discrepancy was that metformin accumulates in the mitochondria in a voltage-dependent manner, reaching millimolar concentrations compared to the micromolar concentrations in the cytosol [95]. However, many authors argue against the hypothesis that metformin accumulates in the mitochondria. Indeed, a major concern is that the mitochondrial inner membrane allows the passage of hydrophilic molecules only through specific transporters but there is no evidence that supports the existence of a carrier specific for metformin. Moreover, the entrance of numerous positive charges in the mitochondria is expected to cause a collapse of mitochondrial membrane potential, while some authors show that metformin is not able to depolarize isolated mitochondria [95,96].

Defects in mitochondrial respiratory chain activity are reported to contribute to the development of insulin resistance and hyperglycemia in T2DM [97–100]. Mitochondria have a peculiar life cycle that includes continuous phases of fusion and fission necessary for the maintenance of their bioenergetic efficiency [101,102]. Impairing these mechanisms leads to defects of the mitochondrial functions and culminates in the decrease of mitochondrial respiration [103,104]. Wang et al. show that micromolar concentrations of metformin (75 µM) not only fail to inhibit complex I activity but also improve mitochondrial respiration by increasing mitochondrial fission through AMPK signaling. The authors suggest that the decrease in ATP levels and oxygen consumption rate observed with supra-pharmacological doses of metformin would rather be a consequence of adenine synthesis inhibition. Insufficient levels of cellular ADP would lead to an inability to utilize the mitochondrial membrane potential to generate ATP. To support this hypothesis, they showed that the enzymatic activity of purified mitochondrial complexes is unchanged after metformin treatment at all concentrations, including 1000 µM [105]. Accordingly, using permeabilized skeletal muscles derived from type II diabetes patients, Larsen and colleagues tested a wide range of metformin concentrations revealing that the minimum concentration needed to appreciate a significant reduction of complex I activity is 3 mM [106].

3.1.2. Redox-Dependent Mechanisms

In an attempt to address the concerns about the dosage, Madiraju and colleagues showed that by administering to rats doses of metformin corresponding to the range used in T2DM patients (20–50 mg/Kg), metformin increased hepatic cytosolic NADH/NAD$^+$ ratio to impair glucose production from redox-dependent substrates (lactate and glycerol), independently of complex I [107]. The authors proposed that this redox alteration is due to inhibition of the mitochondrial glycerol-3-phosphate dehydrogenase (mGPD) activity, a key component of the glycerophosphate shuttle (GPS), which is one of two shuttle systems required to transfer reducing equivalents from the cytosol to the mitochondria (Figure 1). mGPD is localized in the outer face of the inner mitochondrial membrane and oxidizes glycerol-3-phosphate (G3P) to dihydroxyacetone phosphate (DAP) with concurrent reduction of flavin adenine dinucleotide (FAD) to FADH2. Its cytosolic partner cGPD reduces DAP to G3P while oxidizing cytosolic NADH [108].

Acute and chronic metformin treatment elicited a significant decrease in the mitochondrial redox state and an increase in the cytosolic redox state, impairing glucose production from lactate. Furthermore, mGPD knockdown phenocopied metformin activity in vivo and abolished metformin effects [107]. In a further study, the same group showed that metformin inhibits hepatic gluconeogenesis in a redox-dependent manner without affecting mitochondrial citrate synthase flux and hepatic energy charge [27]. They infused awake rats with ^{13}C-labeled lactate or alanine and traced these molecules through the gluconeogenic flux using ^{13}C NMR spectroscopy, finding that metformin impedes the hepatic conversion of reduced substrates (lactate and glycerol), but not oxidized substrates (alanine and pyruvate) into glucose [27].

These observations provided a plausible explanation for the mechanism of action of biguanides at therapeutic doses, although they also raised some criticisms. A first concern regards the role of glycerophosphate shuttle in the liver since it is less relevant than the malate-aspartate shuttle (MAS), the other NADH shuttle. Thus, glycerol-phosphate shuttle (GPS) inhibition may not be sufficient to prevent gluconeogenesis [109]. Indeed, mice with selective disruption of the glycerol–phosphate shuttle showed unchanged fasting blood glucose levels, while knockout of malate–aspartate shuttles resulted in a significant decrease of blood glucose levels that was further reduced in mice with double inactivation of GPS and MAS [110]. Alshawi and coll. [111] found that a low dose of metformin (<2 nmol/mg) caused a more oxidized mitochondrial NADH/NAD$^+$ state and an increase in lactate/pyruvate ratio, supporting previous findings by Madiraju et al. However, in contrast to these authors, they found that metformin prevented gluconeogenesis from both reduced and oxidized substrates and did not inhibit mGPD activity. Instead, they found that metformin accumulates in the mitochondria due to its positive charge, depolarizing the mitochondrial membrane and causing inhibition of citrin, the electrogenic transporter for aspartate, and consequent inhibition of the malate-aspartate shuttle. To compensate for this inhibition, the glycerol-phosphate shuttle is stimulated and leads to a decrease of glycerol-3-phosphate, a potent allosteric inhibitor of phosphofructokinase 1 (PFK1). As a result, decreased G3P stimulates PFK1 and glycolysis and inhibits gluconeogenesis. However, the lack of inhibition by metformin on malate dehydrogenase or aspartate aminotransferase observed by Madiraju et al. [107], argues against this interpretation.

Calza et al. failed to observe a reduction of lactate-induced hepatic glucose output by metformin in rats [112] and MacDonald et al. did not see direct inhibition of mGPD by metformin in biochemical assays [113].

In a very recent publication, LaMoia et al. provided novel evidence to resolve these controversies, supporting mGPD, but not complex I inhibition as a major determinant of metformin inhibition of hepatic gluconeogenesis [114].

They demonstrated that biguanides (metformin, phenformin, galegine) repress hepatic gluconeogenesis from the redox-dependent substrate glycerol by blocking complex IV, which in turn results in inhibition of mGPD activity and increased cytosolic redox state. Inhibition of complex IV was proposed to backlog the electron transport chain (ETC) and cause indirect mGPD inhibition. Conversely, the authors showed that the specific complex I inhibitor piericidin A was unable to prevent gluconeogenesis from glycerol, while the specific complex IV inhibitor KCN phenocopied the effect of biguanides in vitro.

While the issue that mGPD is a direct target of biguanides needs to be properly addressed with compelling biochemical approaches, the authors noted that most of the biochemical assays arguing against mGPD were performed using KCN or other complex IV inhibitors in the reaction buffer. Hence, considering this new finding, it is possible that these inhibitors may have masked the effect of biguanides on GPD2 activity [114].

In another recent article, metformin administered at clinically relevant concentrations was shown to inhibit gluconeogenesis in primary hepatocytes and animal models of type 2 diabetes by activating the let-7/TET3/HNF4α axis in a redox-dependent fashion [115]. They demonstrated that clinically relevant doses of metformin up-regulate microRNA let-7, leading to the downregulation of TET3 and changes in the ratio of HNF4α isoforms, with consequent transcriptional inhibition of the gluconeogenic gene program (Figure 1). Therefore, these observations further support the modulation of the redox state as a determinant of metformin inhibition of hepatic gluconeogenesis.

3.1.3. Lysosomal Mechanisms

Very recently, Ma and colleagues have proposed a further alternative mechanism, whereby low doses of metformin activate AMPK by inhibiting lysosomal v-ATPase, independently of energy charge [23]. Previous observations from the same group demonstrated that AMPK could be activated by low glucose through aldolase, which senses the decrease of fructose-1,6-biphosphate FBP and forms a complex with v-ATPase, Regulator, axin, LKB1 that activates AMPK [116]. Hence, low glucose activates AMPK independently of ATP/AMP ratio, by regulating lysosomal v-ATPase. By performing a proteomic screening of metformin-interacting lysosomal proteins with a biotinylated photoactive probe, the authors identified PEN2 as a direct metformin interacting protein and found that, after binding with the drug, PEN2 associates with ATP6AP1, a member of the v-ATPase complex, thereby causing inhibition of the ATPase complex and activation of AMPK (Figure 1). Of note, loss of hepatic PEN2 abrogated the ability of metformin to lower hepatocyte fat content in mice, while conditional PEN2 knockout in the gut abrogated its glucose-lowering effect.

Together, these data support the idea that AMPK activation by this lysosomal-mediated mechanism is responsible for the therapeutic action of metformin. However, since other studies failed to detect phosphorylation of the AMPK substrate ACC in the liver following metformin administration in mice [27], this novel mechanism requires further investigation.

3.2. Gut as a Target Tissue

Biguanides accumulate in the small intestine at concentrations that are up to 20–300 times greater than plasma [32], suggesting that the gut could be an important site for biguanides action.

Early studies provided evidence that intravenous injection of metformin did not significantly lower glucose levels [117,118], although only acute effects were evaluated in those reports. Also, an increase in metformin concentration in plasma through inhibition of the MATE transporter, which mediates hepatic and renal elimination of the drug, had little effect on circulating glucose levels [119]. Furthermore, a gut-restricted formulation of metformin had greater glucose-lowering efficacy than systemically absorbed formulation [120]. These observations have been linked to a reduction in the rate of glucose absorption in the small intestine [121] and an increase in glucose uptake from the bloodstream and its utilization in metformin-treated enterocytes. Two different studies measured glucose uptake in diabetic patients or healthy volunteers treated with metformin using [18F]-fluoro-2-deoxy-D-glucose (FDG), a non-metabolized glucose analog. PET-computed tomography revealed a three-fold increase in FDG uptake in the small intestine and especially in the colon [122,123].

In addition to the increased glucose uptake and utilization in the enterocytes, in recent years the mechanism of biguanides action in the gut has been also linked to their ability to alter the secretion of some key molecules (GLP1 and GDF15) or to affect the composition of the gut microbiota.

3.2.1. Glp-1

Glucagon-like peptide 1 (GLP1) is an incretin hormone secreted from the intestinal enteroendocrine L cells in response to the presence of nutrients in the intestinal lumen. In healthy individuals, incretins are responsible for up to 70% of insulin secretion after an oral glucose load and their effect is severely impaired in T2DM patients [124]. GLP1 is essential for glucose homeostasis acting through a gut-brain neuronal axis that provides insulin secretion, inhibition of glucagon secretion, slowing of gastric emptying, and a reduction in appetite and food intake.

According to recent studies, metformin may increase the secretion of GLP1 from enteroendocrine L cells by direct and indirect mechanisms and may induce the expression of the GLP1 receptor [125].

In a double-blinded randomized placebo-controlled trial, healthy patients showed an overall increase of 23.4% of GLP1 plasma concentration after treatment with metformin for 18 months compared to placebo [126]. Another landmark study demonstrated that 75% of acute glucose-lowering properties of metformin could be attributed to its direct stimulation of GLP-1 from L cells and that a GLP1 receptor antagonist could prevent the observed decrease of blood glucose [127]. Conversely, other studies demonstrate an indirect effect of metformin on GLP1 levels through the modulation of dipeptidyl peptidase-4 (DPP4) [128], while other authors did not observe any effect on DPP4 [129]. Hence, the actual mechanism and involvement of GLP1 signaling in the response to biguanides are still unclear and need to be further clarified.

3.2.2. Gdf-15

Obesity is one of the main risk factors for T2DM and people with type 2 diabetes show a significant metformin-induced body weight loss [130,131]. This effect has been recently linked to an increased secretion of growth differentiation factor 15 (GDF15) [132,133].

GDF15 is a divergent TGF-β superfamily cytokine that acts through the recently identified orphan receptor GFRAL (GDNF receptor α-like), a member of the glial-cell-derived neurotropic factor family (GDNF), which is expressed in the area postrema in the brainstem of mice, rats, monkeys, and humans [134].

In 2006, it was observed that transgenic mice with ubiquitous expression of the full-length human GDF15 protein showed a significant reduction in body weight compared to non-transgenic littermates [135]. Despite equivalent food intake, transgenic GDF15 mice had less white and brown fat, improved glucose tolerance, lower insulin levels, and were resistant to dietary-and genetic-induced obesity [136]. In wild-type mice, oral metformin increased GDF15 circulating protein levels and GDF15 mRNA in the small intestine, colon, and kidney. Metformin decreased food intake and prevented weight gain in response to a high-fat diet in wild-type mice but not in mice lacking GDF15 or its receptor. In obese mice on a high-fat diet, the effects of metformin to reduce body weight were reversed by a GFRAL-antagonist antibody [132], suggesting that metformin activity could be mediated by GDF-15.

GDF15 is also essential for the increased insulin sensitivity associated with the use of metformin. The pharmacological mechanism underlying the metformin induction of GDF15 seems to involve the integrated stress pathway [132]. In primary mouse hepatocytes, metformin stimulates the secretion of GDF15 by increasing the expression of activating transcription factor 4 (ATF4) and C/EBP homologous protein (CHOP) [133]. The new insight that the lower small intestine and colon are major sites of metformin-induced GDF15 expression, provides further evidence that metformin can mediate its benefits, at least in part, by acting on the intestinal epithelium as a major target.

3.2.3. Gut Microbiota

High interest has been focused on the gut microbiota as a target of metformin action. A double-blind study indicated that metformin can change intestinal microbiota composition in human patients and that glucose tolerance is improved in mice receiving metformin-altered microbiota [121]. Metagenomic and metabolomic analysis of samples from individuals with T2DM and treated with metformin for 3 days, revealed that metformin treatment increased the levels of the bile acid glycoursodeoxycholic acid (GUDCA) in the gut by decreasing the abundance of species of *Bacteroides fragilis*. It was found that GUDCA is a novel antagonist of intestinal FXR, a ligand-activated nuclear receptor that regulates hepatic bile acid biosynthesis, transport, and secretion and may inhibit GLP1 secretion from L cells [137]. In addition, metformin increases the abundance of short-chain fatty acid (SCFA)-producing bacteria and facilitates SCFA-induced GLP1 secretion via signaling through GPR41 and GPR43 in L cells [138]. However, in contrast with all these observations, a different study showed that metformin significantly improved oral glucose tolerance also in GLP1R$^{-/-}$ mice and in wild-type mice fed with a high-fat diet and treated with a GLP1R inhibitor [125].

3.3. Muscle as a Target Tissue

Some studies have suggested that skeletal muscle may be involved in the glucose-lowering properties of metformin. Early studies showed that metformin lowers glucose levels in T2DM patients by increasing insulin-stimulated glucose uptake [80,139,140].

In isolated skeletal muscle, Zhou et al. reported that metformin activated AMPK and concomitantly increased glucose uptake, an effect that was additive with insulin stimulation [86]. These observations led to the conclusion that, by inhibiting complex I and activating AMPK, metformin promotes glucose uptake in muscle [93] and enhances insulin sensitivity [141]. However, this hypothesis has been challenged by a very recent study on the muscle-specific knockout of AMPKα1/α2 mouse models, where it was shown that lack of AMPK activity in skeletal muscle of lean and diet-induced obese mice does not affect the ability of metformin to lower blood glucose levels or improve whole-body glucose tolerance [142]. Moreover, in T2DM patients rendered normoglycemic with 4 weeks of insulin treatment, metformin had no effect on insulin-stimulated peripheral glucose metabolism [143], suggesting that the ability of metformin to increase insulin-stimulated muscle glucose uptake could be secondary to improved glucose homeostasis and reduction of glucose toxicity rather than due to a direct effect.

4. Biguanides and Cancer

The anti-tumor properties of biguanides were unknown until 2005, when Evans et al. [144] identified in diabetic patients an inverse correlation between metformin treatment and cancer occurrence, paving the way for the exploration of biguanides usage in cancer therapy and prevention. Until December 2021, metformin has been investigated in 1901 clinical trials on various types of cancer, and 216 of them are still underway. While studies seem to support the anti-tumor effects of metformin in diabetic patients, less is known about the therapeutic effect of metformin in non-diabetic cancer patients. Many studies have been focused on the understanding of the molecular mechanism underlying the anti-cancer properties of biguanides that led to the identification of a plethora of different molecular targets. Similar to the research on diabetes, in this context, the exact mechanism by which biguanides operate and their target selectivity in different experimental conditions is still controversial, due to the lack of a unifying model.

In general, biguanides are believed to exert their antitumor properties by two main mechanisms: direct, by acting directly on the tumor cells and inhibiting their growth, and indirect, by inducing changes in the body that ultimately affect tumorigenesis.

4.1. Direct Antitumor Effects

The notion that biguanides exert direct antitumor effects comes mostly from the evidence that the growth, proliferation, viability, and/or motility of cultured cancer cells are impaired upon exposure to the drugs. As for the regulation of glucose homeostasis, also in this context, mitochondria are believed to be the main site of biguanides action, and AMPK is a critical mediator of their therapeutic effects.

4.1.1. Mitochondrial Mechanisms

Most studies addressing the mechanism of action of biguanides have been focused on targets localized into the mitochondria (Figure 2). As discussed above, it is widely recognized that metformin is capable of inhibiting complex I of the electron transport chain. Supporting the role of complex I inhibition as an important player in the anti-tumorigenic effect of metformin target in cancer, cells expressing the rotenone-resistant yeast complex I analog NDI1 were no longer inhibited by metformin [145]. Similarly, ectopic expression of NDI1 impaired the ability of phenformin to inhibit cancer cell proliferation and oxygen consumption, although only in cells with complex I mutations [146]. However, while the use of NDI1 overexpression is generally considered relevant evidence to confirm complex I involvement, it has to be noted that NDI1 corrects the $NAD^+/NADH$ ratio, which can be reduced by many alterations in mitochondria other than inhibition of complex I (e.g., see [147]).

Also, the use of NDI1 may have limitations if not carefully controlled. For instance, its exclusive localization in the mitochondria should be verified, the expression levels should be monitored during experimentation, and complex I should be inactivated in cells expressing NDI1, to avoid artifactual results.

Targeting complex I using small molecules has shown anti-cancer efficacy in vitro and in animal models [148,149]. Several observations point to the inhibition of complex I as the main mechanism of action of metformin in cancer cells. In human oral squamous carcinoma KB cells, metformin (0.1–10 mM) specifically inhibits complex I, both in intact cells and after permeabilization [150]. Metformin (3–10 mM) effectively diminished pancreatic cancer stem cells by the inhibition of mitochondrial respiration [151]. In permeabilized human HCT116 $p53^{-/-}$ colorectal carcinoma cells expressing NDI1, metformin (0.25–1 mM) failed to decrease cell proliferation [145], while metformin (1–10 mM) potently inhibited mitochondrial complex I in pancreatic ductal adenocarcinoma cells [152].

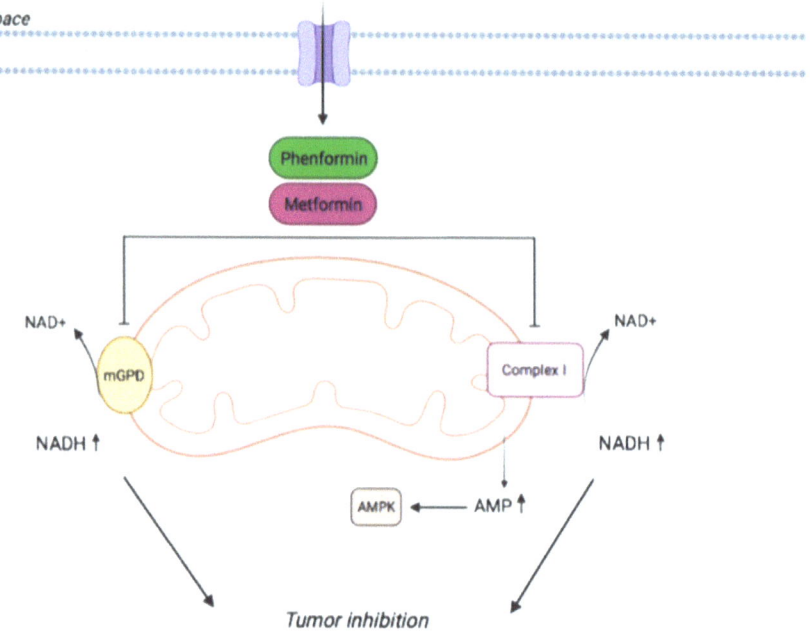

Figure 2. Redox-dependent inhibition of tumor growth by biguanides. Therapeutic doses of biguanides inhibit mGPD in cancer cells, increasing NADH content and redox state and inhibiting tumor growth. Supra-pharmacologic concentrations of biguanides inhibit complex I, increasing NADH content and AMP levels and suppressing tumor growth.

In 2019, Momcilovic and colleagues used 4-(18F) fluorobenzyl-triphenylphosphonium (18F-BnTP PET) imaging to detect in vivo changes in mitochondrial membrane potential in a mouse model of lung cancer. They showed that phenformin decreases the uptake of the tracer, indicating the ability of the drug to lower mitochondrial membrane potential (ψ), a consequence attributed by the authors to complex I inhibition [153], although a decrease of membrane potential can also be caused by inhibition of other mitochondrial targets, such as mGPD [154] or by the accumulation of the positively charged biguanide in the mitochondria.

Since in the majority of the above-mentioned studies biguanides have been used at supraphysiological doses that are unlikely to reflect the actual concentrations measured in humans and animal models [33,155,156], it is generally tempted to believe that other mechanisms, beyond complex I inhibition, may operate on cellular and animal models exposed to therapeutic concentrations of biguanides.

Recent work carried out on Sonic Hedgehog-driven medulloblastoma cells showed that pharmacological phenformin concentrations (1–5 µM) inhibit tumor growth independently of complex I and AMPK, through alterations in cytoplasmic redox potential and increased NADH levels [52], by inhibiting glycerol-3-phosphate dehydrogenase. Elevated NADH levels promote the association between the redox sensor CtBP2 and the transcription factor GLI1, leading to inhibition of Hedgehog-dependent transcriptional output and medulloblastoma growth.

In keeping with these findings, it has been observed that in thyroid cancer cells, metformin inhibits the activity and downregulates the expression of mGPD, decreasing their growth and metabolism [157]. Another work showed that low expression of cGPD correlates with poor responses to metformin in 15 cell lines of various cancer types and that cGPD overexpression enhanced the anticancer activity of metformin, leading to glycerol-3-phosphate overproduction and inhibition of mitochondrial function [158].

In contrast to this study, it was shown that ablation of cGPD enhanced the inhibition of tumor growth mediated by metformin, although the biguanide was given at supraphysiological concentrations [159].

Consistent with redox imbalance as a major alteration underlying the antiproliferative effect of metformin, Gui and collaborators [160] proposed that metformin's antiproliferative effect is due to loss of $NAD^+/NADH$ homeostasis and inhibition of aspartate biosynthesis, an effect that was attributed to the blockade of NADH dehydrogenase activity of complex I rather than to mGPD inhibition and that could be rescued by pyruvate, due to its ability to regenerate NAD^+.

Therefore, these latter studies seem to point at $NADH/NAD^+$ alteration as key mechanisms underlying the antitumor properties of biguanides, although concerns about the primary target need to be properly addressed, as discussed above (Figure 2).

4.1.2. AMPK as a Mediator of the Response to Biguanides in Cancer

Although the activation of the energy sensor AMPK represents one of the most frequently evoked events accompanying biguanides therapeutic action, the role of AMPK in cancer seems to be ambiguous [161]. The discovery that AMPK is the key downstream effector of the tumor suppressor LKB1 and the ability of AMPK to inhibit fatty acid synthesis, mRNA translation, and cell growth support the notion that this kinase acts as a tumor suppressor. However, in different contexts, at different stages of tumor development or under certain conditions (e.g., metabolic stress), AMPK seems to function as a tumor promoter, by activating programs that facilitate cancer progression and survival [162].

In this view, the use of AMPK agonists is now suggested to be more appropriate for cancer prevention, while AMPK inhibitors seem to be better suited for the treatment of established malignancies [161].

Supporting the notion of a tumor-promoting function of AMPK, phenformin was shown to be more effective in reducing lung tumor growth when cells lacked a functional LKB1/AMPK pathway [54].

However, many studies have supported the metformin-mediated activation of AMPK as a tumor-suppressive mechanism (Figure 3). In the "classical" mechanism, metformin inhibits complex I of the mitochondrial respiratory chain and ATP synthase, raising the levels of intracellular AMP/ADP that trigger the activation of AMPK [41]. Alternatively, metformin may activate AMPK through the lysosomal pathway by a non-canonical mechanism [163]. Indeed, AMPK can be activated by low concentrations of metformin through the formation of a complex with Axin and late endosomal/lysosomal adaptor, MAPK, and LAMTOR1. Thus, metformin might also activate AMPK by a mechanism involving the lysosomes, rather than complex I.

Once activated, AMPK is thought to inhibit key substrates involved in cell growth and proliferation, being the most relevant and best-studied the mechanistic Target Of Rapamycin Complex 1 (mTORC1). mTORC1 plays a key role in controlling the metabolism, growth, and proliferation of cancer cells [164,165] mostly by phosphorylating two key targets: S6 Kinase 1 (S6K1) and initiation factor 4E binding protein 1 (4E-BP1) [166,167]. By activating AMPK, biguanides are thought to inhibit mTORC1 through phosphorylation of TSC1, TSC2, and Raptor [168,169]. Additionally, Kalender and collaborators demonstrated that biguanides suppress mTORC1 signaling also independently of AMPK and TSC1/2, by inhibiting Rag GTPases [170].

Besides mTORC1 inhibition, AMPK has been also shown to promote p53 activation via phosphorylation of Ser15, thus promoting cell survival in response to glucose limitation [171] and p53-deficient cancer cells were shown to be more sensitive to metformin treatment [172], indicating that p53 regulates cancer cells survival in response to metformin-induced metabolic changes.

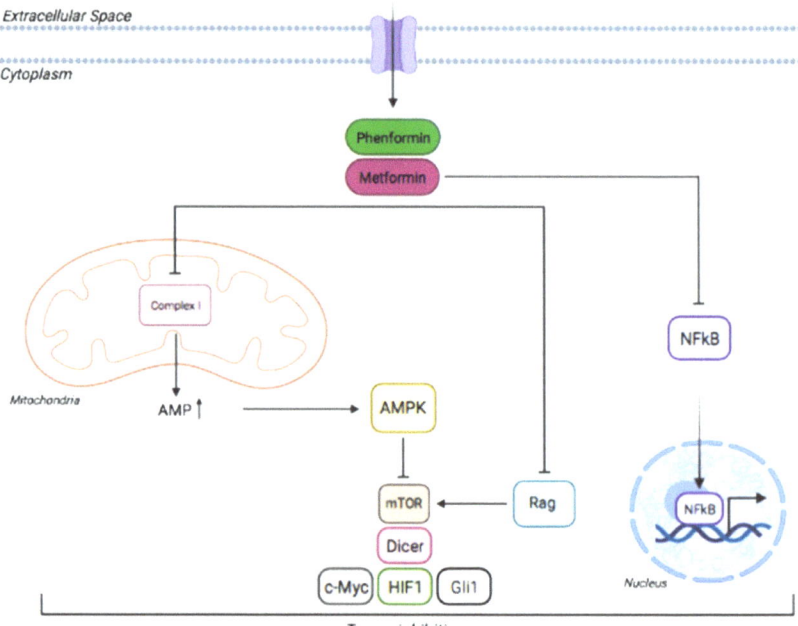

Figure 3. AMPK-dependent and AMPK-independent inhibition of tumor growth by biguanides. Supra-pharmacological concentrations of biguanides inhibit complex I, which increases AMP levels and leads to the activation of AMPK. Alternatively, metformin prevents the activation of NFkB pathway by inhibiting the translocation of NFkB to the nucleus. AMPK regulates DICER, cMyc, HIF1α, and Gli1 activity and inhibits mTOR complex, suppressing tumor growth. Biguanides also inhibit Rag GTPases to suppress mTOR signaling.

Other targets regulated by metformin via AMPK, causing inhibition of cancer cell proliferation by blocking the Warburg effect are DICER, cMyc, HIF1α [173]. Conversely, other works found that metformin inhibits the growth of various cancers by preventing nuclear translocation of the transcription factor NFkB, an effect that was believed to be independent of AMPK [174–177] (Figure 3).

In a work on ovarian cancer patients, it was shown that metformin treatment affects pathways related to mitochondrial metabolism involving nucleotide metabolism, redox, and energy status [178]. More recently, a study in breast cancer patients showed that metformin reduces the levels of mitochondrial metabolites and increases 18-FDG flux in primary breast cancers, without apparent activation of AMPK, arguing against the involvement of this kinase in mediating the effects of metformin in this clinical context [179]. Similarly, in mouse models of SHH medulloblastoma, it was recently shown that phenformin elicited a potent antitumor effect independently of AMPK and of phosphorylation of the AMPK substrate GLI1 [52,180].

Together, all these data suggest that the exact role of AMPK as a mediator of biguanide anticancer action is still unclear and studies using specific loss of function in in vivo models, at different stages of cancer development, are required.

4.2. Indirect Antitumor Effects

4.2.1. Effects on Insulin Signaling

The ability of biguanides to lower blood glucose levels through inhibition of hepatic gluconeogenesis and glucose uptake in muscle is thought to contribute to their antitumor properties. Indeed, owing to their glucose-lowering effects, biguanides also reduce circulating levels of insulin and IGF-1. Both hormones bind to receptors that are often expressed at high levels in cancer cells or in cells from which tumors originate, and that activate the oncogenic PAM (Pi3K-AKT-mTOR) pathway, leading to activation of mTOR and promoting cell proliferation and growth [181,182]. Supporting this notion, patients with type II diabetes, who have insulin resistance and thus higher levels of circulating insulin, are at higher risk for various types of cancers due to the mitogenic effects of insulin. Indeed, it has been observed that there is an increased risk of various cancers, including breast [183,184], prostate [185], and colon [186,187] cancers in hyperinsulinemic and obese patients, compared to normal subjects. In this view, the indirect anticancer properties of biguanides are thought to play a role mostly in patients with hyperinsulinemia rather than in subjects that are not insulin resistant at baseline [188].

4.2.2. Effects on the Immune System

According to emerging studies, many of the antitumoral properties of biguanides may rely on their ability to target different components of the immune cells (CD8$^+$T cells, Tregs, MDSC, TAM) in the tumor microenvironment.

CD8$^+$ T cells: Pearce et al. [189] showed that metformin promotes the generation of CD8$^+$ T cells and increases protective immunity against lymphoma in mice, while Ekawa et al. [190] demonstrated that metformin enhances tumor infiltration of CD8$^+$T cells, protects them from apoptosis, and promotes the production of IL-2, TNFα, INFγ. Metformin was also shown to increase the effect of anti-PD1-therapy in melanoma cells, by alleviating CD8$^+$ T cell suppression through inhibition of cancer cell oxygen consumption and consequent reduction of the hypoxic tumor microenvironment [191]. Additionally, metformin enhances the antitumor immune response of cytotoxic T lymphocytes (CTL) through AMPK-mediated phosphorylation of PD-L1 at S195, which is followed by glycosylation and ERAD-mediated degradation. Therefore, it was shown that the combination of metformin with anti-CTLA4 therapy has a synergistic antitumor effect [192]. Conversely, other studies showed that phenformin decreased INFγ production from CD8$^+$ T cells [193] and did not affect tumor infiltration of CTC cells [194].

Thus, given the divergence of these observations, further studies seem to be required to fully understand the effect of biguanides on CD8$^+$ T cells.

- Tregs: Biguanides modulate the activity of Tregs, which suppress cytotoxic T cell functions required for tumor elimination. The administration of metformin was shown to decrease the infiltration of Tregs and to reprogram the tumor immune microenvironment in patients with esophageal squamous cell carcinoma [195].
- MDSC: MDSCs are myeloid cell precursors that increase cancer and suppress T and NK cells. Recent works have shown that biguanides inhibit the function of MDSCs in different cancer models and with various mechanisms [196–198].
- TAM: Tumor-associated macrophages may contribute to creating an immunosuppressive tumor microenvironment that promotes cancer development. Recent studies have shown that metformin may change the macrophage population toward tumor-suppressive subsets or may inhibit macrophage polarization towards the M2 phenotype in various tumors [199,200].

4.3. Variables Affecting the Response to Biguanides in Cancer

The sensitivity of cancer cells to biguanides depends on genetic and microenvironmental factors that allow adaptation to metabolic dysfunctions. Many studies suggest that biguanides alter substrate utilization in the mitochondria [178]. Cancer cells that strongly depend on mitochondrial metabolism and are poorly capable of engaging compensatory glycolysis would be highly sensitive to biguanides. Conversely, leukemia and lymphoma cells markedly depend on the activation of HIF-1a signaling during exposure to biguanides, being resistant to biguanide-induced complex I dysfunction mediated by HIF1α-regulated transcriptional rewiring of glucose metabolism [201]. Cancer cells with mitochondrial defects show a higher sensitivity to biguanides due to the lack of metabolic flexibility at the mitochondrial level. This hypothesis has been confirmed by the evidence of higher phenformin sensitivity in cells harboring complex I mutations [146,153]. Additionally, cancer cells with a defective PGC-1α axis are more sensitive to metformin as well as cells with impaired AMPK signaling [202–204], being unable to metabolically adapt to the unfavorable conditions of energy depletion.

The metabolic environment seems also to influence the sensitivity to biguanides. Gui et al. [205] demonstrated that culture media alters the sensitivity of cancer cells to metformin, as cells cultured in DMEM required up to 10 mM metformin to inhibit proliferation, while cells cultured in RPMI media required lower metformin doses. In this scenario, pyruvate was proposed to suppress the anti-proliferative effects of metformin, since cells cultured in DMEM without pyruvate showed increased sensitivity to metformin, while cells cultured in RPMI supplemented with 1 mM pyruvate were less sensitive. Authors proposed that pyruvate modulates complex I dependency by providing an alternative pathway for NAD^+ regeneration since it acts as an electron acceptor for NAD^+ regeneration allowing aspartate synthesis [160]. Similarly, glucose availability plays a crucial role in the response to metformin since it was demonstrated that metformin sensitivity in cancer cells was increased upon lowering glucose concentration to 11 mM or upon addition of aspartate (150 µM) in culture media [160]. In another paper from Birsoy and colleagues [146], the authors demonstrated that cancer cells with defects in glucose utilization or complex I function were more sensitive to phenformin. In 0.75 mM glucose media, cell lines with complex I mutations or impaired glucose utilization were 5- to 20-fold more sensitive to phenformin compared to control cancer cell lines. This effect of glucose availability on biguanides sensitivity of cancer cells was further confirmed by another paper where medulloblastoma cells were treated with biguanides in media containing 5.5 mM glucose, corresponding to the average physiological plasma fasting concentration, or 0.75 mM glucose, corresponding to the cancer tissue glucose concentration [52], The authors show that phenformin induced a significant inhibition of cell growth, with a stronger effect at 0.75 mM glucose. While in high glucose conditions the antiproliferative effects of metformin are mediated by the AMPK/LKB1 axis, at low glucose concentrations in the absence of AMPK/LKB1 cells are more sensitive to growth inhibition by metformin, because they are not able to sustain the high energy demand. Dietary limitation through intermittent fasting has been shown to enhance the response to biguanides, and metformin seems to impair tumor growth only when administered during fasting-induced hypoglycemia [205].

Biodistribution and tissue specificity seem also to determine the degree of biguanides accumulation and thus influence their molecular and therapeutical actions. Indeed, the glucose-lowering effect of metformin resulting from inhibition of hepatic gluconeogenesis correlates with the high tissue concentrations that the drug reaches in the liver. Metformin is usually administered orally in diabetic patients, reaching concentrations between 40 and 70 µM in the portal vein, and it accumulates to a larger extent in the gut and liver. This is due to the systemic circulation and to the high level of expression of OCT transporters in these tissues. However, this is not representative of other tissues or organs, where metformin reaches lower micromolar concentrations.

4.4. Clinical Studies

Alteration of cellular metabolism is a hallmark of tumor cells, also believed to represent an attractive target for cancer therapy. The best known metabolic alteration in cancer is represented by the so-called Warburg effect, consisting of the transformation of glucose to lactate, regardless of the presence of extracellular oxygen [206]. In more recent years it has been understood that mitochondria are also essential for tumor growth, mostly because of their biosynthetic role rather than their pro-energetic features [207]. In this view, the ability of metformin to inhibit mitochondrial function seems to play an important role in mediating its anti-cancer effect. However, the low availability of metformin in humans at therapeutic antidiabetic doses has pointed to the need to find strategies aimed to maximize its activity and enhance its toxicity toward cancer cells. In this regard, several groups have improved mitochondrial targeting of metformin to achieve therapeutically effective plasma concentrations in cancer patients by modifying its chemical structure, which resulted in mitochondria-targeted metformin analogs with significantly enhanced anti-tumor potential [208,209].

Clinical studies have been performed in diabetic patients where metformin was shown to reduce the incidence of liver, colorectal, breast, and pancreatic cancers and to increase the survival of colorectal, lung, and prostate cancer patients (Table 2). A meta-analysis of ovarian cancer showed a lower incidence and significantly increased survival in patients with diabetes [210]. Another meta-analysis in diabetic patients estimated the relationship between lung cancer incidence and metformin usage and showed a lower risk of cancer in metformin users if compared to non-users [211].

Table 2. Clinical trials of biguanides in cancer.

No.	NCT-ID	Title	Status	Treatment	Phase
1	NCT01941953	Metformin and 5-fluorouracil for Refractory Colorectal Cancer	Completed	Metformin Fluorouracil	Phase 2
2	NCT02614339	Effect of Adjunctive Metformin on Recurrence of Non-DM Colorectal Cancer Stage II High-risk/III Colorectal Cancer	Recruiting	Metformin	Phase 3
3	NCT01312467	Trial of Metformin for Colorectal Cancer Risk Reduction for History of Colorectal Adenomas and Elevated BMI	Completed	Metformin HCl	Phase 2
4	NCT01926769	A Phase II Study to Determine the Safety and Efficacy of Second-line Treatment with Metformin and Chemotherapy (FOLFOX6 or FOFIRI) in the Second-Line Treatment of Advanced Colorectal Cancer	Terminated	Metformin	Phase 2
5	NCT01523639	A Randomized, Placebo-controlled, Double-blind Phase II Study Evaluating if Glucophage Can Avoid Liver Injury Due to Chemotherapy Associated Steatosis	Terminated	Metformin	Phase 2
6	NCT01816659	An Open-Labeled Pilot Study of Biomarker Response Following Short-Term Exposure to Metformin	Terminated	Metformin ER	Phase 1
7	NCT03800602	Nivolumab and Metformin in Patients with Treatment Refractory MSS Colorectal Cancer	Recruiting	Metformin Nivolumab	Phase 2
8	NCT01930864	Metformin Plus Irinotecan for Refractory Colorectal Cancer	Recruiting	Metformin Irinotecan	Phase 2
9	NCT03047837	A Randomized, 2 × 2 Factorial Design Biomarker Prevention Trial of Low-dose Aspirin and Metformin in Stage I-III Colorectal Cancer Patients	Recruiting	Aspirin Metformin	Phase 2
10	NCT01440127	Impact of Pretreatment with Metformin on Colorectal Cancer Stem Cells (CCSC) and Related Pharmacodynamic Markers	Terminated	Metformin	Phase 1

Table 2. Cont.

No.	NCT-ID	Title	Status	Treatment	Phase
11	NCT01340300	Exercise and Metformin in Colorectal and Breast Cancer Survivors	Completed	Metformin, Exercise training, Educational information	Phase 2
12	NCT04033107	High Dose Vitamin C Combined with Metformin in the Treatment of Malignant Tumors	Recruiting	Vitamin C Metformin	Phase 2
13	NCT01632020	Effect of Metformin on Biomarkers of Colorectal Tumor Cell Growth	Terminated	Metformin	Phase 2
14	NCT03359681	Metformin Treatment for Colon Cancer	Recruiting	Metformin	Phase 2
15	NCT02431676	Survivorship Promotion in Reducing IGF-1 Trial	Completed	Metformin, Coach Directed Behavioral Weight Loss, Self-control weight loss	Phase 2
16	NCT02201381	Study of the Safety, Tolerability, and Efficacy of Metabolic Combination Treatments on Cancer	Recruiting	Metformin Atorvastatin Doxycycline Mebendazole	Phase 3
17	NCT02437656	Combination of Metformin with Neoadjuvant Radiochemotherapy in the Treatment of Locally Advanced (METCAP).	Completed	Metformin	Phase 2
18	NCT03053544	Metformin with Neoadjuvant Chemoradiation to Improve Pathologic Responses in Rectal Cancer	Completed	Metformin	Phase 2
19	NCT02473094	Neoadjuvant Metformin in Association with Chemoradiotherapy for Locally Advanced Rectal Cancer	Terminated	Metformin Capecitabine	Phase 2
20	NCT01620593	Castration Compared to Castration Plus Metformin as First-Line Treatment for Patients with Advanced Prostate Cancer	Completed	Metformin	Phase 2
21	NCT02581137	Metformin Hydrochloride in Preventing Oral Cancer in Patients with an Oral Premalignant Lesion	Active	Metformin	Phase 2
22	NCT01447927	Metformin Hydrochloride in Preventing Esophageal Cancer in Patients with Barrett Esophagus	Completed	Metformin	Phase 2
23	NCT03238495	Randomized Trial of Neo-adjuvant Chemotherapy With or Without Metformin for HER2 Positive Operable Breast Cancer (HERMET)	Recruiting	Taxotere, Carboplatin, Herceptin + Pertuzumab Metformin	Phase 2
24	NCT03026517	Clinical Trial of Phenformin in Combination With BRAF Inhibitor + MEK Inhibitor for Patients With BRAF-mutated	Recruiting	Dabrafenib Trametinib Phenformin	Phase 1

More recently, many clinical trials have been developed to investigate the anti-tumoral potential of metformin in nondiabetic patients. Two perspective trials on metformin combinatorial therapy with platinum-based chemotherapy in advanced NSCLC (Non-Small Cell Lung Cancer) showed a composed median overall survival of 17.5 months for patients with

KRAS mutations with good tolerability, validating metformin clinical efficacy as adjuvant therapy in this setting [65]. One phase I trial of metformin combinatorial treatment with standard therapy in relapsed refractory acute lymphoblastic leukemia showed an overall response rate (complete and partial responses) of 43% [212]. One randomized, phase II clinical trial of metformin in combination with standard chemotherapy in HER2-negative metastatic breast cancer showed no benefit. Another randomized trial combining metformin with neo-adjuvant chemotherapy in HER2-positive breast cancers (NCT03238495) is still underway. One meta-analysis in pancreatic cancer patients evidenced a significant increase in overall survival in patients at stage I–II and at stage I–IV treated with adjuvant metformin, suggesting a potentially available option for the treatment [213]. However, a randomized phase II study of metformin combinatorial treatment with standard systemic therapy in metastatic pancreatic cancer patients did not show any significant improvement in the clinical outcome [214].

Phenformin is currently in phase I clinical trials for combinatorial treatment with dabrafenib and trametinib in patients with BRAFV600E/K-mutated melanoma (NCT03026517).

These studies in normal subjects will unveil the potential of biguanides in oncology, revealing their ability to counteract tumor growth and progression and clarifying the contribution of their systemic effects in the successful clinical outcome that has been observed in diabetic patients treated with this class of drugs.

5. Conclusions

Although metformin is prescribed to more than 120 million patients worldwide and almost 3000 papers on biguanides are published every year, how these drugs exert their therapeutic effects is an open question that still begs conclusive answers.

Based on the topics discussed in this article, some conclusions that will find a broad consensus may be drawn and should be taken as general guidelines in future investigations.

1. While inhibition of complex I activity at millimolar concentrations of biguanides is a reproducible phenomenon in vitro and in cell culture, it remains to be fully clarified if this occurs in animal models or in patients taking standard doses of the drugs and, even in such case, if the degree of inhibition is sufficient to mediate a significant biological response when the drugs are given orally at the therapeutic conditions. Except for some tissues, such as the gut and liver, biguanides have been only found at low micromolar concentrations in the body of people taking therapeutic doses of the drugs. Data obtained with overexpression of the budding yeast NDI1, which is often used to formally demonstrate complex I-dependence, may actually be due to effects on other mitochondrial regulators of $NAD^+/NADH$ ratio and have to be carefully controlled.
2. Activation of AMPK and phosphorylation of its downstream targets are additional well-established events, often believed to be responsible for the therapeutic response to biguanides. As for complex I inhibition, AMPK phosphorylation is generally detected in most cell culture experiments when millimolar doses of biguanides are used. In addition, some data obtained in animal models have shown a certain degree of phosphorylation of AMPK and its targets in response to low levels of biguanides. However, it remains to be fully elucidated if the magnitude of activation reached under therapeutic conditions is biologically meaningful and whether targeted deletion of AMPK truly impairs the response to biguanides in vivo.
3. Any concentration of biguanides, including those that fall within the therapeutic range, causes redox imbalance, with an increased $NADH/NAD^+$ ratio. It is still unclear if this is the consequence of the interaction of biguanides with complex I and/or mGPD and/or complex IV and/or other mechanisms. Regardless of the target involved, it should be carefully evaluated to what extent and how redox alterations affect gluconeogenesis or cancer growth. Approaches directed to the selective targeting of the redox state, possibly without causing energy stress, would be needed to properly address this issue.

4. The anticancer effect of biguanides is dependent on several local variables in the tumor microenvironment: drug concentration, nutrient concentration (glucose, pyruvate, amino acids, etc.), and genetic mutations affecting metabolic processes (e.g., respiration, glucose utilization). These aspects need to be fully characterized and evaluated when treating any cells in vivo and in vitro.
5. Biguanides are typically taken orally, and this implies that their effect could be mediated, at least in part, by the interaction with the cells of the GI tract and the commensal microbiota, which may both release molecules involved in an indirect response to the drug. To date, it is still unclear and debated the exact contribution of the gut to the therapeutic properties of biguanides. This issue should also be considered when administering the drug to animal models, by evaluating the effect after parenteral (i.e., i.p., i.v.) administration.

Author Contributions: Conceptualization: G.C.; Funding acquisition: G.C.; Writing—original draft: L.D.M., F.D.P., R.B. and G.C.; Writing—review and editing: L.D.M., S.C. and G.C. All authors have read and agreed to the published version of the manuscript.

Funding: This work was supported by AIRC, IG 2021, code n. 25833 (G.C.); Istituto Pasteur Italia—Fondazione Cenci Bolognetti, Call 2018 Anna Tramontano (G.C.); Sapienza University of Rome (RG12117A61923A6F), Dipartimenti di Eccellenza—L. 232/2016 and Fondazione Umberto Veronesi (fellowship to LDM).

Data Availability Statement: The data presented in this study are available on request from the corresponding author.

Conflicts of Interest: The authors declare that they have no known competing financial interests or personal relationships that could have appeared to influence the work reported in this paper.

References

1. Bailey, C.J. Metformin: Historical Overview. *Diabetologia* **2017**, *60*, 1566–1576. [CrossRef] [PubMed]
2. Currie, C.J.; Poole, C.D.; Jenkins-Jones, S.; Gale, E.A.M.; Johnson, J.A.; Morgan, C.L. Mortality after Incident Cancer in People with and without Type 2 Diabetes: Impact of Metformin on Survival. *Diabetes Care* **2012**, *35*, 299–304. [CrossRef]
3. Bowker, S.L.; Majumdar, S.R.; Veugelers, P.; Johnson, J.A. Increased Cancer-Related Mortality for Patients with Type 2 Diabetes Who Use Sulfonylureas or Insulin. *Diabetes Care* **2006**, *29*, 254–258. [CrossRef] [PubMed]
4. Decensi, A.; Puntoni, M.; Goodwin, P.; Cazzaniga, M.; Gennari, A.; Bonanni, B.; Gandini, S. Metformin and Cancer Risk in Diabetic Patients: A Systematic Review and Meta-Analysis. *Cancer Prev. Res.* **2010**, *3*, 1451–1461. [CrossRef] [PubMed]
5. Walker, R.S.; Linton, A.L. Phenethyldiguanide: A Dangerous Side-Effect. *Br. Med. J.* **1959**, *2*, 1005–1006. [CrossRef]
6. Luft, D.; Schmülling, R.M.; Eggstein, M. Lactic Acidosis in Biguanide-Treated Diabetics: A Review of 330 Cases. *Diabetologia* **1978**, *14*, 75–87. [CrossRef] [PubMed]
7. Werner, E.A.; Bell, J. CCXIV—The Preparation of Methylguanidine, and of Bβ-Dimethylguanidine by the Interaction of Dicyanodiamide, and Methylammonium and Dimethylammonium Chlorides Respectively. *J. Chem. Soc. Trans.* **1922**, *121*, 1790–1794. [CrossRef]
8. Slotta, K.H.; Tschesche, R. Über Biguanide, II.: Die Blutzucker-Senkende Wirkung Der Biguanide. *Ber. Dtsch. Chem. Ges. (A and B Series)* **1929**, *62*, 1398–1405. [CrossRef]
9. Sterne, J. Du nouveau dans les antidiabetiques. La NN dimethylamine guanyl guanide (NNDG). *Maroc. Med.* **1957**, *36*, 1295–1296.
10. Graham, G.G.; Punt, J.; Arora, M.; Day, R.O.; Doogue, M.P.; Duong, T.J.; Furlong, T.J.; Greenfield, J.R.; Greenup, L.C.; Kirkpatrick, C.M.; et al. Clinical Pharmacokinetics of Metformin. *Clin. Pharm.* **2011**, *50*, 81–98. [CrossRef] [PubMed]
11. Jonker, J.W.; Wagenaar, E.; Mol, C.A.; Buitelaar, M.; Koepsell, H.; Smit, J.W.; Schinkel, A.H. Reduced Hepatic Uptake and Intestinal Excretion of Organic Cations in Mice with a Targeted Disruption of the Organic Cation Transporter 1 (Oct1 [Slc22a1]) Gene. *Mol. Cell Biol.* **2001**, *21*, 5471–5477. [CrossRef]
12. Shu, Y.; Leabman, M.K.; Feng, B.; Mangravite, L.M.; Huang, C.C.; Stryke, D.; Kawamoto, M.; Johns, S.J.; DeYoung, J.; Carlson, E.; et al. Evolutionary Conservation Predicts Function of Variants of the Human Organic Cation Transporter, OCT1. *Proc. Natl. Acad. Sci. USA* **2003**, *100*, 5902–5907. [CrossRef]
13. Nakamichi, N.; Shima, H.; Asano, S.; Ishimoto, T.; Sugiura, T.; Matsubara, K.; Kusuhara, H.; Sugiyama, Y.; Sai, Y.; Miyamoto, K.-I.; et al. Involvement of Carnitine/Organic Cation Transporter OCTN1/SLC22A4 in Gastrointestinal Absorption of Metformin. *J. Pharm. Sci.* **2013**, *102*, 3407–3417. [CrossRef]
14. Zhou, M.; Xia, L.; Wang, J. Metformin Transport by a Newly Cloned Proton-Stimulated Organic Cation Transporter (Plasma Membrane Monoamine Transporter) Expressed in Human Intestine. *Drug Metab. Dispos.* **2007**, *35*, 1956–1962. [CrossRef] [PubMed]

15. Chen, E.C.; Liang, X.; Yee, S.W.; Geier, E.G.; Stocker, S.L.; Chen, L.; Giacomini, K.M. Targeted Disruption of Organic Cation Transporter 3 Attenuates the Pharmacologic Response to Metformin. *Mol. Pharmacol.* **2015**, *88*, 75–83. [CrossRef]
16. Masuda, S.; Terada, T.; Yonezawa, A.; Tanihara, Y.; Kishimoto, K.; Katsura, T.; Ogawa, O.; Inui, K. Identification and Functional Characterization of a New Human Kidney-Specific H+/Organic Cation Antiporter, Kidney-Specific Multidrug and Toxin Extrusion 2. *J. Am. Soc. Nephrol.* **2006**, *17*, 2127–2135. [CrossRef]
17. Xia, L.; Engel, K.; Zhou, M.; Wang, J. Membrane Localization and PH-Dependent Transport of a Newly Cloned Organic Cation Transporter (PMAT) in Kidney Cells. *Am. J. Physiol. Renal. Physiol.* **2007**, *292*, F682–F690. [CrossRef]
18. Choi, M.-K.; Song, I.-S. Organic Cation Transporters and Their Pharmacokinetic and Pharmacodynamic Consequences. *Drug Metab. Pharmacokinet* **2008**, *23*, 243–253. [CrossRef]
19. Hilgendorf, C.; Ahlin, G.; Seithel, A.; Artursson, P.; Ungell, A.-L.; Karlsson, J. Expression of Thirty-Six Drug Transporter Genes in Human Intestine, Liver, Kidney, and Organotypic Cell Lines. *Drug Metab. Dispos.* **2007**, *35*, 1333–1340. [CrossRef] [PubMed]
20. Müller, J.; Lips, K.S.; Metzner, L.; Neubert, R.H.H.; Koepsell, H.; Brandsch, M. Drug Specificity and Intestinal Membrane Localization of Human Organic Cation Transporters (OCT). *Biochem. Pharmacol.* **2005**, *70*, 1851–1860. [CrossRef]
21. Gong, L.; Goswami, S.; Giacomini, K.M.; Altman, R.B.; Klein, T.E. Metformin Pathways: Pharmacokinetics and Pharmacodynamics. *Pharm. Genom.* **2012**, *22*, 820–827. [CrossRef] [PubMed]
22. Chandel, N.S.; Avizonis, D.; Reczek, C.R.; Weinberg, S.E.; Menz, S.; Neuhaus, R.; Christian, S.; Haegebarth, A.; Algire, C.; Pollak, M. Are Metformin Doses Used in Murine Cancer Models Clinically Relevant? *Cell Metab.* **2016**, *23*, 569–570. [CrossRef] [PubMed]
23. Ma, T.; Tian, X.; Zhang, B.; Li, M.; Wang, Y.; Yang, C.; Wu, J.; Wei, X.; Qu, Q.; Yu, Y.; et al. Low-Dose Metformin Targets the Lysosomal AMPK Pathway through PEN2. *Nature* **2022**, *603*, 159–165. [CrossRef] [PubMed]
24. Moonira, T.; Chachra, S.S.; Ford, B.E.; Marin, S.; Alshawi, A.; Adam-Primus, N.S.; Arden, C.; Al-Oanzi, Z.H.; Foretz, M.; Viollet, B.; et al. Metformin Lowers Glucose 6-Phosphate in Hepatocytes by Activation of Glycolysis Downstream of Glucose Phosphorylation. *J. Biol. Chem.* **2020**, *295*, 3330–3346. [CrossRef]
25. Tucker, G.T.; Casey, C.; Phillips, P.J.; Connor, H.; Ward, J.D.; Woods, H.F. Metformin Kinetics in Healthy Subjects and in Patients with Diabetes Mellitus. *Br. J. Clin. Pharmacol.* **1981**, *12*, 235–246. [CrossRef] [PubMed]
26. Lalau, J.-D.; Lacroix, C. Measurement of Metformin Concentration in Erythrocytes: Clinical Implications. *Diabetes Obes. Metab.* **2003**, *5*, 93–98. [CrossRef]
27. Madiraju, A.K.; Qiu, Y.; Perry, R.J.; Rahimi, Y.; Zhang, X.-M.; Zhang, D.; Camporez, J.-P.G.; Cline, G.W.; Butrico, G.M.; Kemp, B.E.; et al. Metformin Inhibits Gluconeogenesis via a Redox-Dependent Mechanism In Vivo. *Nat. Med.* **2018**, *24*, 1384–1394. [CrossRef]
28. Bailey, C.J.; Wilcock, C.; Scarpello, J.H.B. Metformin and the Intestine. *Diabetologia* **2008**, *51*, 1552–1553. [CrossRef]
29. Pentikäinen, P.J.; Neuvonen, P.J.; Penttilä, A. Pharmacokinetics of Metformin after Intravenous and Oral Administration to Man. *Eur. J. Clin. Pharm.* **1979**, *16*, 195–202. [CrossRef]
30. LaMoia, T.E.; Shulman, G.I. Cellular and Molecular Mechanisms of Metformin Action. *Endocr. Rev.* **2021**, *42*, 77–96. [CrossRef] [PubMed]
31. Dowling, R.J.O.; Lam, S.; Bassi, C.; Mouaaz, S.; Aman, A.; Kiyota, T.; Al-Awar, R.; Goodwin, P.J.; Stambolic, V. Metformin Pharmacokinetics in Mouse Tumors: Implications for Human Therapy. *Cell Metab.* **2016**, *23*, 567–568. [CrossRef] [PubMed]
32. Wilcock, C.; Bailey, C.J. Accumulation of Metformin by Tissues of the Normal and Diabetic Mouse. *Xenobiotica* **1994**, *24*, 49–57. [CrossRef]
33. Marchetti, P.; Giannarelli, R.; di Carlo, A.; Navalesi, R. Pharmacokinetic Optimisation of Oral Hypoglycaemic Therapy. *Clin. Pharm.* **1991**, *21*, 308–317. [CrossRef]
34. Schwartz, S.; Fonseca, V.; Berner, B.; Cramer, M.; Chiang, Y.-K.; Lewin, A. Efficacy, Tolerability, and Safety of a Novel Once-Daily Extended-Release Metformin in Patients with Type 2 Diabetes. *Diabetes Care* **2006**, *29*, 759–764. [CrossRef] [PubMed]
35. Ohta, K.; Inoue, K.; Yasujima, T.; Ishimaru, M.; Yuasa, H. Functional Characteristics of Two Human MATE Transporters: Kinetics of Cimetidine Transport and Profiles of Inhibition by Various Compounds. *J. Pharm. Pharm. Sci.* **2009**, *12*, 388–396. [CrossRef] [PubMed]
36. Davidson, M.B.; Peters, A.L. An Overview of Metformin in the Treatment of Type 2 Diabetes Mellitus. *Am. J. Med.* **1997**, *102*, 99–110. [CrossRef]
37. Tanihara, Y.; Masuda, S.; Sato, T.; Katsura, T.; Ogawa, O.; Inui, K.-I. Substrate Specificity of MATE1 and MATE2-K, Human Multidrug and Toxin Extrusions/H+-Organic Cation Antiporters. *Biochem. Pharmacol.* **2007**, *74*, 359–371. [CrossRef]
38. Shapiro, S.L.; Parrino, V.A.; Freedman, L. Hypoglycemic Agents. I.[1] Chemical Properties of β-Phenethylbiguanide.[2] A New Hypoglycemic Agent[3]. *J. Am. Chem. Soc.* **1959**, *81*, 2220–2225. [CrossRef]
39. Appleyard, M.V.C.L.; Murray, K.E.; Coates, P.J.; Wullschleger, S.; Bray, S.E.; Kernohan, N.M.; Fleming, S.; Alessi, D.R.; Thompson, A.M. Phenformin as Prophylaxis and Therapy in Breast Cancer Xenografts. *Br. J. Cancer* **2012**, *106*, 1117–1122. [CrossRef]
40. Daugan, M.; Dufaÿ Wojcicki, A.; d'Hayer, B.; Boudy, V. Metformin: An Anti-Diabetic Drug to Fight Cancer. *Pharmacol. Res.* **2016**, *113*, 675–685. [CrossRef]
41. Hawley, S.A.; Ross, F.A.; Chevtzoff, C.; Green, K.A.; Evans, A.; Fogarty, S.; Towler, M.C.; Brown, L.J.; Ogunbayo, O.A.; Evans, A.M.; et al. Use of Cells Expressing Gamma Subunit Variants to Identify Diverse Mechanisms of AMPK Activation. *Cell Metab.* **2010**, *11*, 554–565. [CrossRef]
42. Shitara, Y.; Nakamichi, N.; Norioka, M.; Shima, H.; Kato, Y.; Horie, T. Role of Organic Cation/Carnitine Transporter 1 in Uptake of Phenformin and Inhibitory Effect on Complex I Respiration in Mitochondria. *Toxicol. Sci.* **2013**, *132*, 32–42. [CrossRef] [PubMed]

43. Bridges, H.R.; Sirviö, V.A.; Agip, A.-N.A.; Hirst, J. Molecular Features of Biguanides Required for Targeting of Mitochondrial Respiratory Complex I and Activation of AMP-Kinase. *BMC Biol.* **2016**, *14*, 65. [CrossRef] [PubMed]
44. Sogame, Y.; Kitamura, A.; Yabuki, M.; Komuro, S.; Takano, M. Transport of Biguanides by Human Organic Cation Transporter OCT2. *Biomed. Pharm.* **2013**, *67*, 425–430. [CrossRef] [PubMed]
45. Beckmann, R. The Fate of Biguanides in Man. *Ann. N. Y. Acad. Sci.* **1968**, *148*, 820–832. [CrossRef] [PubMed]
46. Shah, R.R.; Evans, D.A.; Oates, N.S.; Idle, J.R.; Smith, R.L. The Genetic Control of Phenformin 4-Hydroxylation. *J. Med. Genet* **1985**, *22*, 361–366. [CrossRef]
47. Alkalay, D.; Khemani, L.; Wagner, W.E.; Bartlett, M.F. Pharmacokinetics of Phenformin in Man. *J. Clin. Pharmacol.* **1975**, *15*, 446–448. [CrossRef]
48. Matin, S.B.; Karam, J.H.; Forsham, P.H.; Knight, J.B. Determination of Phenformin in Biological Fluids Using Chemical Ionization Mass Spectrometry. *Biomed. Mass Spectrom.* **1974**, *1*, 320–322. [CrossRef]
49. Nattrass, M.; Sizer, K.; Alberti, K.G. Correlation of Plasma Phenformin Concentration with Metabolic Effects in Normal Subjects. *Clin. Sci.* **1980**, *58*, 153–155. [CrossRef]
50. Marchetti, P.; Navalesi, R. Pharmacokinetic-Pharmacodynamic Relationships of Oral Hypoglycaemic Agents. An Update. *Clin. Pharm.* **1989**, *16*, 100–128. [CrossRef]
51. Karam, J.H.; Matin, S.B.; Forsham, P.H. Antidiabetic Drugs after the University Group Diabetes Program (UGDP). *Annu. Rev. Pharmacol.* **1975**, *15*, 351–366. [CrossRef] [PubMed]
52. Di Magno, L.; Manni, S.; Di Pastena, F.; Coni, S.; Macone, A.; Cairoli, S.; Sambucci, M.; Infante, P.; Moretti, M.; Petroni, M.; et al. Phenformin Inhibits Hedgehog-Dependent Tumor Growth through a Complex I-Independent Redox/Corepressor Module. *Cell Rep.* **2020**, *30*, 1735–1752.e7. [CrossRef] [PubMed]
53. Huang, X.; Wullschleger, S.; Shpiro, N.; McGuire, V.A.; Sakamoto, K.; Woods, Y.L.; McBurnie, W.; Fleming, S.; Alessi, D.R. Important Role of the LKB1-AMPK Pathway in Suppressing Tumorigenesis in PTEN-Deficient Mice. *Biochem. J.* **2008**, *412*, 211–221. [CrossRef]
54. Shackelford, D.B.; Abt, E.; Gerken, L.; Vasquez, D.S.; Seki, A.; Leblanc, M.; Wei, L.; Fishbein, M.C.; Czernin, J.; Mischel, P.S.; et al. LKB1 Inactivation Dictates Therapeutic Response of Non-Small Cell Lung Cancer to the Metabolism Drug Phenformin. *Cancer Cell* **2013**, *23*, 143–158. [CrossRef]
55. Bando, K.; Ochiai, S.; Kunimatsu, T.; Deguchi, J.; Kimura, J.; Funabashi, H.; Seki, T. Comparison of Potential Risks of Lactic Acidosis Induction by Biguanides in Rats. *Regul. Toxicol. Pharmacol.* **2010**, *58*, 155–160. [CrossRef]
56. Wick, A.N.; Bolinger, R.; Shapiro, S.; Clarke, D.W.; Ungar, G.; Kruger, F.A.; Volk, B.W. Laboratory Studies with Phenformin: Panel Discussion. *Diabetes* **1960**, *9*, 178–182. [CrossRef]
57. Sogame, Y.; Kitamura, A.; Yabuki, M.; Komuro, S. Liver Uptake of Biguanides in Rats. *Biomed. Pharm.* **2011**, *65*, 451–455. [CrossRef]
58. Conlay, L.A.; Karam, J.H.; Matin, S.B.; Loewenstein, J.E. Serum Phenformin Concentrations in Patients with Phenformin-Associated Lactic Acidosis. *Diabetes* **1977**, *26*, 628–631. [CrossRef]
59. Bosisio, E.; Kienle, M.G.; Galli, G.; Ciconali, M.; Negri, A.; Sessa, A.; Morosati, S.; Sirtori, C.R. Defective Hydroxylation of Phenformin as a Determinant of Drug Toxicity. *Diabetes* **1981**, *30*, 644–649. [CrossRef]
60. Ungar, G.; Freedman, L.; Shapiro, S.L. Pharmacological Studies of a New Oral Hypoglycemic Drug. *Proc. Soc. Exp. Biol. Med.* **1957**, *95*, 190–192. [CrossRef]
61. Zhu, Z.; Jiang, W.; Thompson, M.D.; Echeverria, D.; McGinley, J.N.; Thompson, H.J. Effects of Metformin, Buformin, and Phenformin on the Post-Initiation Stage of Chemically Induced Mammary Carcinogenesis in the Rat. *Cancer Prev. Res.* **2015**, *8*, 518–527. [CrossRef] [PubMed]
62. Beckmann, R.; Lintz, W.; Schmidt-Böthelt, E. Evaluation of a Sustained Release Form of the Oral Antidiabetic Butylbiguanide (Silubin Retard). *Eur. J. Clin. Pharmacol.* **1971**, *3*, 221–228. [CrossRef] [PubMed]
63. Beckmann, R. The Mechanism of Action of the Biguanides. *Ger. Med. Mon.* **1966**, *11*, 107–112. [PubMed]
64. Beckmann, R.; Hübner, G. On the pharmacokinetics of 1-butyl-biguanide hydrochloride and the prolonged-action form of this substance. *Arzneimittelforschung* **1965**, *15*, 765–770.
65. Garrett, E.R.; Tsau, J.; Hinderling, P.H. Application of Ion-Pair Methods to Drug Extraction from Biological Fluids. II. Quantitative Determination of Biguanides in Biological Fluids and Comparison of Protein Binding Estimates. *J. Pharm. Sci.* **1972**, *61*, 1411–1418. [CrossRef]
66. Lintz, W.; Berger, W.; Aenishaenslin, W.; Kutova, V.; Baerlocher, C.; Kapp, J.P.; Beckmann, R. Butylbiguanide Concentration in Plasma, Liver, and Intestine after Intravenous and Oral Administration to Man. *Eur. J. Clin. Pharmacol.* **1974**, *7*, 433–448. [CrossRef]
67. Yoh, Y.J. Distribution of N-Butylbiguanide-^{14}C Hydrochloride in Mouse Tissues. *Jpn. J. Pharmacol.* **1967**, *17*, 439–449. [CrossRef]
68. Haller, H.; Strauzenberg, S.E. A contribution to the method of determination of biguanides, creatinine and creatine in the urine. *Arztl. Forsch* **1966**, *20*, 415–419.
69. Losert, W.; Kolb, K.H.; Bitterling, G. Distribution of 1-butyl-biguanide- 14 C in rats and guinea pigs. *Arzneimittelforschung* **1972**, *22*, 937–946.
70. Caspary, W.F.; Creutzfeldt, W. Inhibition of Intestinal Amino Acid Transport by Blood Sugar Lowering Biguanides. *Diabetologia* **1973**, *9*, 6–12. [CrossRef]

71. Khan, M.A.B.; Hashim, M.J.; King, J.K.; Govender, R.D.; Mustafa, H.; Al Kaabi, J. Epidemiology of Type 2 Diabetes—Global Burden of Disease and Forecasted Trends. *J. Epidemiol. Glob. Health* **2020**, *10*, 107–111. [CrossRef] [PubMed]
72. Magnusson, I.; Rothman, D.L.; Katz, L.D.; Shulman, R.G.; Shulman, G.I. Increased Rate of Gluconeogenesis in Type II Diabetes Mellitus. A 13C Nuclear Magnetic Resonance Study. *J. Clin. Investig.* **1992**, *90*, 1323–1327. [CrossRef] [PubMed]
73. DeFronzo, R.A.; Ferrannini, E.; Groop, L.; Henry, R.R.; Herman, W.H.; Holst, J.J.; Hu, F.B.; Kahn, C.R.; Raz, I.; Shulman, G.I.; et al. Type 2 Diabetes Mellitus. *Nat. Rev. Dis. Primers* **2015**, *1*, 15019. [CrossRef]
74. He, L.; Wondisford, F.E. Metformin Action: Concentrations Matter. *Cell Metab.* **2015**, *21*, 159–162. [CrossRef]
75. Nasri, H.; Rafieian-Kopaei, M. Metformin: Current Knowledge. *J. Res. Med. Sci.* **2014**, *19*, 658–664.
76. Eisenreich, A.; Leppert, U. Update on the Protective Renal Effects of Metformin in Diabetic Nephropathy. *Curr. Med. Chem.* **2017**, *24*, 3397–3412. [CrossRef]
77. Lord, J.M.; Flight, I.H.K.; Norman, R.J. Metformin in Polycystic Ovary Syndrome: Systematic Review and Meta-Analysis. *BMJ* **2003**, *327*, 951–953. [CrossRef]
78. Selvin, E.; Bolen, S.; Yeh, H.-C.; Wiley, C.; Wilson, L.M.; Marinopoulos, S.S.; Feldman, L.; Vassy, J.; Wilson, R.; Bass, E.B.; et al. Cardiovascular Outcomes in Trials of Oral Diabetes Medications: A Systematic Review. *Arch. Intern. Med.* **2008**, *168*, 2070–2080. [CrossRef]
79. Salvatore, T.; Galiero, R.; Caturano, A.; Vetrano, E.; Rinaldi, L.; Coviello, F.; Di Martino, A.; Albanese, G.; Marfella, R.; Sardu, C.; et al. Effects of Metformin in Heart Failure: From Pathophysiological Rationale to Clinical Evidence. *Biomolecules* **2021**, *11*, 1834. [CrossRef]
80. Hundal, R.S.; Krssak, M.; Dufour, S.; Laurent, D.; Lebon, V.; Chandramouli, V.; Inzucchi, S.E.; Schumann, W.C.; Petersen, K.F.; Landau, B.R.; et al. Mechanism by Which Metformin Reduces Glucose Production in Type 2 Diabetes. *Diabetes* **2000**, *49*, 2063–2069. [CrossRef]
81. El-Mir, M.Y.; Nogueira, V.; Fontaine, E.; Avéret, N.; Rigoulet, M.; Leverve, X. Dimethylbiguanide Inhibits Cell Respiration via an Indirect Effect Targeted on the Respiratory Chain Complex I. *J. Biol. Chem.* **2000**, *275*, 223–228. [CrossRef] [PubMed]
82. Owen, M.R.; Doran, E.; Halestrap, A.P. Evidence That Metformin Exerts Its Anti-Diabetic Effects through Inhibition of Complex 1 of the Mitochondrial Respiratory Chain. *Biochem. J.* **2000**, *348*, 607–614. [CrossRef] [PubMed]
83. Hirst, J. Mitochondrial Complex I. *Annu. Rev. Biochem.* **2013**, *82*, 551–575. [CrossRef] [PubMed]
84. Bridges, H.R.; Jones, A.J.Y.; Pollak, M.N.; Hirst, J. Effects of Metformin and Other Biguanides on Oxidative Phosphorylation in Mitochondria. *Biochem. J.* **2014**, *462*, 475–487. [CrossRef]
85. Stephenne, X.; Foretz, M.; Taleux, N.; van der Zon, G.C.; Sokal, E.; Hue, L.; Viollet, B.; Guigas, B. Metformin Activates AMP-Activated Protein Kinase in Primary Human Hepatocytes by Decreasing Cellular Energy Status. *Diabetologia* **2011**, *54*, 3101–3110. [CrossRef]
86. Zhou, G.; Myers, R.; Li, Y.; Chen, Y.; Shen, X.; Fenyk-Melody, J.; Wu, M.; Ventre, J.; Doebber, T.; Fujii, N.; et al. Role of AMP-Activated Protein Kinase in Mechanism of Metformin Action. *J. Clin. Investig.* **2001**, *108*, 1167–1174. [CrossRef]
87. Shaw, R.J.; Lamia, K.A.; Vasquez, D.; Koo, S.-H.; Bardeesy, N.; Depinho, R.A.; Montminy, M.; Cantley, L.C. The Kinase LKB1 Mediates Glucose Homeostasis in Liver and Therapeutic Effects of Metformin. *Science* **2005**, *310*, 1642–1646. [CrossRef]
88. Foretz, M.; Hébrard, S.; Leclerc, J.; Zarrinpashneh, E.; Soty, M.; Mithieux, G.; Sakamoto, K.; Andreelli, F.; Viollet, B. Metformin Inhibits Hepatic Gluconeogenesis in Mice Independently of the LKB1/AMPK Pathway via a Decrease in Hepatic Energy State. *J. Clin. Investig.* **2010**, *120*, 2355–2369. [CrossRef]
89. Hunter, R.W.; Hughey, C.C.; Lantier, L.; Sundelin, E.I.; Peggie, M.; Zeqiraj, E.; Sicheri, F.; Jessen, N.; Wasserman, D.H.; Sakamoto, K. Metformin Reduces Liver Glucose Production by Inhibition of Fructose-1-6-Bisphosphatase. *Nat. Med.* **2018**, *24*, 1395–1406. [CrossRef]
90. Miller, R.A.; Chu, Q.; Xie, J.; Foretz, M.; Viollet, B.; Birnbaum, M.J. Biguanides Suppress Hepatic Glucagon Signalling by Decreasing Production of Cyclic AMP. *Nature* **2013**, *494*, 256–260. [CrossRef]
91. Hardie, D.G. Metformin-Acting through Cyclic AMP as Well as AMP? *Cell Metab.* **2013**, *17*, 313–314. [CrossRef] [PubMed]
92. Hasenour, C.M.; Ridley, D.E.; Hughey, C.C.; James, F.D.; Donahue, E.P.; Shearer, J.; Viollet, B.; Foretz, M.; Wasserman, D.H. 5-Aminoimidazole-4-Carboxamide-1-β-D-Ribofuranoside (AICAR) Effect on Glucose Production, but Not Energy Metabolism, Is Independent of Hepatic AMPK In Vivo. *J. Biol. Chem.* **2014**, *289*, 5950–5959. [CrossRef] [PubMed]
93. Cokorinos, E.C.; Delmore, J.; Reyes, A.R.; Albuquerque, B.; Kjøbsted, R.; Jørgensen, N.O.; Tran, J.-L.; Jatkar, A.; Cialdea, K.; Esquejo, R.M.; et al. Activation of Skeletal Muscle AMPK Promotes Glucose Disposal and Glucose Lowering in Non-Human Primates and Mice. *Cell Metab.* **2017**, *25*, 1147–1159.e10. [CrossRef]
94. Vial, G.; Detaille, D.; Guigas, B. Role of Mitochondria in the Mechanism(s) of Action of Metformin. *Front. Endocrinol.* **2019**, *10*, 294. [CrossRef] [PubMed]
95. Fontaine, E. Metformin-Induced Mitochondrial Complex I Inhibition: Facts, Uncertainties, and Consequences. *Front. Endocrinol.* **2018**, *9*, 753. [CrossRef] [PubMed]
96. Carvalho, C.; Correia, S.; Santos, M.S.; Seiça, R.; Oliveira, C.R.; Moreira, P.I. Metformin Promotes Isolated Rat Liver Mitochondria Impairment. *Mol. Cell Biochem.* **2008**, *308*, 75–83. [CrossRef] [PubMed]
97. Kelley, D.E.; He, J.; Menshikova, E.V.; Ritov, V.B. Dysfunction of Mitochondria in Human Skeletal Muscle in Type 2 Diabetes. *Diabetes* **2002**, *51*, 2944–2950. [CrossRef]

98. Morino, K.; Petersen, K.F.; Dufour, S.; Befroy, D.; Frattini, J.; Shatzkes, N.; Neschen, S.; White, M.F.; Bilz, S.; Sono, S.; et al. Reduced Mitochondrial Density and Increased IRS-1 Serine Phosphorylation in Muscle of Insulin-Resistant Offspring of Type 2 Diabetic Parents. *J. Clin. Investig.* **2005**, *115*, 3587–3593. [CrossRef]
99. Petersen, K.F.; Dufour, S.; Befroy, D.; Garcia, R.; Shulman, G.I. Impaired Mitochondrial Activity in the Insulin-Resistant Offspring of Patients with Type 2 Diabetes. *N. Engl. J. Med.* **2004**, *350*, 664–671. [CrossRef]
100. Ritov, V.B.; Menshikova, E.V.; He, J.; Ferrell, R.E.; Goodpaster, B.H.; Kelley, D.E. Deficiency of Subsarcolemmal Mitochondria in Obesity and Type 2 Diabetes. *Diabetes* **2005**, *54*, 8–14. [CrossRef]
101. Liesa, M.; Shirihai, O.S. Mitochondrial Dynamics in the Regulation of Nutrient Utilization and Energy Expenditure. *Cell Metab.* **2013**, *17*, 491–506. [CrossRef] [PubMed]
102. Youle, R.J.; van der Bliek, A.M. Mitochondrial Fission, Fusion, and Stress. *Science* **2012**, *337*, 1062–1065. [CrossRef] [PubMed]
103. Twig, G.; Elorza, A.; Molina, A.J.A.; Mohamed, H.; Wikstrom, J.D.; Walzer, G.; Stiles, L.; Haigh, S.E.; Katz, S.; Las, G.; et al. Fission and Selective Fusion Govern Mitochondrial Segregation and Elimination by Autophagy. *EMBO J.* **2008**, *27*, 433–446. [CrossRef] [PubMed]
104. Yamada, T.; Murata, D.; Adachi, Y.; Itoh, K.; Kameoka, S.; Igarashi, A.; Kato, T.; Araki, Y.; Huganir, R.L.; Dawson, T.M.; et al. Mitochondrial Stasis Reveals P62-Mediated Ubiquitination in Parkin-Independent Mitophagy and Mitigates Nonalcoholic Fatty Liver Disease. *Cell Metab.* **2018**, *28*, 588–604.e5. [CrossRef] [PubMed]
105. Wang, Y.; An, H.; Liu, T.; Qin, C.; Sesaki, H.; Guo, S.; Radovick, S.; Hussain, M.; Maheshwari, A.; Wondisford, F.E.; et al. Metformin Improves Mitochondrial Respiratory Activity through Activation of AMPK. *Cell Rep.* **2019**, *29*, 1511–1523.e5. [CrossRef] [PubMed]
106. Larsen, S.; Rabøl, R.; Hansen, C.N.; Madsbad, S.; Helge, J.W.; Dela, F. Metformin-Treated Patients with Type 2 Diabetes Have Normal Mitochondrial Complex I Respiration. *Diabetologia* **2012**, *55*, 443–449. [CrossRef]
107. Madiraju, A.K.; Erion, D.M.; Rahimi, Y.; Zhang, X.-M.; Braddock, D.T.; Albright, R.A.; Prigaro, B.J.; Wood, J.L.; Bhanot, S.; MacDonald, M.J.; et al. Metformin Suppresses Gluconeogenesis by Inhibiting Mitochondrial Glycerophosphate Dehydrogenase. *Nature* **2014**, *510*, 542–546. [CrossRef]
108. Mráček, T.; Drahota, Z.; Houštěk, J. The Function and the Role of the Mitochondrial Glycerol-3-Phosphate Dehydrogenase in Mammalian Tissues. *Biochim. Biophys. Acta* **2013**, *1827*, 401–410. [CrossRef]
109. Baur, J.A.; Birnbaum, M.J. Control of Gluconeogenesis by Metformin: Does Redox Trump Energy Charge? *Cell Metab.* **2014**, *20*, 197–199. [CrossRef]
110. Saheki, T.; Iijima, M.; Li, M.X.; Kobayashi, K.; Horiuchi, M.; Ushikai, M.; Okumura, F.; Meng, X.J.; Inoue, I.; Tajima, A.; et al. Citrin/Mitochondrial Glycerol-3-Phosphate Dehydrogenase Double Knock-out Mice Recapitulate Features of Human Citrin Deficiency. *J. Biol. Chem.* **2007**, *282*, 25041–25052. [CrossRef]
111. Alshawi, A.; Agius, L. Low Metformin Causes a More Oxidized Mitochondrial NADH/NAD Redox State in Hepatocytes and Inhibits Gluconeogenesis by a Redox-Independent Mechanism. *J. Biol. Chem.* **2019**, *294*, 2839–2853. [CrossRef] [PubMed]
112. Calza, G.; Nyberg, E.; Mäkinen, M.; Soliymani, R.; Cascone, A.; Lindholm, D.; Barborini, E.; Baumann, M.; Lalowski, M.; Eriksson, O. Lactate-Induced Glucose Output Is Unchanged by Metformin at a Therapeutic Concentration—A Mass Spectrometry Imaging Study of the Perfused Rat Liver. *Front. Pharmacol.* **2018**, *9*, 141. [CrossRef] [PubMed]
113. MacDonald, M.J.; Ansari, I.-U.H.; Longacre, M.J.; Stoker, S.W. Metformin's Therapeutic Efficacy in the Treatment of Diabetes Does Not Involve Inhibition of Mitochondrial Glycerol Phosphate Dehydrogenase. *Diabetes* **2021**, *70*, 1575–1580. [CrossRef] [PubMed]
114. LaMoia, T.E.; Butrico, G.M.; Kalpage, H.A.; Goedeke, L.; Hubbard, B.T.; Vatner, D.F.; Gaspar, R.C.; Zhang, X.-M.; Cline, G.W.; Nakahara, K.; et al. Metformin, Phenformin, and Galegine Inhibit Complex IV Activity and Reduce Glycerol-Derived Gluconeogenesis. *Proc. Natl. Acad. Sci. USA* **2022**, *119*, e2122287119. [CrossRef]
115. Xie, D.; Chen, F.; Zhang, Y.; Shi, B.; Song, J.; Chaudhari, K.; Yang, S.-H.; Zhang, G.J.; Sun, X.; Taylor, H.S.; et al. Let-7 Underlies Metformin-Induced Inhibition of Hepatic Glucose Production. *Proc. Natl. Acad. Sci. USA* **2022**, *119*, e2122217119. [CrossRef]
116. Zhang, C.-S.; Hawley, S.A.; Zong, Y.; Li, M.; Wang, Z.; Gray, A.; Ma, T.; Cui, J.; Feng, J.-W.; Zhu, M.; et al. Fructose-1,6-Bisphosphate and Aldolase Mediate Glucose Sensing by AMPK. *Nature* **2017**, *548*, 112–116. [CrossRef]
117. Sum, C.F.; Webster, J.M.; Johnson, A.B.; Catalano, C.; Cooper, B.G.; Taylor, R. The Effect of Intravenous Metformin on Glucose Metabolism during Hyperglycaemia in Type 2 Diabetes. *Diabet Med.* **1992**, *9*, 61–65. [CrossRef]
118. Bonora, E.; Cigolini, M.; Bosello, O.; Zancanaro, C.; Capretti, L.; Zavaroni, I.; Coscelli, C.; Butturini, U. Lack of Effect of Intravenous Metformin on Plasma Concentrations of Glucose, Insulin, C-Peptide, Glucagon and Growth Hormone in Non-Diabetic Subjects. *Curr. Med. Res. Opin.* **1984**, *9*, 47–51. [CrossRef]
119. Oh, J.; Chung, H.; Park, S.-I.; Yi, S.J.; Jang, K.; Kim, A.H.; Yoon, J.; Cho, J.-Y.; Yoon, S.H.; Jang, I.-J.; et al. Inhibition of the Multidrug and Toxin Extrusion (MATE) Transporter by Pyrimethamine Increases the Plasma Concentration of Metformin but Does Not Increase Antihyperglycaemic Activity in Humans. *Diabetes Obes. Metab.* **2016**, *18*, 104–108. [CrossRef]
120. Buse, J.B.; DeFronzo, R.A.; Rosenstock, J.; Kim, T.; Burns, C.; Skare, S.; Baron, A.; Fineman, M. The Primary Glucose-Lowering Effect of Metformin Resides in the Gut, Not the Circulation: Results From Short-Term Pharmacokinetic and 12-Week Dose-Ranging Studies. *Diabetes Care* **2016**, *39*, 198–205. [CrossRef]
121. Wu, H.; Esteve, E.; Tremaroli, V.; Khan, M.T.; Caesar, R.; Mannerås-Holm, L.; Ståhlman, M.; Olsson, L.M.; Serino, M.; Planas-Fèlix, M.; et al. Metformin Alters the Gut Microbiome of Individuals with Treatment-Naive Type 2 Diabetes, Contributing to the Therapeutic Effects of the Drug. *Nat. Med.* **2017**, *23*, 850–858. [CrossRef]

122. Koffert, J.P.; Mikkola, K.; Virtanen, K.A.; Andersson, A.-M.D.; Faxius, L.; Hällsten, K.; Heglind, M.; Guiducci, L.; Pham, T.; Silvola, J.M.U.; et al. Metformin Treatment Significantly Enhances Intestinal Glucose Uptake in Patients with Type 2 Diabetes: Results from a Randomized Clinical Trial. *Diabetes Res. Clin. Pract.* **2017**, *131*, 208–216. [CrossRef]
123. Bahler, L.; Holleman, F.; Chan, M.-W.; Booij, J.; Hoekstra, J.B.; Verberne, H.J. 18F-FDG Uptake in the Colon Is Modulated by Metformin but Not Associated with Core Body Temperature and Energy Expenditure. *PLoS ONE* **2017**, *12*, e0176242. [CrossRef]
124. Andersen, A.; Lund, A.; Knop, F.K.; Vilsbøll, T. Glucagon-like Peptide 1 in Health and Disease. *Nat. Rev. Endocrinol.* **2018**, *14*, 390–403. [CrossRef]
125. Maida, A.; Lamont, B.J.; Cao, X.; Drucker, D.J. Metformin Regulates the Incretin Receptor Axis via a Pathway Dependent on Peroxisome Proliferator-Activated Receptor-α in Mice. *Diabetologia* **2011**, *54*, 339–349. [CrossRef]
126. Preiss, D.; Dawed, A.; Welsh, P.; Heggie, A.; Jones, A.G.; Dekker, J.; Koivula, R.; Hansen, T.H.; Stewart, C.; Holman, R.R.; et al. Sustained Influence of Metformin Therapy on Circulating Glucagon-like Peptide-1 Levels in Individuals with and without Type 2 Diabetes. *Diabetes Obes. Metab.* **2017**, *19*, 356–363. [CrossRef]
127. Bahne, E.; Sun, E.W.L.; Young, R.L.; Hansen, M.; Sonne, D.P.; Hansen, J.S.; Rohde, U.; Liou, A.P.; Jackson, M.L.; de Fontgalland, D.; et al. Metformin-Induced Glucagon-like Peptide-1 Secretion Contributes to the Actions of Metformin in Type 2 Diabetes. *JCI Insight* **2018**, *3*, 93936. [CrossRef]
128. Migoya, E.M.; Bergeron, R.; Miller, J.L.; Snyder, R.N.K.; Tanen, M.; Hilliard, D.; Weiss, B.; Larson, P.; Gutierrez, M.; Jiang, G.; et al. Dipeptidyl Peptidase-4 Inhibitors Administered in Combination with Metformin Result in an Additive Increase in the Plasma Concentration of Active GLP-1. *Clin. Pharmacol. Ther.* **2010**, *88*, 801–808. [CrossRef]
129. Wu, T.; Thazhath, S.S.; Bound, M.J.; Jones, K.L.; Horowitz, M.; Rayner, C.K. Mechanism of Increase in Plasma Intact GLP-1 by Metformin in Type 2 Diabetes: Stimulation of GLP-1 Secretion or Reduction in Plasma DPP-4 Activity? *Diabetes Res. Clin. Pract.* **2014**, *106*, e3–e6. [CrossRef]
130. Golay, A. Metformin and Body Weight. *Int. J. Obes.* **2008**, *32*, 61–72. [CrossRef]
131. Lee, A.; Morley, J.E. Metformin Decreases Food Consumption and Induces Weight Loss in Subjects with Obesity with Type II Non-Insulin-Dependent Diabetes. *Obes. Res.* **1998**, *6*, 47–53. [CrossRef]
132. Coll, A.P.; Chen, M.; Taskar, P.; Rimmington, D.; Patel, S.; Tadross, J.A.; Cimino, I.; Yang, M.; Welsh, P.; Virtue, S.; et al. GDF15 Mediates the Effects of Metformin on Body Weight and Energy Balance. *Nature* **2020**, *578*, 444–448. [CrossRef]
133. Day, E.A.; Ford, R.J.; Smith, B.K.; Mohammadi-Shemirani, P.; Morrow, M.R.; Gutgesell, R.M.; Lu, R.; Raphenya, A.R.; Kabiri, M.; McArthur, A.G.; et al. Metformin-Induced Increases in GDF15 Are Important for Suppressing Appetite and Promoting Weight Loss. *Nat. Metab.* **2019**, *1*, 1202–1208. [CrossRef]
134. Baek, S.J.; Eling, T. Growth Differentiation Factor 15 (GDF15): A Survival Protein with Therapeutic Potential in Metabolic Diseases. *Pharmacol. Ther.* **2019**, *198*, 46–58. [CrossRef]
135. Baek, S.J.; Okazaki, R.; Lee, S.-H.; Martinez, J.; Kim, J.-S.; Yamaguchi, K.; Mishina, Y.; Martin, D.W.; Shoieb, A.; McEntee, M.F.; et al. Nonsteroidal Anti-Inflammatory Drug-Activated Gene-1 over Expression in Transgenic Mice Suppresses Intestinal Neoplasia. *Gastroenterology* **2006**, *131*, 1553–1560. [CrossRef]
136. Chrysovergis, K.; Wang, X.; Kosak, J.; Lee, S.-H.; Kim, J.S.; Foley, J.F.; Travlos, G.; Singh, S.; Baek, S.J.; Eling, T.E. NAG-1/GDF-15 Prevents Obesity by Increasing Thermogenesis, Lipolysis and Oxidative Metabolism. *Int. J. Obes.* **2014**, *38*, 1555–1564. [CrossRef]
137. Sun, L.; Xie, C.; Wang, G.; Wu, Y.; Wu, Q.; Wang, X.; Liu, J.; Deng, Y.; Xia, J.; Chen, B.; et al. Gut Microbiota and Intestinal FXR Mediate the Clinical Benefits of Metformin. *Nat. Med.* **2018**, *24*, 1919–1929. [CrossRef]
138. Forslund, K.; Hildebrand, F.; Nielsen, T.; Falony, G.; Le Chatelier, E.; Sunagawa, S.; Prifti, E.; Vieira-Silva, S.; Gudmundsdottir, V.; Pedersen, H.K.; et al. Disentangling Type 2 Diabetes and Metformin Treatment Signatures in the Human Gut Microbiota. *Nature* **2015**, *528*, 262–266. [CrossRef]
139. Nosadini, R.; Avogaro, A.; Trevisan, R.; Valerio, A.; Tessari, P.; Duner, E.; Tiengo, A.; Velussi, M.; Del Prato, S.; De Kreutzenberg, S. Effect of Metformin on Insulin-Stimulated Glucose Turnover and Insulin Binding to Receptors in Type II Diabetes. *Diabetes Care* **1987**, *10*, 62–67. [CrossRef]
140. Galuska, D.; Nolte, L.A.; Zierath, J.R.; Wallberg-Henriksson, H. Effect of Metformin on Insulin-Stimulated Glucose Transport in Isolated Skeletal Muscle Obtained from Patients with NIDDM. *Diabetologia* **1994**, *37*, 826–832. [CrossRef]
141. Kjøbsted, R.; Munk-Hansen, N.; Birk, J.B.; Foretz, M.; Viollet, B.; Björnholm, M.; Zierath, J.R.; Treebak, J.T.; Wojtaszewski, J.F.P. Enhanced Muscle Insulin Sensitivity after Contraction/Exercise Is Mediated by AMPK. *Diabetes* **2017**, *66*, 598–612. [CrossRef]
142. Kjøbsted, R.; Kristensen, J.M.; Birk, J.B.; Eskesen, N.O.; Kido, K.; Andersen, N.R.; Larsen, J.K.; Foretz, M.; Viollet, B.; Nielsen, F.; et al. Metformin Improves Glycemia Independently of Skeletal Muscle AMPK via Enhanced Intestinal Glucose Clearance. *bioRxiv* **2022**. [CrossRef]
143. Yu, J.G.; Kruszynska, Y.T.; Mulford, M.I.; Olefsky, J.M. A Comparison of Troglitazone and Metformin on Insulin Requirements in Euglycemic Intensively Insulin-Treated Type 2 Diabetic Patients. *Diabetes* **1999**, *48*, 2414–2421. [CrossRef]
144. Evans, J.M.M.; Donnelly, L.A.; Emslie-Smith, A.M.; Alessi, D.R.; Morris, A.D. Metformin and Reduced Risk of Cancer in Diabetic Patients. *BMJ* **2005**, *330*, 1304–1305. [CrossRef]
145. Wheaton, W.W.; Weinberg, S.E.; Hamanaka, R.B.; Soberanes, S.; Sullivan, L.B.; Anso, E.; Glasauer, A.; Dufour, E.; Mutlu, G.M.; Budigner, G.S.; et al. Metformin Inhibits Mitochondrial Complex I of Cancer Cells to Reduce Tumorigenesis. *eLife* **2014**, *3*, e02242. [CrossRef]

146. Birsoy, K.; Possemato, R.; Lorbeer, F.K.; Bayraktar, E.C.; Thiru, P.; Yucel, B.; Wang, T.; Chen, W.W.; Clish, C.B.; Sabatini, D.M. Metabolic Determinants of Cancer Cell Sensitivity to Glucose Limitation and Biguanides. *Nature* **2014**, *508*, 108–112. [CrossRef]
147. Igelmann, S.; Lessard, F.; Uchenunu, O.; Bouchard, J.; Fernandez-Ruiz, A.; Rowell, M.-C.; Lopes-Paciencia, S.; Papadopoli, D.; Fouillen, A.; Ponce, K.J.; et al. A Hydride Transfer Complex Reprograms NAD Metabolism and Bypasses Senescence. *Mol. Cell* **2021**, *81*, 3848–3865.e19. [CrossRef]
148. Schöckel, L.; Glasauer, A.; Basit, F.; Bitschar, K.; Truong, H.; Erdmann, G.; Algire, C.; Hägebarth, A.; Willems, P.H.; Kopitz, C.; et al. Targeting Mitochondrial Complex I Using BAY 87-2243 Reduces Melanoma Tumor Growth. *Cancer Metab* **2015**, *3*, 11. [CrossRef]
149. Zhang, C.-S.; Jiang, B.; Li, M.; Zhu, M.; Peng, Y.; Zhang, Y.-L.; Wu, Y.-Q.; Li, T.Y.; Liang, Y.; Lu, Z.; et al. The Lysosomal V-ATPase-Ragulator Complex Is a Common Activator for AMPK and MTORC1, Acting as a Switch between Catabolism and Anabolism. *Cell Metab.* **2014**, *20*, 526–540. [CrossRef]
150. Guigas, B.; Detaille, D.; Chauvin, C.; Batandier, C.; De Oliveira, F.; Fontaine, E.; Leverve, X. Metformin Inhibits Mitochondrial Permeability Transition and Cell Death: A Pharmacological In Vitro Study. *Biochem. J.* **2004**, *382*, 877–884. [CrossRef]
151. Sancho, P.; Burgos-Ramos, E.; Tavera, A.; Bou Kheir, T.; Jagust, P.; Schoenhals, M.; Barneda, D.; Sellers, K.; Campos-Olivas, R.; Graña, O.; et al. MYC/PGC-1α Balance Determines the Metabolic Phenotype and Plasticity of Pancreatic Cancer Stem Cells. *Cell Metab.* **2015**, *22*, 590–605. [CrossRef]
152. Cheng, G.; Zielonka, J.; Ouari, O.; Lopez, M.; McAllister, D.; Boyle, K.; Barrios, C.S.; Weber, J.J.; Johnson, B.D.; Hardy, M.; et al. Mitochondria-Targeted Analogues of Metformin Exhibit Enhanced Antiproliferative and Radiosensitizing Effects in Pancreatic Cancer Cells. *Cancer Res.* **2016**, *76*, 3904–3915. [CrossRef]
153. Momcilovic, M.; Jones, A.; Bailey, S.T.; Waldmann, C.M.; Li, R.; Lee, J.T.; Abdelhady, G.; Gomez, A.; Holloway, T.; Schmid, E.; et al. In Vivo Imaging of Mitochondrial Membrane Potential in Non-Small-Cell Lung Cancer. *Nature* **2019**, *575*, 380–384. [CrossRef]
154. Orr, A.L.; Ashok, D.; Sarantos, M.R.; Ng, R.; Shi, T.; Gerencser, A.A.; Hughes, R.E.; Brand, M.D. Novel Inhibitors of Mitochondrial Sn-Glycerol 3-Phosphate Dehydrogenase. *PLoS ONE* **2014**, *9*, e89938. [CrossRef]
155. Christensen, M.M.H.; Brasch-Andersen, C.; Green, H.; Nielsen, F.; Damkier, P.; Beck-Nielsen, H.; Brosen, K. The Pharmacogenetics of Metformin and Its Impact on Plasma Metformin Steady-State Levels and Glycosylated Hemoglobin A1c. *Pharm. Genom.* **2011**, *21*, 837–850. [CrossRef]
156. Scheen, A.J. Clinical Pharmacokinetics of Metformin. *Clin. Pharm.* **1996**, *30*, 359–371. [CrossRef]
157. Thakur, S.; Daley, B.; Gaskins, K.; Vasko, V.V.; Boufraqech, M.; Patel, D.; Sourbier, C.; Reece, J.; Cheng, S.-Y.; Kebebew, E.; et al. Metformin Targets Mitochondrial Glycerophosphate Dehydrogenase to Control Rate of Oxidative Phosphorylation and Growth of Thyroid Cancer In Vitro and In Vivo. *Clin. Cancer Res.* **2018**, *24*, 4030–4043. [CrossRef]
158. Xie, J.; Ye, J.; Cai, Z.; Luo, Y.; Zhu, X.; Deng, Y.; Feng, Y.; Liang, Y.; Liu, R.; Han, Z.; et al. GPD1 Enhances the Anticancer Effects of Metformin by Synergistically Increasing Total Cellular Glycerol-3-Phosphate. *Cancer Res.* **2020**, *80*, 2150–2162. [CrossRef]
159. Liu, S.; Fu, S.; Wang, G.; Cao, Y.; Li, L.; Li, X.; Yang, J.; Li, N.; Shan, Y.; Cao, Y.; et al. Glycerol-3-Phosphate Biosynthesis Regenerates Cytosolic NAD$^+$ to Alleviate Mitochondrial Disease. *Cell Metab.* **2021**, *33*, 1974–1987.e9. [CrossRef]
160. Gui, D.Y.; Sullivan, L.B.; Luengo, A.; Hosios, A.M.; Bush, L.N.; Gitego, N.; Davidson, S.M.; Freinkman, E.; Thomas, C.J.; Vander Heiden, M.G. Environment Dictates Dependence on Mitochondrial Complex I for NAD$^+$ and Aspartate Production and Determines Cancer Cell Sensitivity to Metformin. *Cell Metab.* **2016**, *24*, 716–727. [CrossRef]
161. Vara-Ciruelos, D.; Dandapani, M.; Hardie, D.G. AMP-Activated Protein Kinase: Friend or Foe in Cancer? *Annu. Rev. Cancer Biol.* **2020**, *4*, 1–16. [CrossRef]
162. Eichner, L.J.; Brun, S.N.; Herzig, S.; Young, N.P.; Curtis, S.D.; Shackelford, D.B.; Shokhirev, M.N.; Leblanc, M.; Vera, L.I.; Hutchins, A.; et al. Genetic Analysis Reveals AMPK Is Required to Support Tumor Growth in Murine Kras-Dependent Lung Cancer Models. *Cell Metab.* **2019**, *29*, 285–302.e7. [CrossRef]
163. Zhang, C.-S.; Li, M.; Ma, T.; Zong, Y.; Cui, J.; Feng, J.-W.; Wu, Y.-Q.; Lin, S.-Y.; Lin, S.-C. Metformin Activates AMPK through the Lysosomal Pathway. *Cell Metab.* **2016**, *24*, 521–522. [CrossRef]
164. Zou, Z.; Tao, T.; Li, H.; Zhu, X. MTOR Signaling Pathway and MTOR Inhibitors in Cancer: Progress and Challenges. *Cell Biosci.* **2020**, *10*, 31. [CrossRef]
165. Sabatini, D.M. MTOR and Cancer: Insights into a Complex Relationship. *Nat. Rev. Cancer* **2006**, *6*, 729–734. [CrossRef]
166. Um, S.H.; D'Alessio, D.; Thomas, G. Nutrient Overload, Insulin Resistance, and Ribosomal Protein S6 Kinase 1, S6K1. *Cell Metab.* **2006**, *3*, 393–402. [CrossRef]
167. Wullschleger, S.; Loewith, R.; Hall, M.N. TOR Signaling in Growth and Metabolism. *Cell* **2006**, *124*, 471–484. [CrossRef]
168. Dowling, R.J.O.; Zakikhani, M.; Fantus, I.G.; Pollak, M.; Sonenberg, N. Metformin Inhibits Mammalian Target of Rapamycin-Dependent Translation Initiation in Breast Cancer Cells. *Cancer Res.* **2007**, *67*, 10804–10812. [CrossRef]
169. Gwinn, D.M.; Shackelford, D.B.; Egan, D.F.; Mihaylova, M.M.; Mery, A.; Vasquez, D.S.; Turk, B.E.; Shaw, R.J. AMPK Phosphorylation of Raptor Mediates a Metabolic Checkpoint. *Mol. Cell* **2008**, *30*, 214–226. [CrossRef]
170. Kalender, A.; Selvaraj, A.; Kim, S.Y.; Gulati, P.; Brûlé, S.; Viollet, B.; Kemp, B.E.; Bardeesy, N.; Dennis, P.; Schlager, J.J.; et al. Metformin, Independent of AMPK, Inhibits MTORC1 in a Rag GTPase-Dependent Manner. *Cell Metab.* **2010**, *11*, 390–401. [CrossRef]
171. Jones, R.G.; Plas, D.R.; Kubek, S.; Buzzai, M.; Mu, J.; Xu, Y.; Birnbaum, M.J.; Thompson, C.B. AMP-Activated Protein Kinase Induces a P53-Dependent Metabolic Checkpoint. *Mol. Cell* **2005**, *18*, 283–293. [CrossRef]

172. Buzzai, M.; Jones, R.G.; Amaravadi, R.K.; Lum, J.J.; DeBerardinis, R.J.; Zhao, F.; Viollet, B.; Thompson, C.B. Systemic Treatment with the Antidiabetic Drug Metformin Selectively Impairs P53-Deficient Tumor Cell Growth. *Cancer Res.* **2007**, *67*, 6745–6752. [CrossRef]
173. Faubert, B.; Boily, G.; Izreig, S.; Griss, T.; Samborska, B.; Dong, Z.; Dupuy, F.; Chambers, C.; Fuerth, B.J.; Viollet, B.; et al. AMPK Is a Negative Regulator of the Warburg Effect and Suppresses Tumor Growth In Vivo. *Cell Metab.* **2013**, *17*, 113–124. [CrossRef]
174. Moiseeva, O.; Deschênes-Simard, X.; St-Germain, E.; Igelmann, S.; Huot, G.; Cadar, A.E.; Bourdeau, V.; Pollak, M.N.; Ferbeyre, G. Metformin Inhibits the Senescence-Associated Secretory Phenotype by Interfering with IKK/NF-KB Activation. *Aging Cell* **2013**, *12*, 489–498. [CrossRef]
175. Hirsch, H.A.; Iliopoulos, D.; Struhl, K. Metformin Inhibits the Inflammatory Response Associated with Cellular Transformation and Cancer Stem Cell Growth. *Proc. Natl. Acad. Sci. USA* **2013**, *110*, 972–977. [CrossRef]
176. Tan, X.-L.; Bhattacharyya, K.K.; Dutta, S.K.; Bamlet, W.R.; Rabe, K.G.; Wang, E.; Smyrk, T.C.; Oberg, A.L.; Petersen, G.M.; Mukhopadhyay, D. Metformin Suppresses Pancreatic Tumor Growth with Inhibition of NFκB/STAT3 Inflammatory Signaling. *Pancreas* **2015**, *44*, 636–647. [CrossRef]
177. Qi, X.; Xu, W.; Xie, J.; Wang, Y.; Han, S.; Wei, Z.; Ni, Y.; Dong, Y.; Han, W. Metformin Sensitizes the Response of Oral Squamous Cell Carcinoma to Cisplatin Treatment through Inhibition of NF-κB/HIF-1α Signal Axis. *Sci. Rep.* **2016**, *6*, 35788. [CrossRef]
178. Liu, X.; Romero, I.L.; Litchfield, L.M.; Lengyel, E.; Locasale, J.W. Metformin Targets Central Carbon Metabolism and Reveals Mitochondrial Requirements in Human Cancers. *Cell Metab.* **2016**, *24*, 728–739. [CrossRef]
179. Lord, S.R.; Cheng, W.-C.; Liu, D.; Gaude, E.; Haider, S.; Metcalf, T.; Patel, N.; Teoh, E.J.; Gleeson, F.; Bradley, K.; et al. Integrated Pharmacodynamic Analysis Identifies Two Metabolic Adaption Pathways to Metformin in Breast Cancer. *Cell Metab.* **2018**, *28*, 679–688.e4. [CrossRef]
180. Di Magno, L.; Basile, A.; Coni, S.; Manni, S.; Sdruscia, G.; D'Amico, D.; Antonucci, L.; Infante, P.; De Smaele, E.; Cucchi, D.; et al. The Energy Sensor AMPK Regulates Hedgehog Signaling in Human Cells through a Unique Gli1 Metabolic Checkpoint. *Oncotarget* **2016**, *7*, 9538–9549. [CrossRef]
181. Schultze, S.M.; Hemmings, B.A.; Niessen, M.; Tschopp, O. PI3K/AKT, MAPK and AMPK Signalling: Protein Kinases in Glucose Homeostasis. *Expert Rev. Mol. Med.* **2012**, *14*, e1. [CrossRef]
182. Latres, E.; Amini, A.R.; Amini, A.A.; Griffiths, J.; Martin, F.J.; Wei, Y.; Lin, H.C.; Yancopoulos, G.D.; Glass, D.J. Insulin-like Growth Factor-1 (IGF-1) Inversely Regulates Atrophy-Induced Genes via the Phosphatidylinositol 3-Kinase/Akt/Mammalian Target of Rapamycin (PI3K/Akt/MTOR) Pathway. *J. Biol. Chem.* **2005**, *280*, 2737–2744. [CrossRef]
183. Pritchard, K.I.; Shepherd, L.E.; Chapman, J.-A.W.; Norris, B.D.; Cantin, J.; Goss, P.E.; Dent, S.F.; Walde, D.; Vandenberg, T.A.; Findlay, B.; et al. Randomized Trial of Tamoxifen versus Combined Tamoxifen and Octreotide LAR Therapy in the Adjuvant Treatment of Early-Stage Breast Cancer in Postmenopausal Women: NCIC CTG MA.14. *J. Clin. Oncol.* **2011**, *29*, 3869–3876. [CrossRef]
184. Goodwin, P.J.; Ennis, M.; Pritchard, K.I.; Trudeau, M.E.; Koo, J.; Taylor, S.K.; Hood, N. Insulin- and Obesity-Related Variables in Early-Stage Breast Cancer: Correlations and Time Course of Prognostic Associations. *J. Clin. Oncol.* **2012**, *30*, 164–171. [CrossRef]
185. Di Sebastiano, K.M.; Pinthus, J.H.; Duivenvoorden, W.C.M.; Mourtzakis, M. Glucose Impairments and Insulin Resistance in Prostate Cancer: The Role of Obesity, Nutrition and Exercise. *Obes. Rev.* **2018**, *19*, 1008–1016. [CrossRef]
186. Ma, J.; Giovannucci, E.; Pollak, M.; Leavitt, A.; Tao, Y.; Gaziano, J.M.; Stampfer, M.J. A Prospective Study of Plasma C-Peptide and Colorectal Cancer Risk in Men. *J. Natl. Cancer Inst.* **2004**, *96*, 546–553. [CrossRef]
187. Wolpin, B.M.; Meyerhardt, J.A.; Chan, A.T.; Ng, K.; Chan, J.A.; Wu, K.; Pollak, M.N.; Giovannucci, E.L.; Fuchs, C.S. Insulin, the Insulin-like Growth Factor Axis, and Mortality in Patients with Nonmetastatic Colorectal Cancer. *J. Clin. Oncol.* **2009**, *27*, 176–185. [CrossRef]
188. Campagnoli, C.; Pasanisi, P.; Abbà, C.; Ambroggio, S.; Biglia, N.; Brucato, T.; Colombero, R.; Danese, S.; Donadio, M.; Venturelli, E.; et al. Effect of Different Doses of Metformin on Serum Testosterone and Insulin in Non-Diabetic Women with Breast Cancer: A Randomized Study. *Clin. Breast Cancer* **2012**, *12*, 175–182. [CrossRef]
189. Pearce, E.L.; Walsh, M.C.; Cejas, P.J.; Harms, G.M.; Shen, H.; Wang, L.-S.; Jones, R.G.; Choi, Y. Enhancing CD8 T-Cell Memory by Modulating Fatty Acid Metabolism. *Nature* **2009**, *460*, 103–107. [CrossRef]
190. Eikawa, S.; Nishida, M.; Mizukami, S.; Yamazaki, C.; Nakayama, E.; Udono, H. Immune-Mediated Antitumor Effect by Type 2 Diabetes Drug, Metformin. *Proc. Natl. Acad. Sci. USA* **2015**, *112*, 1809–1814. [CrossRef]
191. Scharping, N.E.; Menk, A.V.; Whetstone, R.D.; Zeng, X.; Delgoffe, G.M. Efficacy of PD-1 Blockade Is Potentiated by Metformin-Induced Reduction of Tumor Hypoxia. *Cancer Immunol. Res.* **2017**, *5*, 9–16. [CrossRef] [PubMed]
192. Cha, J.-H.; Yang, W.-H.; Xia, W.; Wei, Y.; Chan, L.-C.; Lim, S.-O.; Li, C.-W.; Kim, T.; Chang, S.-S.; Lee, H.-H.; et al. Metformin Promotes Antitumor Immunity via Endoplasmic-Reticulum-Associated Degradation of PD-L1. *Mol. Cell* **2018**, *71*, 606–620.e7. [CrossRef] [PubMed]
193. Blagih, J.; Coulombe, F.; Vincent, E.E.; Dupuy, F.; Galicia-Vázquez, G.; Yurchenko, E.; Raissi, T.C.; van der Windt, G.J.W.; Viollet, B.; Pearce, E.L.; et al. The Energy Sensor AMPK Regulates T Cell Metabolic Adaptation and Effector Responses In Vivo. *Immunity* **2015**, *42*, 41–54. [CrossRef] [PubMed]
194. Kim, S.H.; Li, M.; Trousil, S.; Zhang, Y.; Pasca di Magliano, M.; Swanson, K.D.; Zheng, B. Phenformin Inhibits Myeloid-Derived Suppressor Cells and Enhances the Anti-Tumor Activity of PD-1 Blockade in Melanoma. *J. Investig. Dermatol.* **2017**, *137*, 1740–1748. [CrossRef]

195. Wang, S.; Lin, Y.; Xiong, X.; Wang, L.; Guo, Y.; Chen, Y.; Chen, S.; Wang, G.; Lin, P.; Chen, H.; et al. Low-Dose Metformin Reprograms the Tumor Immune Microenvironment in Human Esophageal Cancer: Results of a Phase II Clinical Trial. *Clin. Cancer Res.* **2020**, *26*, 4921–4932. [CrossRef]
196. Baumann, T.; Dunkel, A.; Schmid, C.; Schmitt, S.; Hiltensperger, M.; Lohr, K.; Laketa, V.; Donakonda, S.; Ahting, U.; Lorenz-Depiereux, B.; et al. Regulatory Myeloid Cells Paralyze T Cells through Cell-Cell Transfer of the Metabolite Methylglyoxal. *Nat. Immunol.* **2020**, *21*, 555–566. [CrossRef]
197. Uehara, T.; Eikawa, S.; Nishida, M.; Kunisada, Y.; Yoshida, A.; Fujiwara, T.; Kunisada, T.; Ozaki, T.; Udono, H. Metformin Induces CD11b$^+$-Cell-Mediated Growth Inhibition of an Osteosarcoma: Implications for Metabolic Reprogramming of Myeloid Cells and Anti-Tumor Effects. *Int. Immunol.* **2019**, *31*, 187–198. [CrossRef]
198. Xu, P.; Yin, K.; Tang, X.; Tian, J.; Zhang, Y.; Ma, J.; Xu, H.; Xu, Q.; Wang, S. Metformin Inhibits the Function of Granulocytic Myeloid-Derived Suppressor Cells in Tumor-Bearing Mice. *Biomed. Pharm.* **2019**, *120*, 109458. [CrossRef]
199. Ma, Q.; Gu, J.-T.; Wang, B.; Feng, J.; Yang, L.; Kang, X.-W.; Duan, P.; Sun, X.; Liu, P.-J.; Wang, J.-C. PlGF Signaling and Macrophage Repolarization Contribute to the Anti-Neoplastic Effect of Metformin. *Eur. J. Pharmacol.* **2019**, *863*, 172696. [CrossRef]
200. Sloot, Y.J.E.; Rabold, K.; Netea, M.G.; Smit, J.W.A.; Hoogerbrugge, N.; Netea-Maier, R.T. Effect of PTEN Inactivating Germline Mutations on Innate Immune Cell Function and Thyroid Cancer-Induced Macrophages in Patients with PTEN Hamartoma Tumor Syndrome. *Oncogene* **2019**, *38*, 3743–3755. [CrossRef]
201. Khan, H.; Anshu, A.; Prasad, A.; Roy, S.; Jeffery, J.; Kittipongdaja, W.; Yang, D.T.; Schieke, S.M. Metabolic Rewiring in Response to Biguanides Is Mediated by MROS/HIF-1a in Malignant Lymphocytes. *Cell Rep.* **2019**, *29*, 3009–3018.e4. [CrossRef] [PubMed]
202. Deblois, G.; St-Pierre, J.; Giguère, V. The PGC-1/ERR Signaling Axis in Cancer. *Oncogene* **2013**, *32*, 3483–3490. [CrossRef] [PubMed]
203. Audet-Walsh, É.; Papadopoli, D.J.; Gravel, S.-P.; Yee, T.; Bridon, G.; Caron, M.; Bourque, G.; Giguère, V.; St-Pierre, J. The PGC-1α/ERRα Axis Represses One-Carbon Metabolism and Promotes Sensitivity to Anti-Folate Therapy in Breast Cancer. *Cell Rep.* **2016**, *14*, 920–931. [CrossRef] [PubMed]
204. Chaube, B.; Malvi, P.; Singh, S.V.; Mohammad, N.; Meena, A.S.; Bhat, M.K. Targeting Metabolic Flexibility by Simultaneously Inhibiting Respiratory Complex I and Lactate Generation Retards Melanoma Progression. *Oncotarget* **2015**, *6*, 37281–37299. [CrossRef] [PubMed]
205. Elgendy, M.; Cirò, M.; Hosseini, A.; Weiszmann, J.; Mazzarella, L.; Ferrari, E.; Cazzoli, R.; Curigliano, G.; DeCensi, A.; Bonanni, B.; et al. Combination of Hypoglycemia and Metformin Impairs Tumor Metabolic Plasticity and Growth by Modulating the PP2A-GSK3β-MCL-1 Axis. *Cancer Cell* **2019**, *35*, 798–815.e5. [CrossRef] [PubMed]
206. Liberti, M.V.; Locasale, J.W. The Warburg Effect: How Does It Benefit Cancer Cells? *Trends Biochem. Sci.* **2016**, *41*, 211–218. [CrossRef] [PubMed]
207. Missiroli, S.; Perrone, M.; Genovese, I.; Pinton, P.; Giorgi, C. Cancer Metabolism and Mitochondria: Finding Novel Mechanisms to Fight Tumours. *EBioMedicine* **2020**, *59*, 102943. [CrossRef]
208. Kalyanaraman, B.; Cheng, G.; Hardy, M.; Ouari, O.; Sikora, A.; Zielonka, J.; Dwinell, M. Mitochondria-Targeted Metformins: Anti-Tumour and Redox Signalling Mechanisms. *Interface Focus* **2017**, *7*, 20160109. [CrossRef]
209. Boyle, K.A.; Van Wickle, J.; Hill, R.B.; Marchese, A.; Kalyanaraman, B.; Dwinell, M.B. Mitochondria-Targeted Drugs Stimulate Mitophagy and Abrogate Colon Cancer Cell Proliferation. *J. Biol. Chem.* **2018**, *293*, 14891–14904. [CrossRef]
210. Shih, A.J.; Menzin, A.; Whyte, J.; Lovecchio, J.; Liew, A.; Khalili, H.; Bhuiya, T.; Gregersen, P.K.; Lee, A.T. Identification of Grade and Origin Specific Cell Populations in Serous Epithelial Ovarian Cancer by Single Cell RNA-Seq. *PLoS ONE* **2018**, *13*, e0206785. [CrossRef]
211. Yao, L.; Liu, M.; Huang, Y.; Wu, K.; Huang, X.; Zhao, Y.; He, W.; Zhang, R. Metformin Use and Lung Cancer Risk in Diabetic Patients: A Systematic Review and Meta-Analysis. *Dis. Markers* **2019**, *2019*, 6230162. [CrossRef] [PubMed]
212. Trucco, M.; Barredo, J.C.; Goldberg, J.; Leclerc, G.M.; Hale, G.A.; Gill, J.; Setty, B.; Smith, T.; Lush, R.; Lee, J.K.; et al. A Phase I Window, Dose Escalating and Safety Trial of Metformin in Combination with Induction Chemotherapy in Relapsed Refractory Acute Lymphoblastic Leukemia: Metformin with Induction Chemotherapy of Vincristine, Dexamethasone, PEG-Asparaginase, and Doxorubicin. *Pediatr. Blood Cancer* **2018**, *65*, e27224. [CrossRef] [PubMed]
213. Wan, G.; Sun, X.; Li, F.; Wang, X.; Li, C.; Li, H.; Yu, X.; Cao, F. Survival Benefit of Metformin Adjuvant Treatment for Pancreatic Cancer Patients: A Systematic Review and Meta-Analysis. *Cell Physiol. Biochem.* **2018**, *49*, 837–847. [CrossRef] [PubMed]
214. Reni, M.; Dugnani, E.; Cereda, S.; Belli, C.; Balzano, G.; Nicoletti, R.; Liberati, D.; Pasquale, V.; Scavini, M.; Maggiora, P.; et al. (Ir)Relevance of Metformin Treatment in Patients with Metastatic Pancreatic Cancer: An Open-Label, Randomized Phase II Trial. *Clin. Cancer Res.* **2016**, *22*, 1076–1085. [CrossRef]

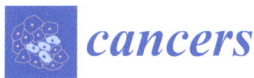

Correction

Correction: Zheng et al. Glycolysis-Related SLC2A1 Is a Potential Pan-Cancer Biomarker for Prognosis and Immunotherapy. *Cancers* 2022, *14*, 5344

Haosheng Zheng [1,†], Guojie Long [2,3,†], Yuzhen Zheng [1], Xingping Yang [1], Weijie Cai [1], Shiyun He [1], Xianyu Qin [1,*] and Hongying Liao [1,*]

[1] Department of Thoracic Surgery, Thoracic Cancer Center, The Sixth Affiliated Hospital, Sun Yat-sen University, Guangzhou 510655, China
[2] Guangdong Research Institute of Gastroenterology, The Sixth Affiliated Hospital, Sun Yat-sen University, Guangzhou 510655, China
[3] Department of Pancreatic Hepatobiliary Surgery, The Sixth Affiliated Hospital of Sun Yat-sen University, Guangzhou 510655, China
* Correspondence: qinxy27@mail.sysu.edu.cn (X.Q.); liaohy2@mail.sysu.edu.cn (H.L.); Tel.: +86-139-2884-5885 (H.L.)
† These authors contributed equally to this work.

The authors wish to make the following corrections to this paper [1]:

In the published version, there were mistakes in "3.9. Immune Cell Infiltration Analysis of SLC2A1" of page 14 and Figure 10.

On page 14, in the Section "3.9. Immune Cell Infiltration Analysis of SLC2A1".

The sentence "SLC2A1 expression is negatively correlated with CD8+ T cells in 12 types of cancers (STES, TGCT, ESCA, LUSC, SKCM, LUAD, BLCA, HNSC, CESC, LAMLC, THYM, and GBM), but positively with CD8+ T cells in 5 types of cancers (PRAD, KIPAN, KIRP, CHOL, and LIHC) (Figure 13A)." should be changed to "SLC2A1 expression is negatively correlated with CD8+ T cells in 9 types of cancers (LUSC, TGCT, HNSC, CESC, LUAD, LAML, SKCM, THYM, and GBM), but positively with CD8+ T cells in 4 types of cancers (PRAD, KIPAN, UVM, and CHOL) (Figure 13A)."

The sentence "SLC2A1 expression is negatively correlated with CD8+ T cells in 12 types of cancers (LUSC, TGCT, THYM, HNSC, BRCA, SKCM, STES, GBMLGG, GBM, PAAD, ALL, and ESCA), but positively correlated with CD8+ T cells in 5 types of cancers (KIPAN, LIHC, LAML, PCPG, and CHOL) (Figure 13B)." should be changed to "SLC2A1 expression is negatively correlated with CD8+ T cells in 11 types of cancers (LUSC, TGCT, THYM, HNSC, BRCA, SKCM, STES, GBMLGG, GBM, PAAD, and ESCA), but positively with CD8+ T cells in 5 types of cancers (KIPAN, LIHC, LAML, PCPG, and CHOL) (Figure 13B)."

The gene symbols of Figure 10 were not correct. The corrected Figure 10 appears below.

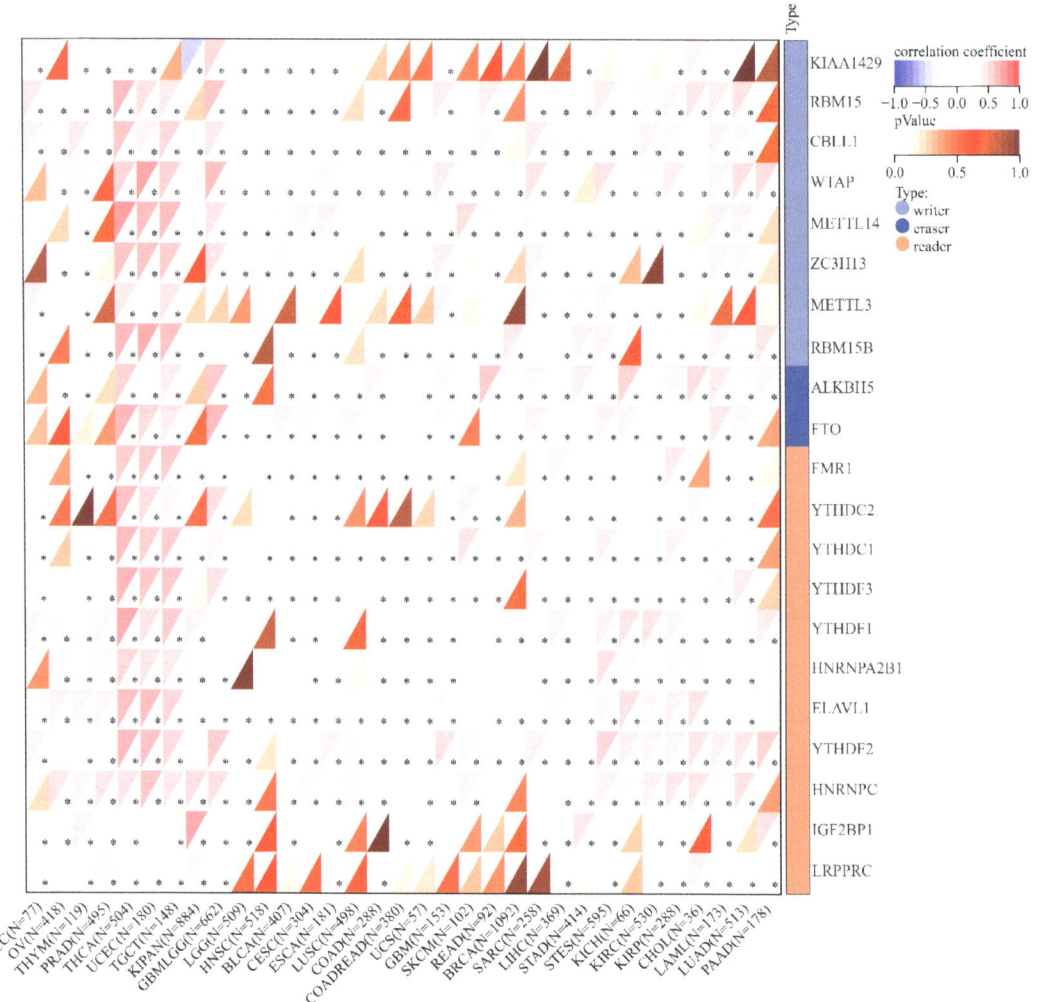

Figure 10. Relationship between SLC2A1 expression and RNA m6A-methylation-related genes in pan-cancer (*, $p < 0.05$).

The authors emphasize that the mistakes were entirely due to human error and oversight. The corrections do not affect the main scientific results and the final conclusions of this manuscript. The authors would like to apologize for any inconvenience caused. The original article has been updated.

Reference

1. Zheng, H.; Long, G.; Zheng, Y.; Yang, X.; Cai, W.; He, S.; Qin, X.; Liao, H. Glycolysis-Related SLC2A1 Is a Potential Pan-Cancer Biomarker for Prognosis and Immunotherapy. *Cancers* **2022**, *14*, 5344. [CrossRef] [PubMed]

Disclaimer/Publisher's Note: The statements, opinions and data contained in all publications are solely those of the individual author(s) and contributor(s) and not of MDPI and/or the editor(s). MDPI and/or the editor(s) disclaim responsibility for any injury to people or property resulting from any ideas, methods, instructions or products referred to in the content.

MDPI AG
Grosspeteranlage 5
4052 Basel
Switzerland
Tel.: +41 61 683 77 34

Cancers Editorial Office
E-mail: cancers@mdpi.com
www.mdpi.com/journal/cancers

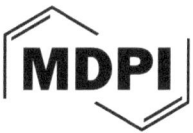

Disclaimer/Publisher's Note: The title and front matter of this reprint are at the discretion of the Guest Editor. The publisher is not responsible for their content or any associated concerns. The statements, opinions and data contained in all individual articles are solely those of the individual Editor and contributors and not of MDPI. MDPI disclaims responsibility for any injury to people or property resulting from any ideas, methods, instructions or products referred to in the content.

www.ingramcontent.com/pod-product-compliance
Lightning Source LLC
LaVergne TN
LVHW072343090526
838202LV00019B/2471